MEDICAL TERMINOLOGY DEMYSTIFIED

Demystified Series

Advanced Statistics Demystified
Algebra Demystified
Anatomy Demystified
asp.net Demystified
Astronomy Demystified
Biology Demystified
Business Calculus Demystified
Business Statistics Demystified
C++ Demystified
Calculus Demystified
Chemistry Demystified
College Algebra Demystified
Data Structures Demystified
Databases Demystified
Differential Equations Demystified
Digital Electronics Demystified
Earth Science Demystified
Electricity Demystified
Electronics Demystified
Environmental Science Demystified
Everyday Math Demystified
Genetics Demystified
Geometry Demystified
Home Networking Demystified
Investing Demystified
Java Demystified
JavaScript Demystified
Linear Algebra Demystified
Macroeconomics Demystified
Math Proofs Demystified
Math Word Problems Demystified
Medical Terminology Demystified
Meteorology Demystified
Microbiology Demystified
OOP Demystified
Options Demystified
Organic Chemistry Demystified
Personal Computing Demystified
Pharmacology Demystified

Physics Demystified
Physiology Demystified
Pre-Algebra Demystified
Precalculus Demystified
Probability Demystified
Project Management Demystified
Quality Management Demystified
Quantum Mechanics Demystified
Relativity Demystified
Robotics Demystified
Six Sigma Demystified
sql Demystified
Statistics Demystified
Trigonometry Demystified
uml Demystified
Visual Basic 2005 Demystified
Visual C# 2005 Demystified
xml Demystified

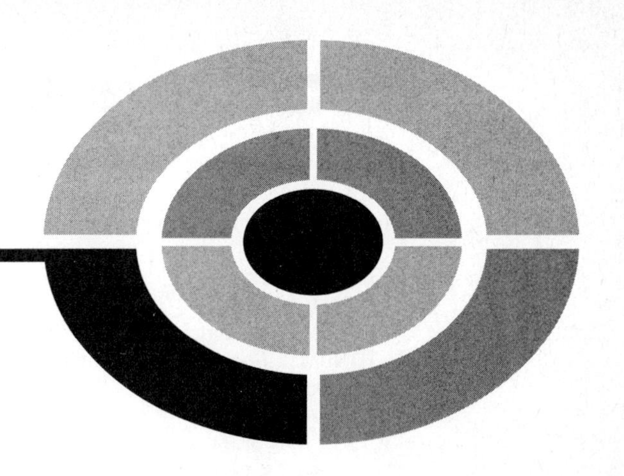

MEDICAL TERMINOLOGY DEMYSTIFIED

The Hon. Dr. Dale Pierre Layman, Ph.D.,
Grand Ph.D. in Medicine (Belgium)

McGRAW-HILL
New York Chicago San Francisco Lisbon London
Madrid Mexico City Milan New Delhi San Juan
Seoul Singapore Sydney Toronto

The McGraw-Hill Companies

Library of Congress Cataloging-in-Publication Data

Layman, Dale Pierre.
Medical terminology demystified / Dale Pierre Layman.
p. cm.
Includes index.
ISBN 0-07-146104-3 (alk. paper)
1. Medicine—Terminology. I. Title.
[DNLM: 1. Medicine—Terminology—English. W 15 L427m 2006]
R123.L363 2006
610.1′4—dc22

2005058417

5 6 7 8 9 0 DOC/DOC 0 1 0 9

ISBN 0-07-146104-3

The sponsoring editor for this book was Judy Bass and the production supervisor was Pamela A. Pelton. It was set in Times Roman by TechBooks. The art director for the cover was Margaret Webster-Shapiro; the cover designer was Handel Low.

Printed and bound by RR Donnelley.

This book is fondly dedicated to ***J. D. Ross***, the President of Joliet Junior College; to ***Dr. Michael Lee***, Chairman of the Natural Sciences Department; and to College Trustee ***Dick Dystrup*** (representing ***Eleanor McGuan-Boza*** and the entire Joliet Junior College Board of Trustees). This dedication is in due recognition of their efforts in successfully establishing a professorial ranking system at Joliet Junior College (located in Joliet, Illinois) in the Millennial Year, 2000. From now on, the first and oldest public community college in the United States will honor its teachers with the rank of Professor! For this historic success, these fine people will have my everlasting thanks!

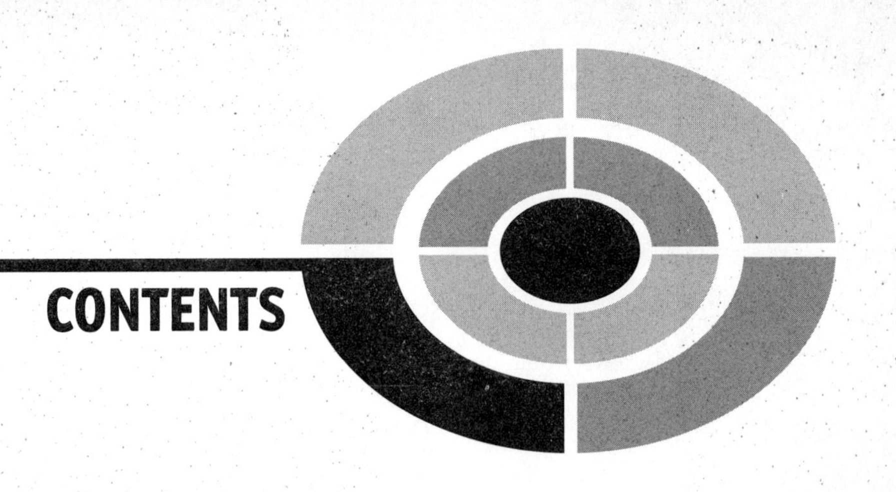

CONTENTS

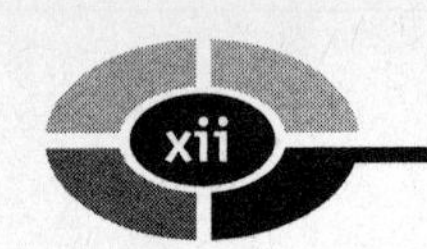

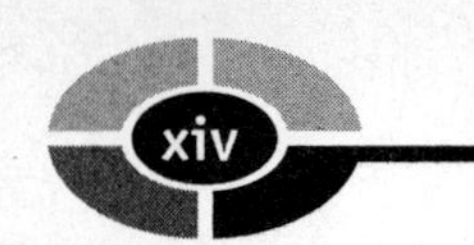

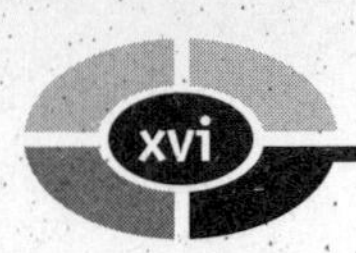

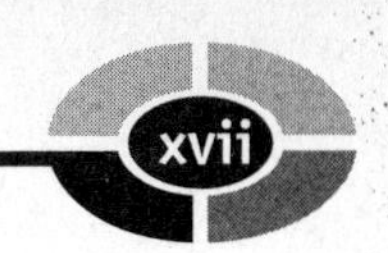
xvii

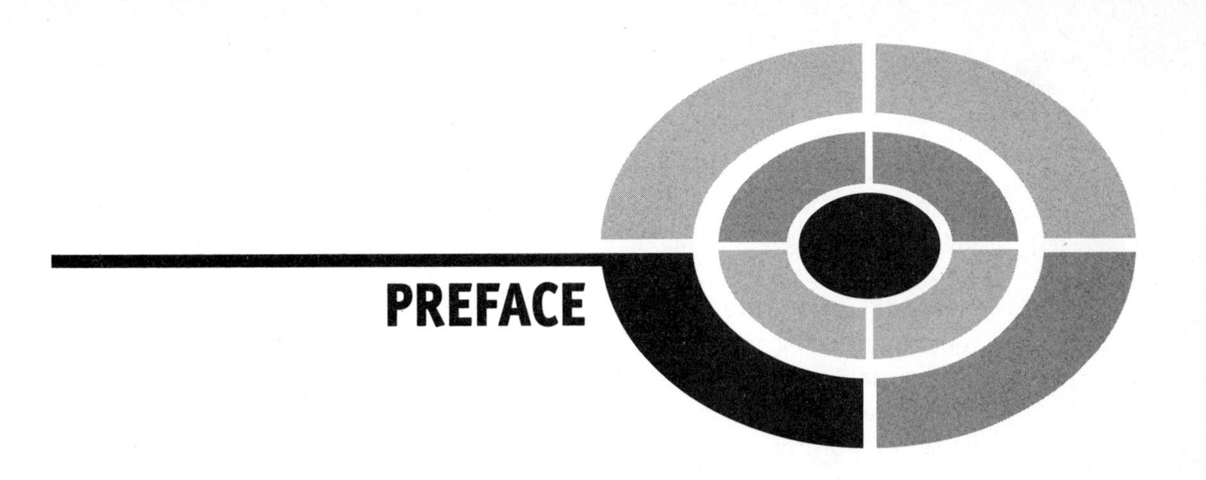

PREFACE

This book is for people who want to get acquainted with the basic concepts of medical terminology without having to take a formal course. It can also serve as a supplemental text in a classroom, tutored, or home-schooling environment. It should also be useful for career changers who need to refresh their knowledge of the subject. I recommend that you start at the beginning of this book and go straight through.

There are 5 icons (cartoon pictures) that repeatedly appear in the page margins of every chapter. Each icon takes the form of a "Memory Pill"—a key fact for you to write down and remember in a "Memory Pillbox" (handy numbered grid) at chapter end. An *Anatomy* icon indicates a key fact about *normal body structure*. Conversely, a *Physiology* icon labels an important fact about *normal body function*. Knowing some of these key structure-function facts in the *normal* body helps you to understand their associated *disease* and *disorders* within the *abnormal* body.

The medical terminology of the book provides key facts tagged as *Disease* icons and other facts as *Treatment/Therapy* icons. Finally, there are numerous *Background and History* icons that identify critical people and historical events behind the development of medical terminology. A special icon is that of *Hippocrates* (pronounced as hih-**PAHK**-rah-**tees**). Hippocrates was an ancient Greek physician who is considered the Father of Modern Medicine. For this reason, *MEDICAL TERMINOLOGY DEMYSTIFIED* is subtitled as "A Visit with Hippocrates." The Ghost of Hippocrates is our narrator, who guides us along throughout the book. He is occasionally assisted by both Professor Joe, the Talking Skeleton (from *ANATOMY DEMYSTIFIED* and *PHYSIOLOGY DEMYSTIFIED*), and by Baby Heinie (his mischievous little sidekick). The goal is to provide some meaningful "edu-tainment"—"education" plus "entertainment"—for the reader.

There are many highly imaginative illustrations in the text that feature both normal and abnormal body states, as well as fascinating historical landmarks in the evolution of medical language. The etymology (original Latin-Greek source) for many words is provided, often with accompanying figures.

Words are frequently broken down into their component word parts—prefixes, roots, combining vowels, and suffixes—soon after they are introduced. And within each chapter, Summary Tables provide the reader with repeated practice in medical word translation. The reader is given a particular term, along with its set of word parts. The reader is then directed to write the exact meanings of these key words in regular English. By this means, the reader acquires skill in transforming strange, unfamiliar medical terms into comfortable, familiar, Common English.

A Medical Case History ends most of the chapters. This Case History provides a real-life, "you-are-there" feeling for the reader, who is introduced to the practical uses of the modern medical language for injured or diseased patients.

Each chapter has a multiple choice quiz. Every section of the book has its own 25-question test. And at the end, a comprehensive Final Exam with 100 multiple-choice questions drills the reader to recall essential elements from all the book chapters. Answers for these quizzes and tests are listed in the back of the book.

In short, everything you need is provided to help you master the Medical Language on your own! Our wise guide and mentor, the Ghost of Noble Hippocrates, is here to help you succeed!

Best of luck! And be sure to have fun!

The Hon. Dr. Dale Pierre Layman, Ph.D.,
Grand Ph.D. in Medicine

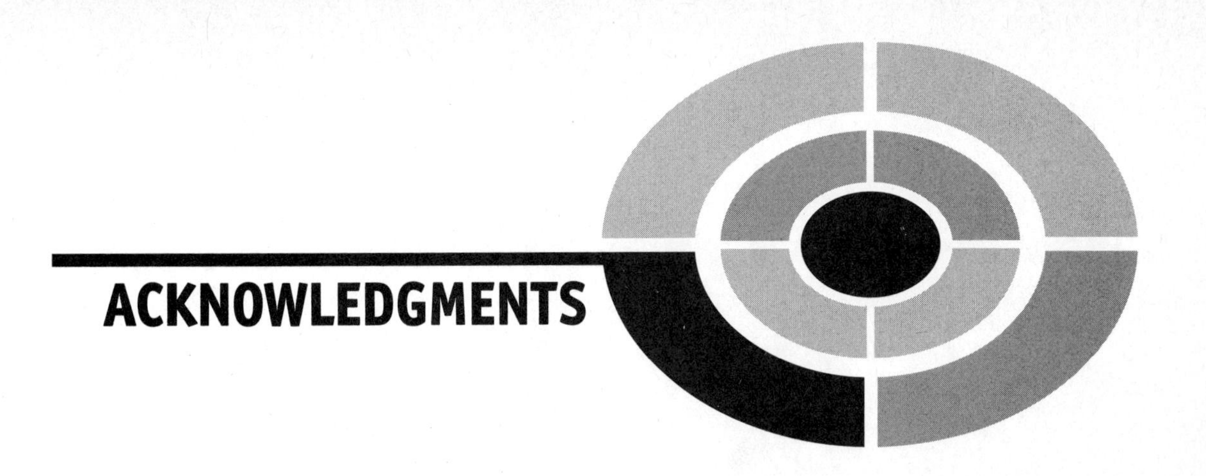

ACKNOWLEDGMENTS

I wish to acknowledge the great help of one of my artistically talented daughters, Allison Victoria Layman, for her critical role in generating much of the artwork for this book. And my ever-dependable wife, Kathy, also played a vital supporting function. I can ***always*** depend upon ***her***! (That's why I call her ***The Rock***!)

Emma Previato of Boston University provided assistance with technical editing of the manuscript.

Thanks are also due to Stephanie Lentz and her staff at TechBooks, who kept bringing the work out to me at a fast pace (thereby getting it ***done***!).

Finally, I wish to acknowledge the trust of my editor at McGraw-Hill, Judy Bass, who believes in the quality of my work.

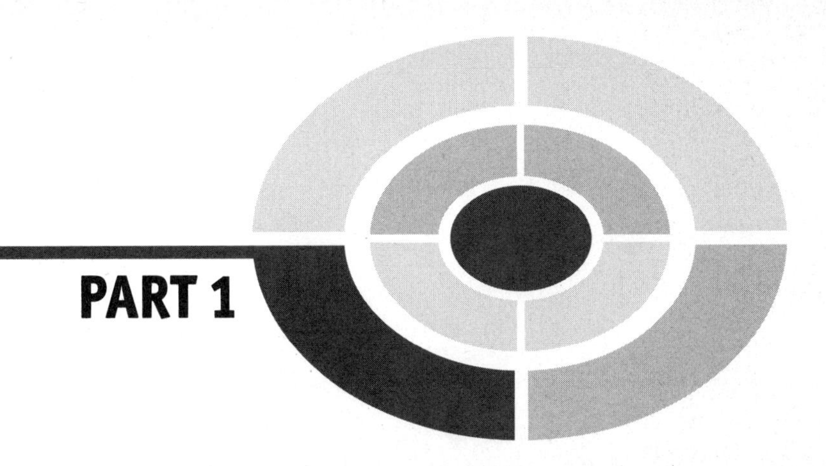

PART 1

The Foundations of Medical Terminology

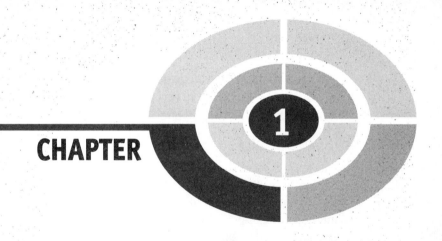

CHAPTER 1

The Basic Ideas, or "Hey! It's Just *Greek* (or *Latin*) to Me!"

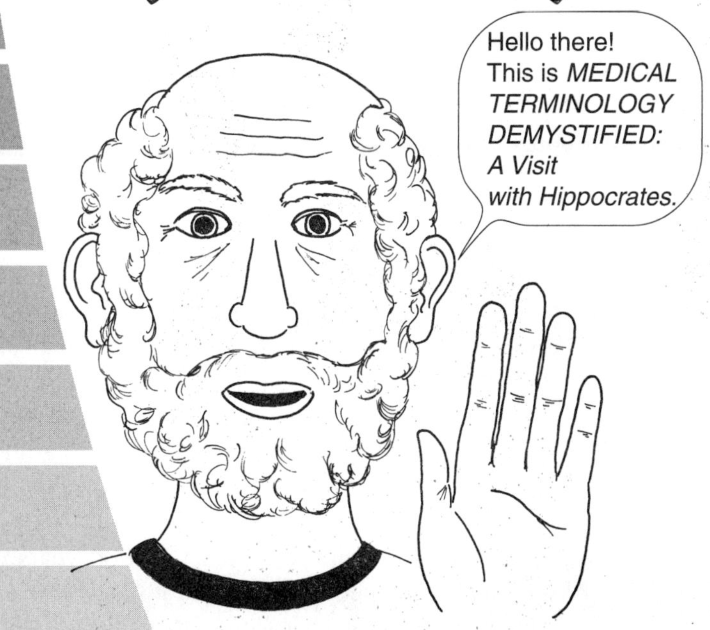

A greeting from Hippocrates, the father of Modern Medicine.

I am *Hippocrates* (pronounced as hih-**PAHK**-rah-**tees**), the Father of Modern Medicine. Welcome to my world—the world of Ancient Greece and Rome. It is here that we begin our introduction to medical terminology. Our approach is much different from that taken by a medical dictionary, where you merely look up a particular medical word, try to correctly pronounce and spell it, and then attempt to memorize its definition. How dry, dull, and *boring*!

You, my Lucky Friend, have finally found an orderly, logical system or method for better learning, understanding, and correctly using those strange medical words you may have encountered! In short, you have entered the vibrant pages of *MEDICAL TERMINOLOGY DEMYSTIFIED: A Visit with Hippocrates*.

Background and History

Another major weakness of medical dictionaries (and many books on medical terminology) is a lack of emphasis upon *medical background and history*. "How can you and I thoroughly understand and appreciate the medical terms we encounter if we don't know the background or history lying behind them?" the reasonable person could intelligently ask.

I, Hippocrates, will be standing and pointing to key facts about medical background and history within each chapter of this book. You will see me again and again as a small icon or picture-symbol in the page margins (see Figure 1.1). After the icon will be the letter *H*, for *HISTORY*. As each key historical fact is labeled with my picture-symbol, it will be numbered in sequence. My picture followed by *H1*, for example, will indicate that this is "key fact #1 of medical history" in a particular chapter.

Please notice also (Figure 1.1) that my picture is surrounded by an oval capsule—really a *pill capsule!* This means it is tagging a certain key fact in the book that serves as an important "Memory Pill" for medical history! This icon is a response to what you may have actually said to a relative or friend when they just couldn't *remember* something! Now, what did you say? Why, you told them, "Go take a *pill!*" And in this book, that's exactly what we're going to do! We're going to be taking Memory Pills for key text facts—lots and lots of them, to help us remember what we have read!

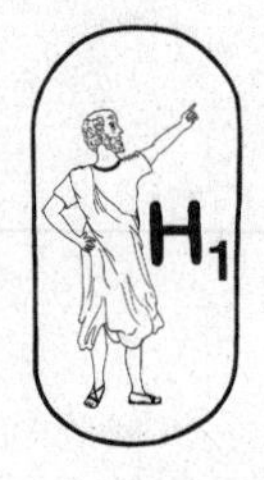

So, here we go! Now, primitive medicine is at least 10,000 years old. We know this is true, because paintings of people performing surgery and various other types of therapies have been found scrawled upon the walls of long-buried ancient cities.

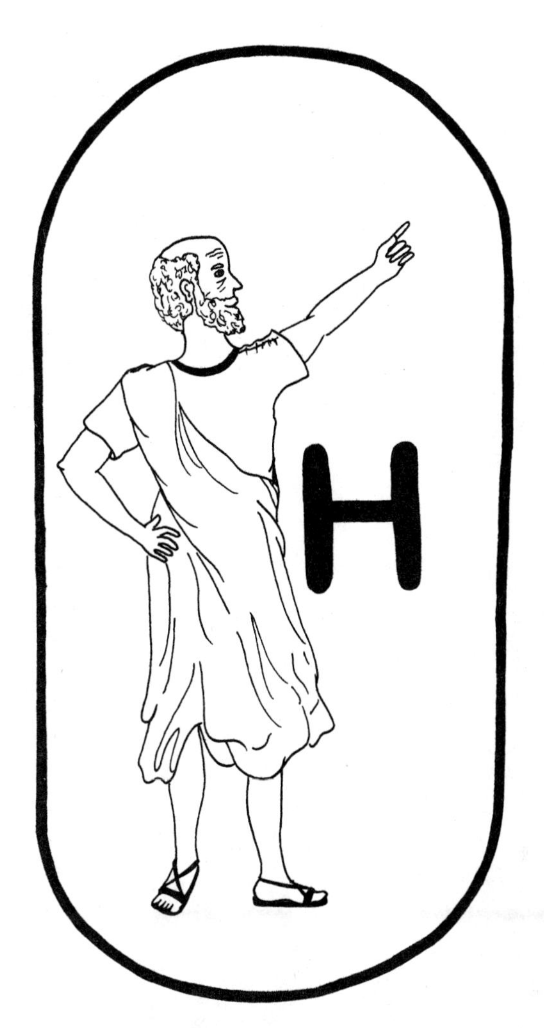

Fig. 1.1 The "memory pill" icon for key facts about medical history (*H*).

In early times, very few scientific facts were known, so death and disease were often regarded as supernatural, rather than natural, occurrences. So if you were sick, it was because you had offended the gods!

But even a very primitive form of medicine required a certain language. Terms for sicknesses and diseases had to be invented, and the tools and techniques used to treat these diseases had to be described. Thus, medical terminology was born with medicine itself, and is probably just as old.

As diseases were recognized, they had to be named and described in terms which were very different from ordinary daily language. When various treatments and therapies were developed, they had to be explained and communicated to others across the gap of generations. Soon a massive, complex medical language evolved, and it was known and used mainly by people involved in the healing arts.

EARLY MEDICAL LAWS: THE CODE OF HAMMURABI

One of the first major bodies of medical rules and language occurred around 1780 BC in ancient *Mesopotamia* (**mes**-uh-puh-**TAY**-me-uh). In Greek, the word *Mesopotamia* actually means "between the rivers." Much of this region

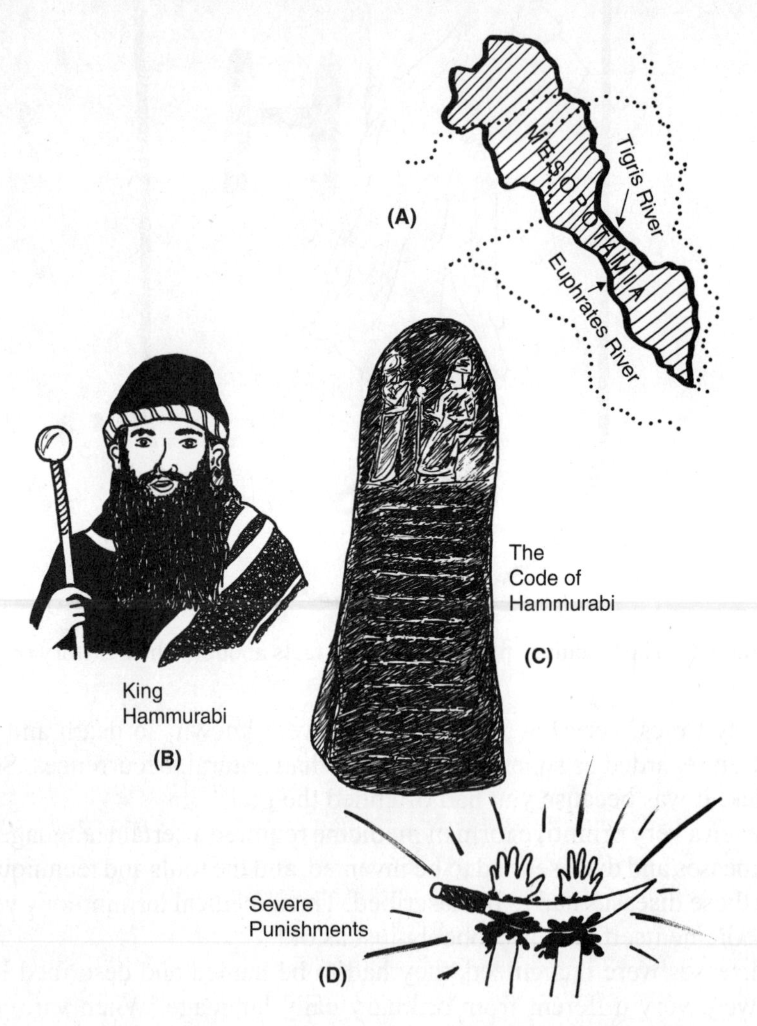

Fig. 1.2 The Code of Hammurabi and its severe punishments.

is now known as Iraq. [**Study suggestion:** Look carefully at the map drawn in Figure 1.2 A. What two rivers, specifically, did Mesopotamia occur between?]

In this fertile land "between the rivers," a great civilization developed. *King Hammurabi* (ham-uh-**RAH**-bee) was an efficient ruler who created a great new system of laws for Mesopotamia. These laws thus became known as the *Code of Hammurabi*. The Code was carved upon a spooky-looking black stone monument that was 8 feet high. (See Figure 1.2 C.)

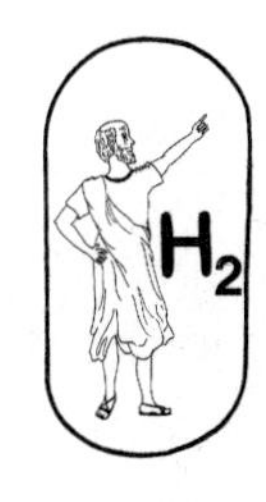

The stone was probably erected in a public square, where everyone could see it plainly. A modern translation of this Code reveals why citizens really needed to pay attention to it! The Code of Hammurabi provided a set of laws that governed all kinds of citizen conduct, including those of early physicians. But even more important, it included a precise listing of severe punishments for breaking these laws! Consider these examples: "If a man put out the eye of another man, his eye shall be put out. [An eye for an eye]. If a man knock out the teeth of his equal, his teeth shall be knocked out. [A tooth for a tooth]. If he break another man's bone, his bone shall be broken. If a man give his child to a nurse and the child die in her hands, but the nurse unbeknown to the father and mother nurse another child, then they shall convict her of having nursed another child without the knowledge of the father and mother, and her breasts shall be cut off."

Laws and punishments for physicians accused of misconduct were no less severe under the Code. We have, for instance, this frightening directive: "If a physician make a large incision with the operating knife, and kill him, or open a tumor with the operating knife, and cut out the eye, his hands shall be cut off." (Review Figure 1.2 D.) Quite obviously, then, there was no need for malpractice insurance in those days!

HEALING, NOT HURTING: ENTER THE ANCIENT GREEKS AND ASCLEPIUS

While the Code of Hammurabi was a strict and merciless body of laws governing the conduct of healers, it seemed to actually promote *hurting* more than *healing*, didn't it? Perhaps this is why our main tradition of healing in Western Medicine has largely come down from the Ancient Greeks, who worshipped many gods of healing.

Greek myths of healing due to divine intervention by the gods were eventually mixed in with the curing work of real people. One of the most important of these was *Asclepius* (as-**KLEE**-pea-us), a famous physician who practiced in Greece around 1200 BC. He was very skillful in his use of natural herbs and surgery, and soon founded a large order of priest-physicians. They controlled the sacred

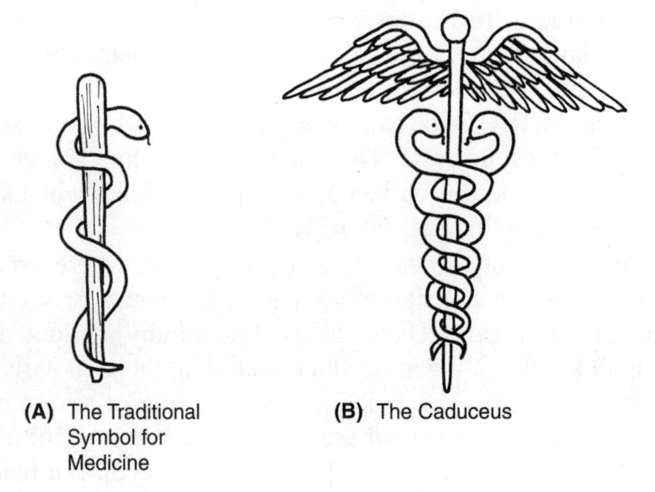

Fig. 1.3 Two common symbols for medicine.

secrets of healing and passed them on, from father to son. Eventually, temples of Asclepius were built throughout Greece, and they spread to Rome and much of Italy. At such temples, sick pilgrims would come to sleep, rest, and be prayed over by the priest-physicians.

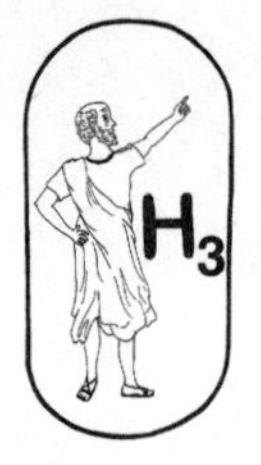

Asclepius adopted the sacred snake as his symbol for healing. This was because the snake periodically sheds its skin, which is then regrown or "healed." Thus, every temple of Asclepius had many sacred snakes slithering through its hallways—and probably crawling over the bodies of the sleeping pilgrims! Over time, a single snake coiled around a wooden staff carried by Asclepius became the traditional symbol for medicine (Figure 1.3 A).

Interestingly, this symbol differs from the *caduceus* (kuh-**DEW**-see-us) or "staff of Mercury" (Figure 1.3 B). The caduceus is composed of a central staff with two snakes entwined in opposite directions around it, with a pair of wings placed on top. The caduceus was carried by *Mercury,* the winged "Messenger of the gods." It is sometimes used as an emblem of the medical profession, because the two snakes can represent the struggle between the powers of Life and Death.

The Romans made statues of Asclepius holding a staff with its single serpent. Eventually, the fame of Asclepius became so great that, legend has it, *Zeus* (ZOOS), the Father of the Gods and the People, became angry and jealous. *Hades* (**HAY**-deez), God of the Underworld, also complained to Zeus that Asclepius was healing far too many mortals and even bringing some back from the dead, thereby reducing the population of the Underworld! Zeus therefore struck Asclepius down with a bolt of lightning (Greek myth says) to eliminate his excessive skill as a great physician (Figure 1.4). As far as we know, Asclepius

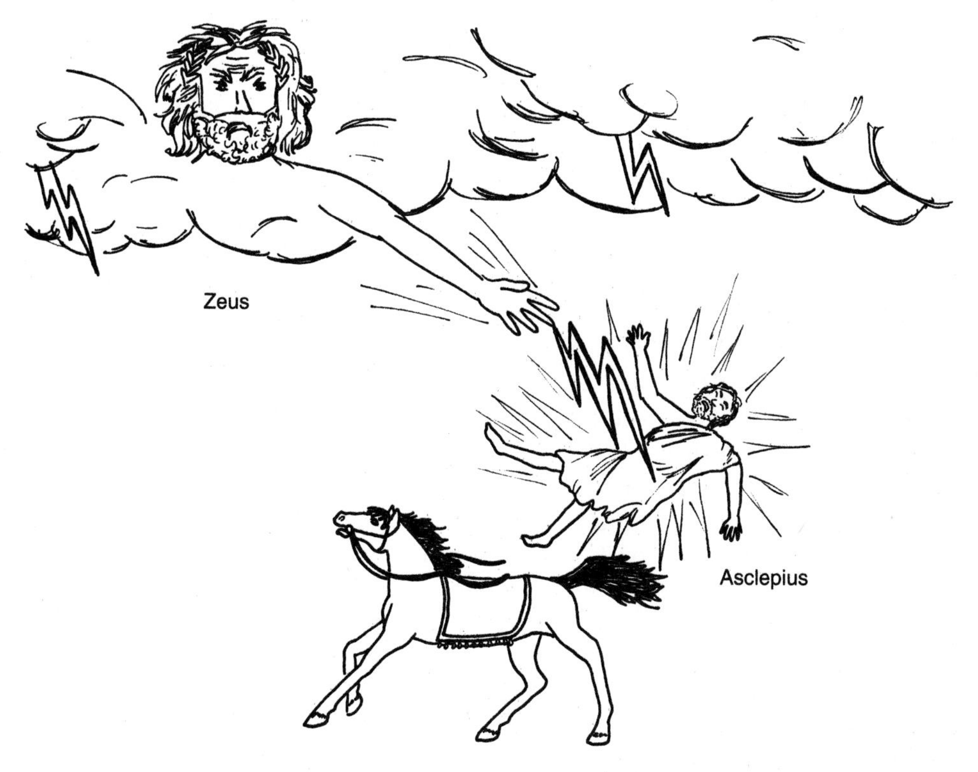

Fig. 1.4 Zeus striking down Asclepius with a lightning bolt.

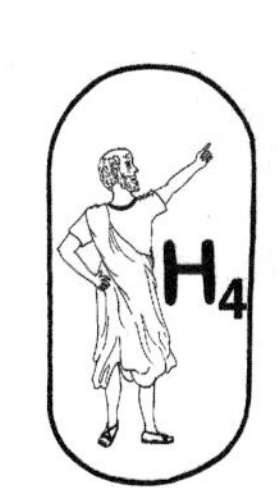

(the real mortal man) may actually have been killed by a lightning bolt while wandering through the countryside.

After his death, this myth of Asclepius grew until he finally became known as the God of Healing. The temples of Asclepius continued to spread throughout much of the Roman empire. Every night for more than a thousand years, sick pilgrims would come and sleep in the temples, where the priest-physicians would give them herbal remedies and pray to Asclepius (the God of Healing) for supernatural intervention.

THE GREEK FOUNDATION OF MODERN MEDICINE: HIPPOCRATES

Asclepius and his followers emphasized *supernatural* remedies for healing, such as that of fasting and praying to the Greek gods. Yet, while Asclepius was still alive, another Greek physician, Hippocrates, began to take a different route. Hippocrates, as we have mentioned, is considered the Father of Modern

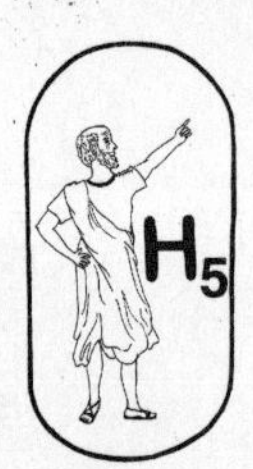

Medicine because he emphasized a logical and *natural* route to wellness. He believed that medical treatment should assist nature in healing the body. He considered changes in diet first, then turned to drugs and surgery as a last resort. He liked to feed his patients a watery *gruel* (**GROO**-el) or "meal" of thin porridge containing barley. His main medicine was honey: "The drink to be employed should there be any pain is vinegar and honey. If there be great thirst, give water and honey." He made many important observations that are as true today as they were in his own time. For example, his saying that "Fat persons are more exposed to sudden death than the slender" reflects what we know today about the relationship between obesity and increased risk for heart disease.

Perhaps most important, Hippocrates turned to love and kindness in his dealings with patients: "For where there is the love of man, there is also the love of the Art." This central concern for the patient's welfare is reflected in the *Hippocratic* (**hip**-uh-**KRAT**-ik) *Oath*. The Oath provided kindly guidelines for future physicians, such as this line: "I will follow that method of treatment which, according to my ability and judgment, I consider for the benefit of my patients, and abstain from whatever is deleterious and mischievous." Even today, the Hippocratic Oath is sworn by many graduating medical students.

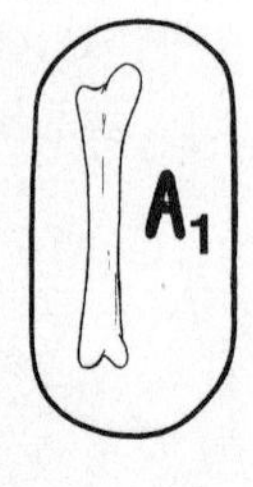

Hippocrates became fairly knowledgeable in the subject of *anatomy* (**ah**-**NAT**-oh-me). We can define anatomy as body structure, and the study of body structures. Because Hippocrates was able to heal fractured bones by forcing the broken ends back together in the proper way, for instance, he must have had some expertise in bone anatomy.

In this book, many of the chapters will have background information on related *normal anatomy* of the healthy, uninjured human body. [**Special note:** A closely related book in this series, *ANATOMY DEMYSTIFIED*, discusses body structures in great detail.] To help us identify a certain key fact about normal anatomy, an icon of a normal *long* bone will be shown in the nearby page margin. In addition, a black capital letter *A* will indicate that the fact is about anatomy. (Figure 1.5 shows such an Anatomy Memory Pill.) A picture of a long bone followed by *A1*, for example, will indicate "anatomy, key fact #1."

PHYSIOLOGY AND GALEN

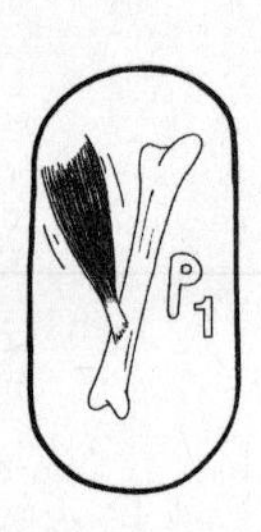

To be sure, Hippocrates and other Greek healers had some significant knowledge about the anatomy of the body parts they treated. "But what good is *treating* injured or diseased body structures if they don't *do* what they did *before* their anatomy was disturbed in the first place?" the impatient reader might feel a need to ask.

In essence, such an impatient reader would be asking a question about *human physiology* (**fih**-zee-**AHL**-uh-jee). By the word *physiology*, we mean body

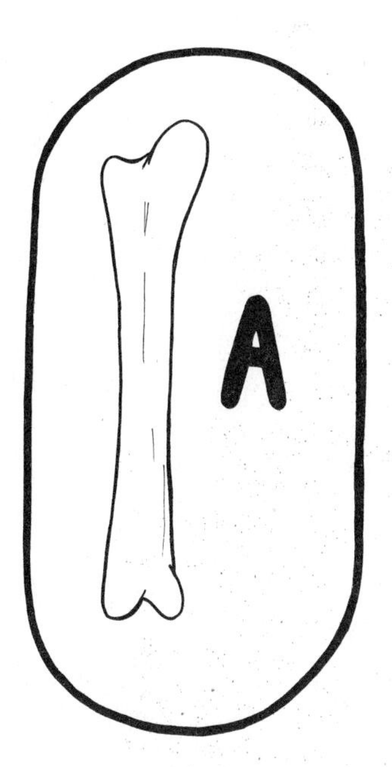

Fig. 1.5 An intact long bone serves as an Anatomy Memory Pill to emphasize key facts about normal body structure.

functions and the study of body functions. "What is a body function?" A body function is something that a particular body structure *does*, or something that is *done to* a body structure. [Another close relative, *PHYSIOLOGY DEMYSTIFIED*, handles body functions in considerable depth.] For the bones, we can consider the physiology of the various *skeletal* (**SKEL**-uh-**tal**) *muscles*, which are attached to the bones of the skeleton.

Whenever a certain skeletal muscle shortens or contracts, it carries out the body function (physiology) of pulling upon its attached bone (Figure 1.6). When the bone is pulled upon hard enough, part of the body moves. [**Study suggestion:** When looking at Figure 1.6, ask yourself, "What does the skeletal muscle *itself* represent—anatomy, or physiology?"]

Since Figure 1.6 shows the *physiology* of body movement, we will use it as our general symbol or icon to label key text facts representing various examples of physiology. (Specifically, we shall use it as our Physiology Memory Pill!) As the physiology icon in a page margin, the contracting muscle and its moving bone will be accompanied by a white capital letter *P*, denoting physiology. A picture of contracting muscle pulling upon its bone, followed by *P1*, for instance, will indicate "physiology, key fact #1."

"Who was it, in history, who *first* really developed this concept of physiology or study of body function?" the interested reader might now question. The

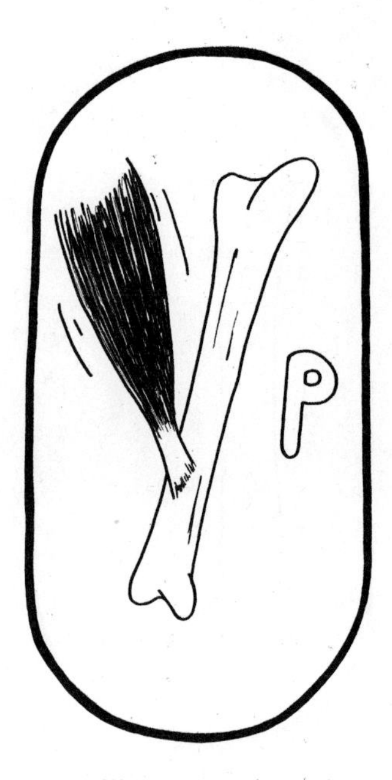

Fig. 1.6 The Physiology Memory Pill: Contraction (shortening) of a skeletal muscle produces the function of body movement.

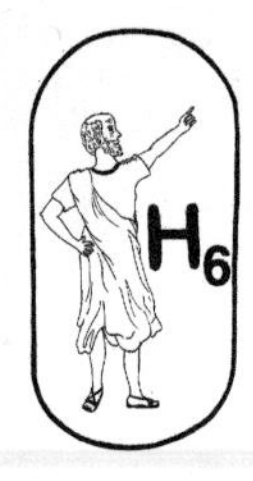

answer is a man named *Claudius Galen* (**GAY**-lun). Galen lived in Greece and Rome from AD 130 to 200, several hundred years after Hippocrates. Galen was both a philosopher and a physician. He is often called the Father of Experimental Physiology.

As shown in Figure 1.7, Galen dissected or cut apart *living* animals (such as pigs) to discover their body functions. Blood spurted out of the cut Galen made in the wall of the living pig's heart as it pumped the blood. Therefore, the pumping of the blood by the living heart during Galen's experiment was a prime example of physiology (body function).

VESALIUS: THE FOUNDER OF MODERN ANATOMY

As we have seen, Hippocrates, the Father of Modern Medicine, had considerable knowledge about anatomy. His successor, Galen, as the Father of Experimental Physiology, added significantly more information about normal body functions. He discovered, for example, that *arteries* actually contained blood, rather than air (as had been thought by earlier Greeks). Most unfortunately, however, Galen made numerous errors in his writings. He knew that the heart set the blood into motion, yet he failed to realize that the blood actually *circulated* throughout the body! For hundreds of years, even into the Middle Ages of Europe, scholars

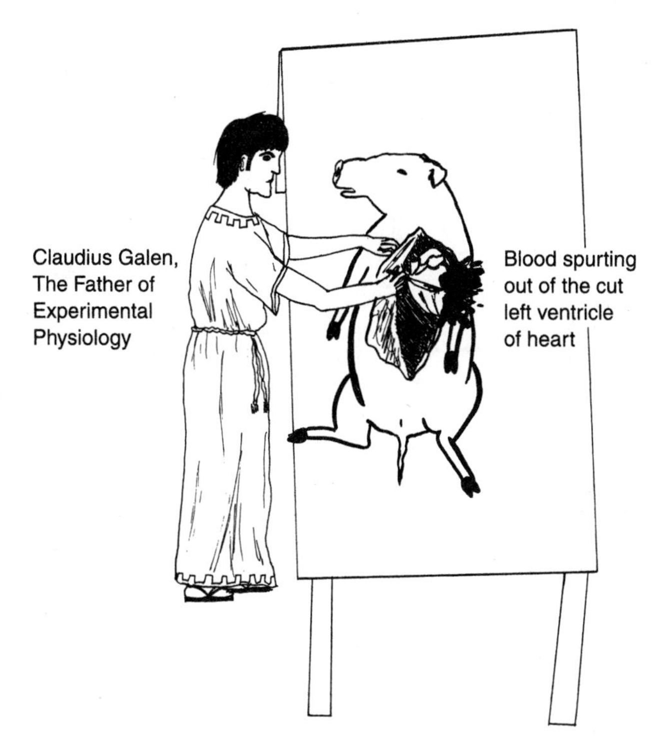

Fig. 1.7 Galen shows the pumping physiology of a living pig heart.

simply "took as gospel" whatever Galen had written—including his errors about the true nature of the blood circulation!

Part of the problem was a reluctance to challenge the authority of the Father of Experimental Physiology. Another problem was a great fear of dissecting human *cadavers* (kuh-**DAV**-ers)—bodies that have "fallen dead" (*cadav*). Galen had been a surgeon to the Roman gladiators, but even *their* bodies were considered sacred vessels of the soul. Thus, it was not considered morally proper to dissect them!

A definite advance came between 1514 and 1564 with the work of an Italian professor named *Andreas* (an-**DRAY**-us) *Vesalius* (vih-**SAY**-lee-**us**). Unwilling to blindly follow the teachings of Galen, Vesalius pioneered the really thorough dissection of cadavers to discover the truth for himself. Quite often, the source of bodies for dissection was the hangman's noose! Vesalius would frequently cut the hanging bodies of dead criminals from the gallows, and then examine them on his dissection table (Figure 1.8). Artists would make careful sketches of the body's inner anatomy while Vesalius went about his work. The resulting books were of great value and established Vesalius as the Father of Anatomy.

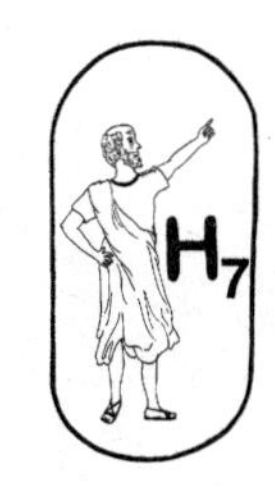

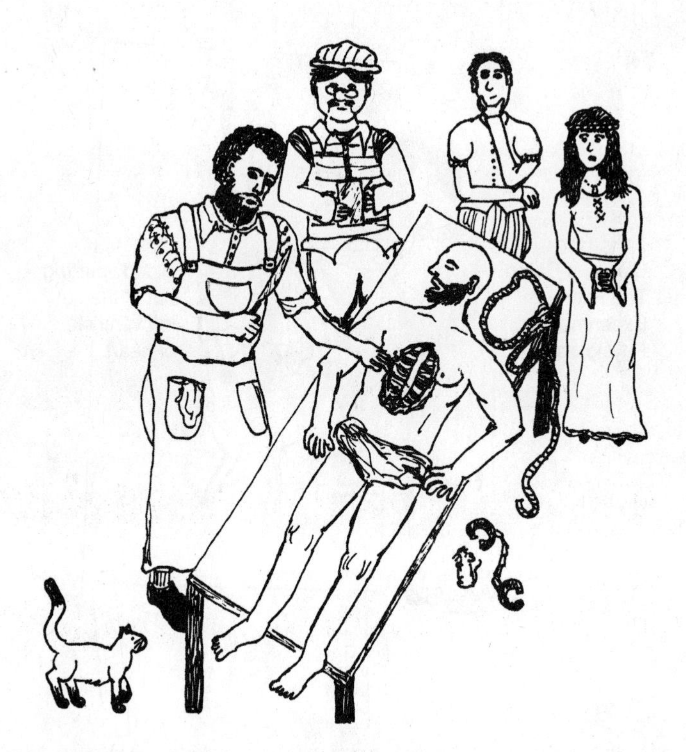

Fig. 1.8 Vesalius pioneers the thorough dissection of cadavers.

Diseases, Injuries, and Therapies

Sometimes neither anatomy (body structure) nor physiology (living body functions) is normal. In such cases, we have a *disease* or *injury*. An example that immediately comes to mind is a *fractured* (broken) bone. When we discuss key terms of disease or injury in this book, therefore, we will tag them with a *broken bone* and a spotted capital *D* (for *Disease*). This will give us a good Disease Memory Pill (Figure 1.9). [**Study suggestion:** Why do you think we have made this disease icon a *spotted* capital D?]

Finally, we should remember that this book teaches us about *medical* terminology. We can dissect or "cut up" the Latin word *medical* by inserting a slash (/) into it. This gives us *medic / al*. Now, *medic* literally (exactly) means "healing," while *-al* means "pertaining to." Hence, the Latin word *medical* literally translates to mean "pertaining to healing" in common English.

We can now ask ourselves, "What word should we use to indicate a treatment that will help promote the healing of a disease or injury?" [**Hint:** This medical term, like the word *treatment*, starts with the letter t. What is it? Take a guess, and then check your answer as you read on!]

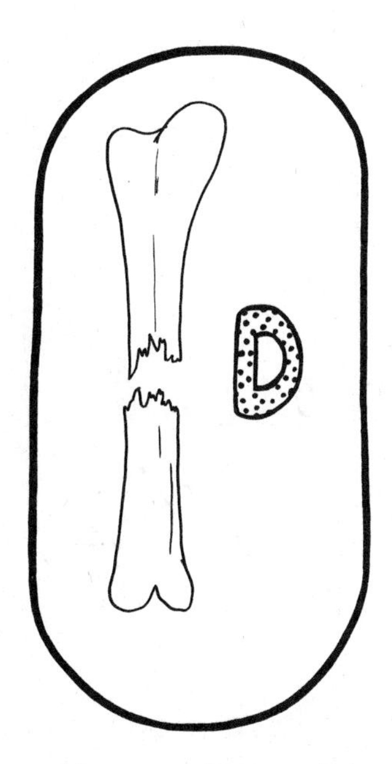

Fig. 1.9 A fractured bone as a "Disease/Injury Memory Pill."

The answer, of course, is *therapy*. A *therapy* is some particular type of medical treatment. When you think of getting some treatment or therapy, doesn't a syringe with a needle come to mind? That's why Figure 1.10 serves as our Therapy or Treatment Memory Pill. The syringe is filled with medicine, and the needle delivers the therapy or treatment via an injection. The cross-hatched capital *T*, of course, is an abbreviation for either *Treatment* or *Therapy.*

"So, Just *Where* Do We Put Our *'Memory Pills'*?"

So far in this chapter, we have been introducing a large amount of information about medical background and history (including normal anatomy and physiology), as well as an overview of diseases, injuries, and therapies.

"Okay, but just *where* should we be putting these key text facts (tagged in the margins as Memory Pills)?" The answer should be quite obvious. [**Hint:** When you are away from home, traveling, what do you use to carry a few days of vitamins and other pills?] Figure 1.11 provides the container: a "Memory Pillbox!"

So that we don't get our "pills" (key facts) mixed up, we will store each type within its own "pillbox"! Specifically, we will have five different types of memory pill boxes: History Pillboxes, Anatomy Pillboxes, Physiology Pillboxes,

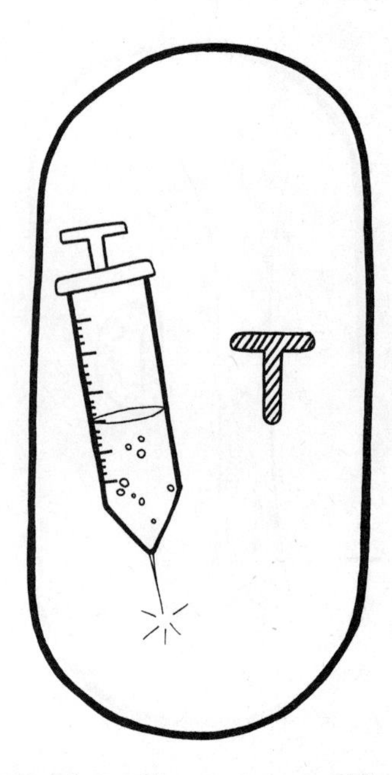

Fig. 1.10 A syringe and needle serves as our Therapy Memory Pill.

Disease/Injury Pillboxes, and Therapy Pillboxes. In other words, these are the five basic categories of medical knowledge, which are to be "filled" with key facts from each chapter. And each of these rectangle-shaped "pillboxes" will open up as a grid or *matrix* (**MAY**-tricks) consisting of four numbered cells or squared regions (Figure 1.12). It is within each of these four smaller regions of each grid that you should write a brief summary of the key facts labeled in the chapter. [*NOTE*: These grids or "pillboxes" are provided in a special section at the end of each chapter.]

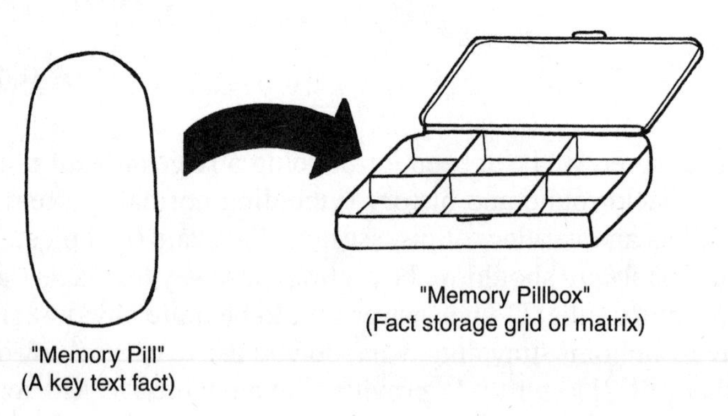

Fig. 1.11 A memory "pillbox" that can store key facts (memory pills) covered in each chapter.

1	2
3	4

Fig. 1.12 The actual four-unit grid or matrix within which you should briefly write a summary of each key text fact.

Medical Terms and Word Parts

Each medical term contains one or more *roots*. A *root* is the main idea or concept of a word. It is called a root because it fixes or anchors a word in the ground of meaning. (In this way, the word root is somewhat like a *real* root that anchors a tree into the ground, isn't it?) Remember that we earlier dissected or "cut up" the Latin term, *medical*. Its root (main idea) is ________, which means "healing" in common English. [**Study suggestion:** Try to fill in this blank from memory, then check your answer as you read.]

The root in *medical* is *medic*, which means "healing." You know, as long as we're comparing a medical term to the parts of a tree, why not compare it to the parts of the human body as well? In this case, we can think of the root or main idea of a medical word as being like the *trunk* or *torso* (**TOR**-soh) of the human body. As Figure 1.13 shows, the trunk or torso represents the main mass of the human body—that is, the part not including the head or limbs (arms and legs). This is very interesting, because the word *torso* literally means "stem" in Latin. Therefore, the trunk (torso) is the main "stem" of the human body, just as *medic* is the root or main part of the word *medical.*

In humans, the trunk or torso consists of the *thorax* (**THOR**-aks) or "chest," the *abdomen* (**AB**-doh-**men**) or "body midsection," and the *pelvis* (**PEL**-vis) or "bowl present" between the two hip bones. Coming before the trunk (torso), we find the head and neck. And coming after the bottom of the trunk (torso), of course, we find the legs.

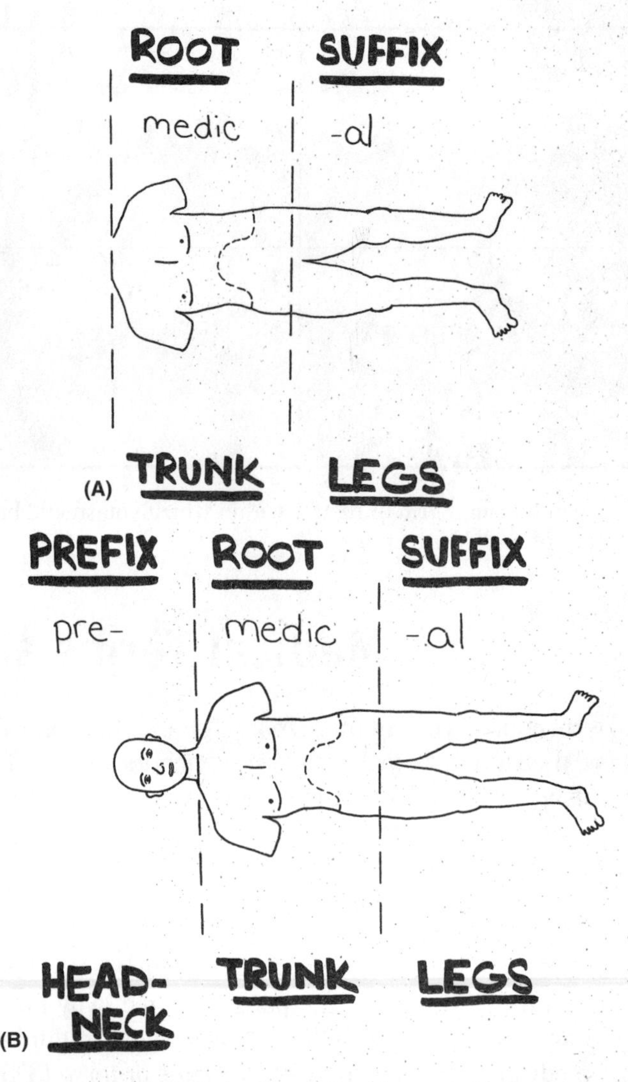

Fig. 1.13 Two different kinds of dissection or "cutting apart": one of the human body, and one of a medical term. (**A**) The root is to the suffix in *medic/al* as the body trunk (stem) is to the legs. (**B**) The *prefix* comes before the word *root* in *pre/medic/al*, like the *head* comes before the *trunk* of the body, and the *suffix* comes after the word *root* in *pre/medic/al*, like *legs* come after the body *trunk*.

WORD DISSECTION OR ANALYSIS

If we *dissect* (cut up) or analyze the whole human body, we obtain its three main parts—the head, trunk (torso), and limbs. Likewise, *word dissection* or *analysis* is the cutting up of a medical term into its component *word parts*. For the word *medical*, you may recall that these were *medic* (the root for "healing") plus *-al*. The word part *-al* is called a *suffix*. A suffix is a letter or letters that follows the root and modifies the meaning of a word. Now, the suffix *-al* means "____________" in regular English. [**Study suggestion:** Try to fill in the preceding blank from previous info in this chapter, then check your answer as you read further.]

WORD TRANSLATION

When we dissect a medical term, we insert one or more slashes (/) into it. In contrast, we dissect the human body using knives or *scalpels* (**SKAL**-pulls). After we have cut up the term, we can do a *word translation*. This is the rewriting of a medical term into its literal (exact) common English meaning. The word *medical*, for instance, literally translates to mean "____________" in common English. [**Study suggestion:** Again, try to fill-in the preceding blank, then check as you read.]

Did you get the right answer? Of course, *medic/al* literally "pertains to" (*-al*) "healing" (*medic*). Note that the meaning of the suffix almost always comes *first* in the common English translation of a medical term.

WORD BUILDING OR SYNTHESIS

Another important skill in medical terminology is *medical word building* or *synthesis*. This is the building up or synthesis of a new medical word by combining two or more word parts together. If we glance back at Figure 1.13, for example, we see a new term, *premedical* (pree-**MED**-ih-**kal**). To build this term, we must add *pre-*, a *prefix*, before the root *medic*. A prefix is a letter or group of letters that comes before a root, thereby modifying the meaning of a word. In *premedical*, the prefix *pre-* means "before." And we still keep the suffix *-al*. Putting all of these word parts together via word building results in the new term:

Prefix + *Root* + *Suffix* = *A new medical term*
PRE- + MEDIC + -AL = PREMEDICAL

Now, after we have built a new term, we can cross-check its meaning by going in reverse. That is, we dissect the newly built word by inserting one or more slashes and labeling the resulting word parts as either a prefix, root, or suffix:

	Prefix	*Root*	*Suffix*
PREMEDICAL⟶	PRE/	MEDIC/	AL
	"Before"	"Healing"	"Pertaining to"

The complete translation of *premedical* thus becomes, "pertaining to (the period) before healing." Note that, once again, the meaning of the suffix (*-al*) comes first in the literal (exact) English translation of the term. We have also been somewhat liberal in our translation, adding "(the period)" or something similar within parentheses, so that the translation sounds smoother.

SUMMARY OF WORD PARTS

In summary, there are three main types of word parts that make up medical terms: prefixes, roots, and suffixes. **Every single medical term has at least one root and a suffix, but not every medical term has a prefix!** To illustrate this important rule, just consider two of our example words used thus far: *medical* and *premedical*. If you dissect each of these words with slashes, once again, you will find that both *medical* and *premedical* contain a root (*medic*) and the suffix *-al*. However, only *premedical* contains a prefix—in this case, *pre-*.

Revising the idea shown back in Figure 1.13, each medical term always has a trunk or torso (word root) and attached body limbs (especially the legs) coming after it (a suffix). But some words (like some of the poor citizens of Ancient Mesopotamia who suffered severe punishments under the Code of Hammurabi) have lost their heads (prefixes)!

THE MAGIC OF THE COMBINING VOWEL: "A SPOONFUL OF SUGAR HELPS THE MEDICINE GO DOWN!"

Now that we have discussed the three major types of word parts—prefixes, roots, and suffixes—it is time to introduce their frequent helpmate, the *combining vowel*. A combining vowel is a vowel (usually the letter o) added between word parts to make word pronunciation easier. Or as that old saying goes, "A spoonful of sugar (the combining vowel) helps the medical (term) go down (into your brain)!"

The phrase *combining vowel* indicates that the vowel is used to smooth the connection or transition between two neighboring word parts when they are placed together within a term. It is somewhat like the fitting together of adjacent

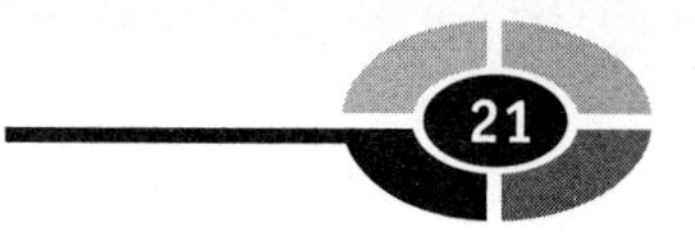

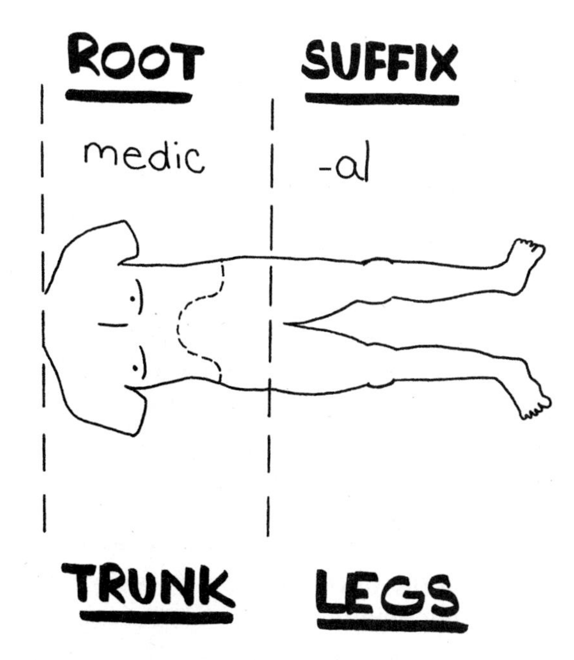

Body trunk and legs without a head compared to a word without a prefix.

bones in anatomy (Figure 1.14). Consider the root *oste* (**ahs**-tee) connecting to the suffix *-on*. Carrying out the process of word-building (synthesis), we get:

oste	+	*-on*	=	*osteon*
"bone"	+	"presence of"	=	"presence of bone"

Note that *osteon* is smoothly pronounced as **AHS**-tee-ahn. Therefore, the fit of its two component word parts is like a smooth *joint* between two bones—no *cartilage* (**KAR**-tih-**laj**) or "gristle" is required. (See Figure 1.14 A.)

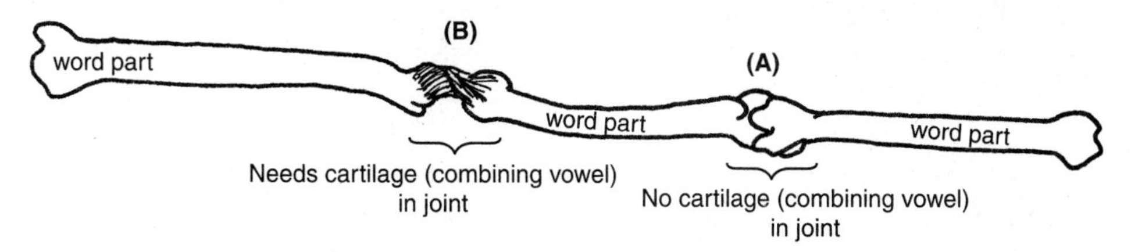

Fig. 1.14 Bone-and-joint metaphors to illustrate the need for a combining vowel. (**A**) "Smooth fit": No combining vowel (no cartilage or gristle) is required between joining word parts (or bones). (**B**) "Rough fit": A combining vowel (like cartilage or gristle) is required between joining word parts (or bones).

Consider, in marked contrast, the important instrument on the dashboard of your car:

speed + *o*		+ -meter	=	*speedometer*
	combining	+ "an instrument	=	"an instrument used
	vowel	used to measure"		to measure speed"

As you can see from Figure 1.14 B, the combination of *speed* with the suffix *-meter*, is a rough fit: The two consonants (*d* at the end of *speed* and *m* at the start of *–meter)* seem to rub and grate harshly against one another when you pronounce them. This is like a rough-fitting joint between two bones, such that some cartilage or gristle is needed to soften their contact. Just pronounce these two words: *speedmeter* and *speedometer*. From this, you can hear for yourself the truth in the old saying that, "A spoonful of sugar helps the 'med term' go down!"

In general, whenever you are building a new medical term, adding a combining vowel between the word parts never really hurts anything, and it may help make the pronunciation easier! So, go right ahead and do it, if the word sounds better to you!

Quiz

Refer to the text in this chapter if necessary. A good score is at least 8 correct answers out of these 10 questions. The answers are listed in the back of this book.

1. Primitive medicine is at least ______ years old.
   (a) 500
   (b) 1,000
   (c) 5,000
   (d) 10,000

2. The Code of Hammurabi was important because it:
   (a) Described special monetary rewards for good behavior of doctors
   (b) Established a set of laws and specific consequences for bad medical practice
   (c) Stated for the first time the clear importance of human life
   (d) Removed any doubts that Zeus was "King of the Gods"

3. Asclepius adopted the sacred snake as his symbol for healing, owing to the fact that:
   (a) The bites of poisonous snakes are always fatal
   (b) Snake venom was shown to be a great cure-all in ancient times

(c) The snake periodically sheds, regrows, and in a sense, "heals" its skin
(d) Mercury was the winged Messenger of the Gods

4. The Greek physician frequently labeled as the Father of Modern Medicine:
(a) Hippocrates
(b) Hades
(c) Dr. Lucifer
(d) Asclepius

5. The study of normal body structure:
(a) Physiology
(b) Medical terminology
(c) Morbidity
(d) Anatomy

6. Galen is commonly credited with being The Father of _____:
(a) Modern medicine
(b) Nursing care and treatment
(c) Radiotherapy
(d) Experimental physiology

7. In the word, *premedical*, the part serving as the root:
(a) -al
(b) pre-
(c) emedical
(d) medic

8. Body functions and the study of body functions:
(a) Etymology
(b) Terminology
(c) Physiology
(d) Geology

9. _____ is the prefix in premedical.
(a) Pre-
(b) -al
(c) Remedi
(d) Eme-

10. _____ is the suffix in premedical.
(a) -dical
(b) -al
(c) Pred-
(d) -medical

Memory Pillboxes for Chapter 1

Several key facts were tagged with numbered icons in the page margins of this chapter. Write a short summary of each of these key facts into a numbered cell or compartment within the appropriate type of Memory Pillbox that appears below.

Background and History **Pillboxes for Chapter 1:**

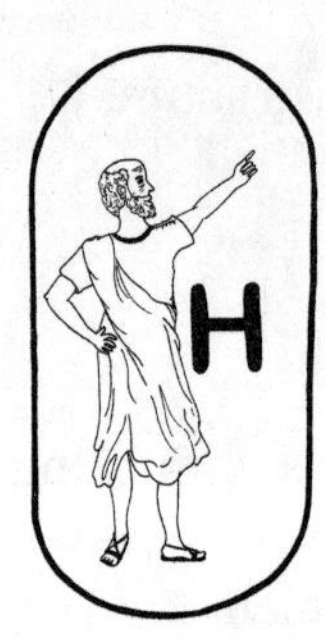

1	2
3	4

5	6

7

***Anatomy* Pillbox for Chapter 1:**

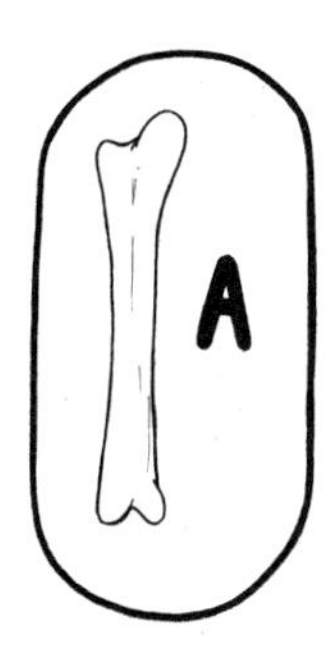

1

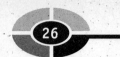

***Physiology* Pillbox for Chapter 1:**

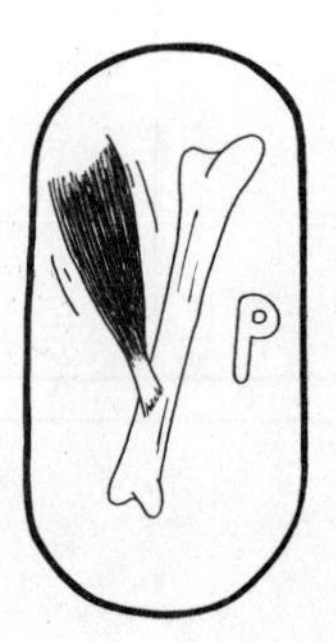

1

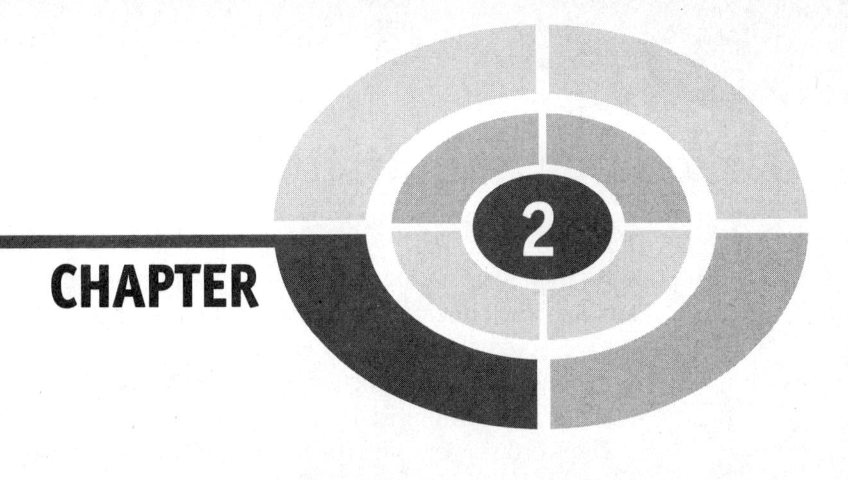

CHAPTER 2

Terms of Anatomy, Anesthesia, and Surgery

Chapter 1 provided us with a general introduction to the basic ideas or themes in this book. Now, starting with Chapter 2, we will begin to focus upon the main "meat" of medical terminology: lists of medical words grouped by their topic or area of study.

In particular, Chapter 2 will focus upon some key terms in the areas of anatomy, anesthesia, and surgery. We will work and practice with these words as we progress through the chapter. In this way, we shall "demystify" the terms and really come to *know* them!

Background and History

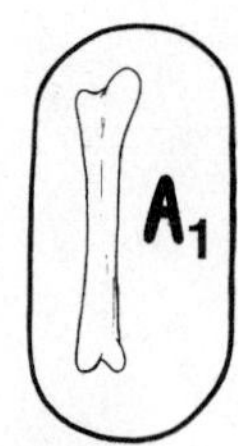

Chapter 1 informed us that medicine is at least 10,000 years old. How do we know this? Part of the proof comes from unearthing ancient fossils of human remains. The bones of the human skeleton—particularly those of the skull—can survive as fossils for many centuries! Thus, when *surgery* was performed upon such bones, the resulting *anatomical* (**an**-ah-**TAHM**-ih-kul) changes in their structure were often preserved.

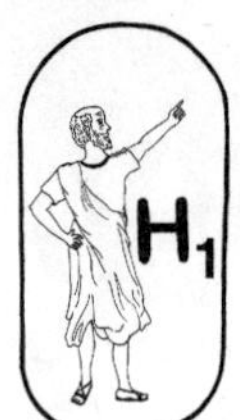

The word *surgery* derives from early Greek and literally means "hand work." Basically, the "hand work" of surgery involves treating various diseases, deformities, and injuries by means of *operations*. Such operations are more formally called *operative procedures*. An operation is a "process of working." Therefore, *operative* (**AHP**-er-ah-tiv) literally "pertains to" (*-ive*) "work" (*operat*). And it is quite appropriate to consider surgery as "hand work," because operations involve *surgeons* working with their hands. In summary, since operations (operative procedures) are performed by surgeons, they can technically be called *surgical* (**SUR**-jih-kul) *procedures*. This is because they "pertain to" (*-ical*) "hand work" (*surgic*).

TREPHINATION: ONE OF THE EARLIEST FORMS OF SURGERY WAS "HOLE-ISTIC MEDICINE"!

Evidence of such intricate surgical "hand work" has appeared in human fossils that are *prehistoric* (**pree**-hiss-**TOR**-ik). [**Study suggestion:** Using the Chapter 1 example of *premedical*, identify the *prefix* in the word *prehistoric*. Now, note that the *suffix* is *-ic*, which, according to Chapter 1, means what? Employing this information, you would translate *prehistoric* to exactly mean "____________." The root in *prehistoric*, __________, obviously means "history." After you write in the answers for these blanks, check them against the text that follows.]

By *prehistoric*, we literally mean "pertaining to" (*-ic*) something that happened "before" (*pre-*) recorded "history" (*histor*). In this case, we mean an operation or surgical procedure that occurred prior to recorded (written) history. The skulls and bones of prehistoric peoples, while they cannot talk, certainly provide distinct anatomical testimony that such cutting did, indeed, take place!

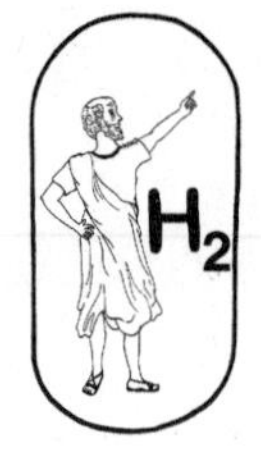

Among the oldest prehistoric surgical fossils ever found are the skulls of the ancient *Peruvian* (peh-**ROO**-vee-an) Indians. These *cranial* (**KRAY**-nee-al) or "pertaining to" (*-al*) "skull" (*crani*) operations may date back 10,000 years! Like many early peoples, the Indians of Peru developed a

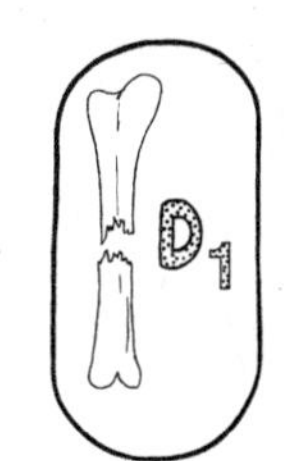

sophisticated type of surgery called *trephination* (**tref**-uh-**NAY**-shun) or *trepanation* (**trep**-uh-**NA**-shun).

Trephination (or trepanation) literally means "the process of" (*-tion*) "boring" (*trephin* or *trepan*). Among these ancient Indians, skull fractures were very common, mostly because people fought each other with slingshots and heavy clubs. When a person's skull is fractured, fluid often builds up within the area *superior* (soo-**PEER**-ee-or) to the brain. This is a particular anatomical area—"one which" (*-or*) is located "above" (*superi*) the brain. Trephination (trepanation) was probably done most often, therefore, to bore a hole in the fractured skull and relieve trapped fluid. This excessive fluid pressure upon the soft, fragile brain often creates a monstrous headache for its victims. Such heavy pressure, if left untreated, can result in permanent brain damage.

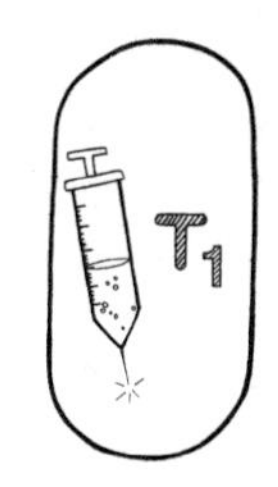

The coming of anesthesia

Imagine an ancient Indian, with a severe skull fracture, crying and thrashing with severe pain. Before any operation could be done, the person would have to be *sedated* (seh-**DAY**-ted) or "quieted down." Such a *sedation* (seh-**DAY**-shun) or "process of" (*-ion*) "quieting" (*sedat*), is also a normal part of modern *preoperative* (**pree-AHP**-er-ah-tiv) care. This care occurs "before" (*pre-*) an operation.

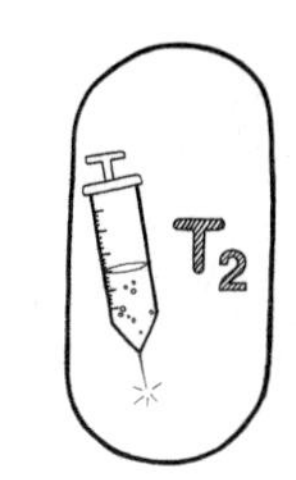

Sedation is often an early part of a schedule of *anesthesia* (**an**-es-**THEE**-zhee-uh) for patients nowadays that eventually results in a "condition" (*-ia*) "without" (*an-*) "feeling" (*esthes*). The Indians had to use natural sources of anesthesia that were available locally. These natural sources included the *coca* (**KOH**-kah) plant, which grows as shrubs on the sides of South American mountains. The coca leaves are chewed until softened, after which the juices are sucked out and swallowed.

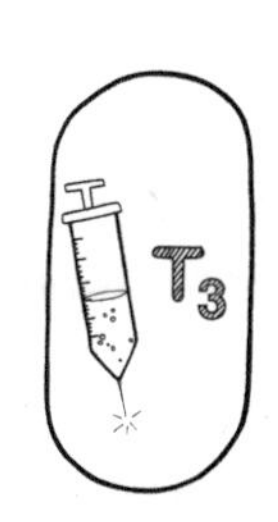

Coca leaves are the natural source of *cocaine* (koh-**KAYN**), an extremely powerful *narcotic* (nar-**KAHT**-ik) drug. The word *narcotic* "pertains to" (*-ic*) "sleepiness or numbness" (*narc*). By chewing and sucking coca leaves, therefore, the natural narcotic cocaine acts to *narcotize* or "produce" (*-ize*) a state of "benumbing" (*narcot*) in the injured patient. And as the skull-fractured Indian chewed the coca leaves as part of his preoperative treatment, a progressive *narcosis* (nar-**KOH**-sis)—"abnormal condition of" (*-osis*) "benumbing" (*narc*)—would occur. (Consult Figure 2.1, A.) Using modern terminology, we could say that the narcotized Indian was undergoing a natural regimen of *preop* (preoperative) anesthesia.

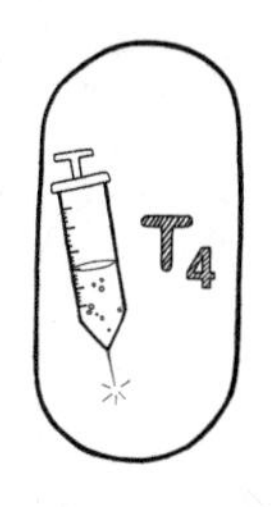

After the distressed patient was sufficiently narcotized and sedated, the actual operative phase of trephination (trepanation) could proceed. (See Figure 2.1, B.) Various types of *scalpels* (**SKAL**-pels) or surgical "knives" were

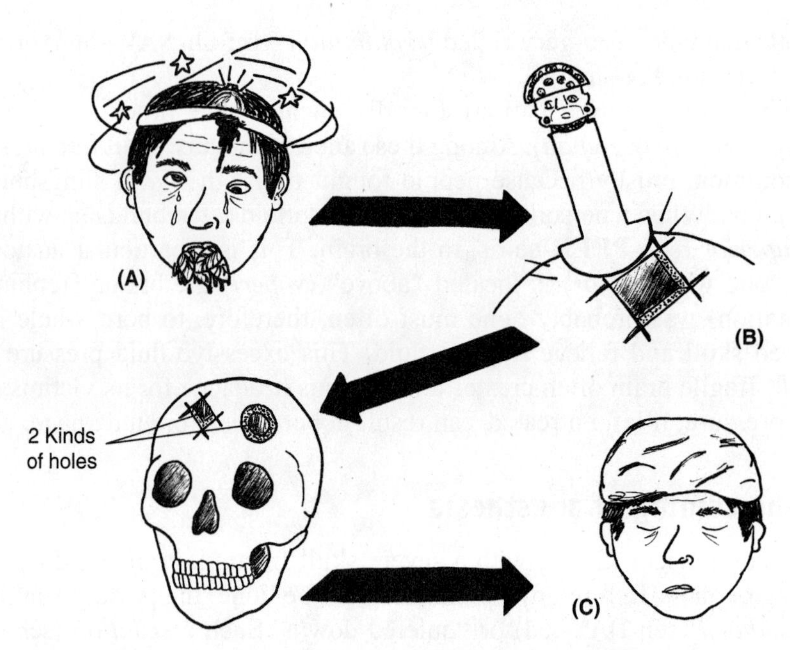

Fig. 2.1 Trephination (trephination) among the ancient Peruvian Indians. (**A**) Preoperative anethesia is induced by narcotics. (**B**) Trephination/ trephination: A scalpel (surgical knife) is used to make a hole in the skull. (**C**) Postoperatively, the wound was covered by a shell or gourd to assist healing.

employed. The first of these knives was used to *incise* (in-**SIZE**) or "cut into" the scalp, which was then "drawn back" by a crude *retractor* (ree-**TRAKT**-er). After the initial *incision* (in-**SIZH**-un) ("process of cutting into") was made, special *trepanation scalpels* carved a variety of openings into the skull, itself. The scalpel-cut openings were usually fairly square. Other instruments drilled rounded holes within the top of the *cranium* (**KRAY**-nee-um) or *skull.* The accumulated fluid lying *inferior* (in-**FEAR**-ee-or) to—that is, "below"—the skull surface, was then released.

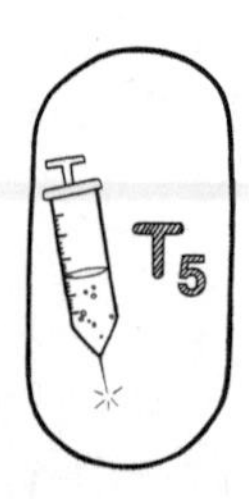

When the operation was over, the head wound was covered with a shell or gourd to protect it during healing (Figure 2.1, C). This was part of the *postop* or *postoperative* (**pohst-AHP**-er-ah-tiv) healing regimen, which literally occurred "after" (*post-*) the operation. An extremely large number of fossil skulls have been found with trephination holes that were at least partially filled in with new bone tissue. Thus, we can conclude that this dramatic operation had a high success rate, even in ancient times. In other words, the Peruvian Indians were very skilled in the practice of "hole-istic" medicine!

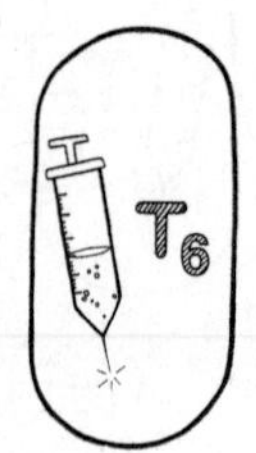

SUMMARY TABLE 2.1

Consult Summary Table 2.1 for a quick review of some important words and word parts.

Summary Table 2.1 Words and Word Parts
Write in the *exact* meaning (literal English translation) for up to 10 key terms selected from the preceding block of text. After you are done, check your word meanings with the correct answers, which are given at the end of this chapter.

Key Terms	Prefixes	Roots	Suffixes	Exact Meanings
operative	(none)	operat "work"	-ive "pertaining to"	1. ________
surgical	(none)	surgic "hand work"	-al "pertaining to"	2. ________
cranial	(none)	crani "skull"	-al "pertaining to"	3. ________
trephination, trepanation	(none)	trephin, trepan "boring"	-tion "the process of"	4. ________
superior	(none)	superi "above"	-or "one which"	5. ________
sedation	(none)	sedat "quieting"	-ion	6. ________
preoperative	pre- "before"	operat	-ive	7. ________
anesthesia	an- "without"	esthes "feeling"	-ia "condition"	8. ________
narcosis	(none)	narc "benumbing"	-osis "abnormal condition of"	9. ________
postoperative	post- "after"	operat	-ive	10. ________

JOHN HUNTER: THE FATHER OF SCIENTIFIC SURGERY HAD NIGHT VISITS FROM GRAVE ROBBERS!

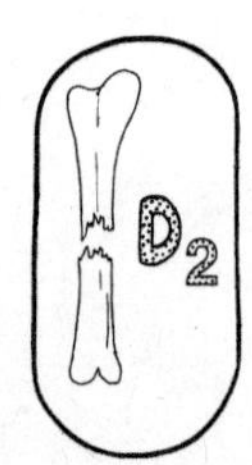

Of great value in performing surgery is a correct knowledge of anatomy. Far too often in ancient times, surgery (especially of the thorax and abdomen) led to a quick death for the unfortunate patient, because his surgeon would accidentally hit a major blood vessel or other vital body part! Eventually, *ligatures* (**LIG**-uh-churs) were developed. Ligatures consist of thread or wire that is "tied" (*ligat*) tightly around a cut blood vessel, thereby stopping heavy bleeding. In addition, the technique of *suturing* (**SOO**-chur-ing) was perfected, in which "seam"-like *sutures* (**SOO**-churs) were created by stitching two cut surfaces back together.

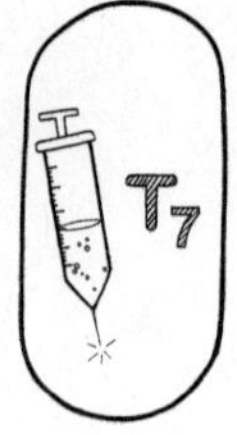

However, *ligation* (lie-**GAY**-shun)—the "process of" (*-ion*) "tying" (*ligat*) and narrowing a blood vessel or other structure—and suturing (creating stitched "seams") simply cannot substitute for advanced anatomical knowledge! Vesalius (whom we introduced in Chapter 1) began the thorough dissection of human cadavers in the 1500s, but this beginning of precise anatomical knowledge had to be greatly expanded before surgery could become scientific. By *scientific*, we literally mean "pertaining to" (*-ic*) "making knowledge" (*scientif*). Specifically, this is the *anatomical* type of scientific knowledge, which is best gained by "cutting" (*tom*) the body "up or apart" (*ana-*). With precise anatomical knowledge, obviously, the surgeon knows exactly *where* to cut (or where *not* to cut) during an operation!

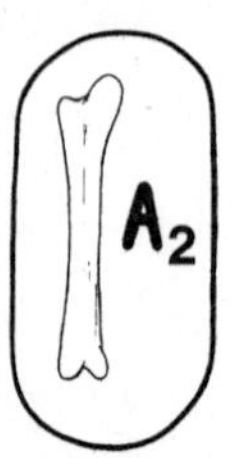

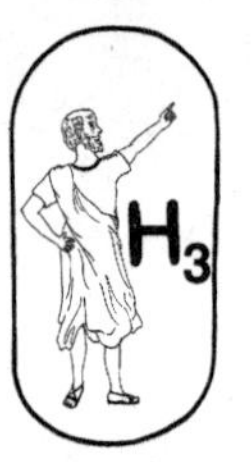

John Hunter, for instance, was a Scottish-born surgeon and *anatomist* (ah-**NAT**-oh-mist)—"one who specializes in" (*-ist*) "cutting" (*tom*) the body "up or apart" (*ana-*). Working in England during the mid-1700s, Hunter helped make surgery scientific (hence more respectable and reliable) by basing it upon careful *autopsies* (**AW**-tahp-sees). An *autopsy* is "the process of" (-y) "seeing" (*ops*) a dead body personally, for your own "self" (*auto-*). Hunter carried out more than 2,000 autopsies on corpses, thereby seeing for himself the exact anatomical changes that were behind many diseases. Most unfortunately, however, Hunter was so eager to carry out autopsies that he utilized the services of grave robbers, who visited cemeteries by night and dug up the corpses of the recently buried!

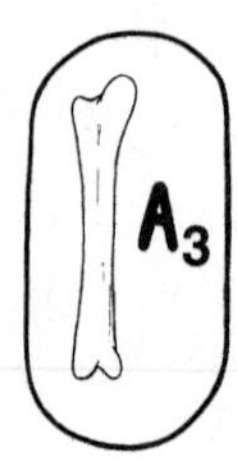

Hunter also carried out dissections on living animals, using no anesthesia, while he took numerous *biopsies* (**BUY**-ahp-sees)! A *biopsy* is "the process of" (-y) "seeing" (*ops*) the tissues of a "living" (*bi*) thing. After a scalpel is used to make an incision into an area of living tissue, a pair of *forceps* (**FOR**-seps) or "tongs" is employed to grab the edge of cut tissue. The isolated tissue is then *excised* (ek-**SIZED**)—"cut" (*cis*) "out of" (*ex*) the body.

To prevent heavy bleeding, the cut vessels left behind after tissue *excision* are often *cauterized* (**KAW**-ter-**eyezd**), that is, burned and sealed off. Originally this was done with a hot "burner" or "burning iron." *Cauterization*

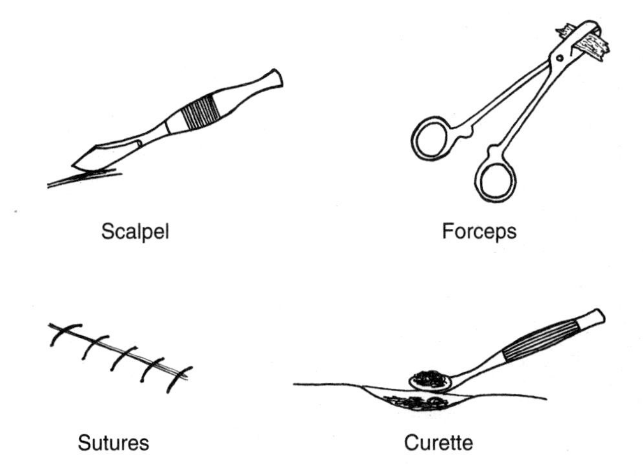

Fig. 2.2 Examples of simple surgical materials and instruments.

(**kaw**-ter-ih-**ZAY**-shun)—the "process of" (*-tion*) "burning" (*cauter*)—now generally involves the use of an electric *cautery* (**KAW**-ter-ee).

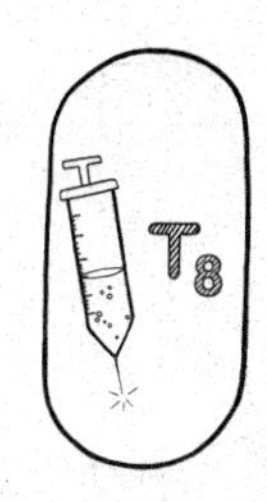

If the biopsy involves the *excision* of a tissue sample from a body cavity, a *curette* (koo-**RET**)—a scoop-ended "scraper" or "cleanser"—may remove bleeding material from the cavity interior. (Figure 2.2 displays some examples of the types of surgical instruments mentioned in this chapter.)

SUMMARY TABLE 2.2

Consult Summary Table 2.2 for a quick review of some important words and word parts.

WILLIAM MORTON: ANESTHESIA GETS "REAL"

We have already mentioned cocaine as a natural narcotic used to induce a state of anesthesia in Ancient Peruvian Indians. Such drug-created narcosis was part of a preoperative technique leading to trephination (trepanation). Natural narcotic substances, such as cocaine and *opium*, have also been used to create *analgesia* since ancient times.

It is very important to distinguish between the two separate medical terms: *anesthesia* and *analgesia* (**an**-al-**JEE**-zee-uh). [**Study suggestion:** Right now, try to give the exact English translation of *anesthesia*. If you can't remember it, go back and quickly review past info in this chapter.] Anesthesia, you may recall, is a body condition where the person lacks feeling or sensation of *any* kind—including the sense of pain.

Summary Table 2.2 Words and Word Parts

Write in the *exact* meaning (literal English translation) for up to 10 key terms selected from the preceding block of text. After you are done, check your word meanings with the correct answers, which are given at the end of this chapter.

Key Terms	Prefixes	Roots	Suffixes	Exact Meanings
ligature	(none)	ligat "ties, tying"	-ure "one which"	1. ________
ligation	(none)	ligat	-ion "process of"	2. ________
anatomical	ana- "up, apart"	tom "cutting"	-ical "pertaining to"	3. ________
anatomist	ana-	tom	-ist "one who specilizes in"	4. ________
autopsy	auto- "self"	-ops "seeing"	-y "process of"	5. ________
biopsy	(none)	bi "living"; ops "seeing"	-y	6. ________
cauterization	(none)	cauteriz "burning"	-tion "process of"	7. ________

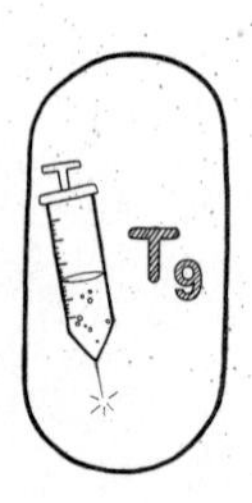

In many instances, however, it is desirable to produce only *analgesia*, which is "a condition" (*-ia*) "without" (*an-*) "pain" (*alges*). For example, many people suffering the constant agony of low back pain try to obtain a good *analgesic* (**an**-al-**JEE**-zik) effect. This only "pertains to" (*-ic*) creating a lack of pain sense. They could achieve this analgesic effect by taking an aspirin, say, or maybe by applying heat or ice packs to the low back area. They would certainly not want to create a much more potent *anesthetic* (**an**-es-**THET**-ik) effect, because such an effect "pertains to" (*ic*) the loss of *all* types of body "feelings or sensations" (*esthet*). Wouldn't it be a foolish example of overkill to totally *anesthetize* (an-**ES**-thuh-**teyez**) or "cause (a person) to" (*-ize*) become completely numb, when all they were suffering was low back pain?

35

In summary, we need to remember that:

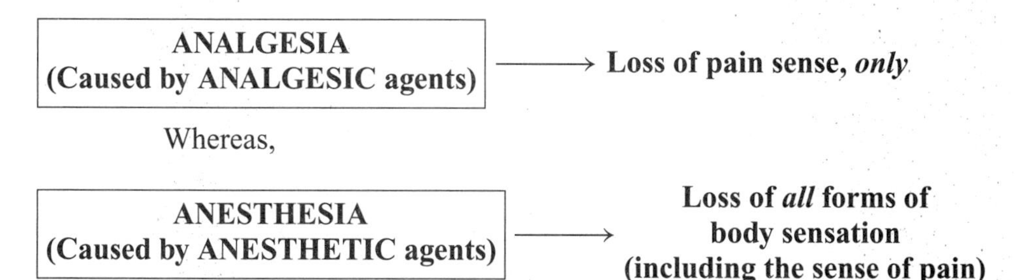
ANALGESIA
(Caused by ANALGESIC agents)
Loss of pain sense, only
Whereas,
ANESTHESIA
(Caused by ANESTHETIC agents)
Loss of all forms of body sensation (including the sense of pain)

The modern story of anesthesia really began with the work of *William Morton*, a Boston dentist. On October 16, 1846, Dr. Morton acted as perhaps the first professional *anesthesiologist* (**an**-es-**thee**-zee-**AHL**-uh-jist). This is literally "one who studies" (*-ologist*) the "lack of" (*an*) "feeling" (*thesi*). Dr. Morton successfully anesthetized a patient who was having a tumor removed from his jaw by a surgeon. Morton had the patient inhale *ether* (**EE**-thur) through a glass flask placed over his face.

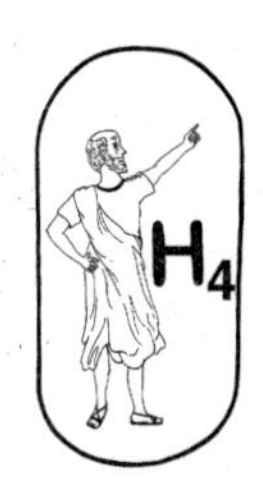
H_4

The patient quickly became unconscious, thereby inducing a state of *general* or *surgical anesthesia*. In this broadly acting type of anesthesia, the patient undergoing surgery loses consciousness and also experiences total loss of all types of body sensation (including pain). "Gentlemen, this is no humbug!" exclaimed a physician who was amazed at how effectively the ether anesthetized the patient.

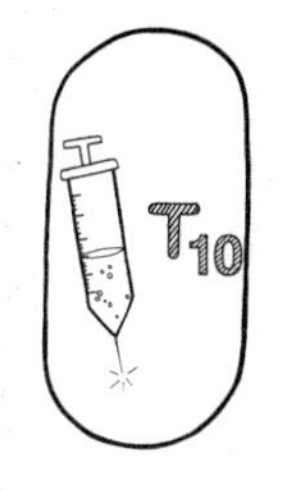
T_{10}

Another major type of anesthesia is called *local anesthesia*. Here, a small amount of some anesthetic is injected into the patient (usually into a skeletal muscle). The local (nearby) area around the injection site quickly becomes numb. You have probably had a local anesthetic injected into the side of your face, for instance, during dental surgery or tooth extraction.

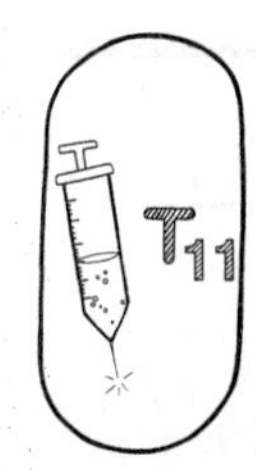
T_{11}

During major surgery, however, anesthetics are typically administered by an *anesthetist* (an-**ES**-theh-**tist**)—"one who specializes in" (*-ist*) this field. Because of ether's sometimes unpredictable effects, nowadays other general anesthetics are usually used in place of it. Various narcotics are often injected and produce excellent analgesia. If given at much higher doses, narcotics not only remove pain but also induce a deep general (surgical) anesthesia.

SUMMARY TABLE 2.3

Consult Summary Table 2.3 for a quick review of some important words and word parts.

Summary Table 2.3 Words and Word Parts
Write in the *exact* meaning (literal English translation) for up to 10 key terms selected from the preceding block of text. After you are done, check your word meanings with the correct answers, which are given at the end of this chapter.

Key Terms	Prefixes	Roots	Suffixes	Exact Meanings
analgesia	an- "without"	alges "pain"	-ia "a condition"	1. ________
analgesic	an-	alges	-ic "pertaining to"	2. ________
anesthetic	an-	esthet "feelings or sensations"	-ic	3. ________
anesthetize	an-	esthet	-ize "cause to"	4. ________
anesthesiologist	an-	-esthesi "feeling"	-ologist "one who studies"	5. ________
anesthetist	an-	esthet	-ist "one who specializes in"	6. ________

Quiz

Refer to the text in this chapter if necessary. A good score is at least 8 correct answers out of these 10 questions. The answers are listed in the back of this book.

1. The word, *surgery*, literally means:
   (a) "One who cuts"
   (b) "The process of cutting (something) up or apart"
   (c) "Hand work"
   (d) "Foot work"
2. *Pretrephination* (pree-**tref**-uh-**NAY**-shun) means that:
   (a) A kid has already gotten a hole cut into his head!
   (b) There is a process of preparation occurring before the cranium is incised

(c) No further pain or bodily sensations will occur
(d) There is an action occurring that follows incision into the cranium

3. The exact opposite of sedation is:
(a) Quieting
(b) Perimeter
(c) Narcotizing
(d) Stimulating

4. A bone lying inferior to the heart would be located:
(a) Behind it
(b) Beside it
(c) Above it
(d) Below it

5. Both ligation and cauterization are similar because:
(a) Each procedure removes warty growths
(b) Neither is based upon solid scientific principles
(c) Both processes increase blood loss from wounds
(d) They generally stabilize and reduce blood loss

6. Surgical knives are called
(a) Scalpels
(b) Cauteries
(c) Curettes
(d) Retractors

7. These professionals actually administer the drugs that reduce or eliminate body sensations:
(a) Zoologists and cosmetologists
(b) Anarchists and separatists
(c) Surgeons and anatomists
(d) Anesthesiologists and anesthetists

8. The Father of Scientific Surgery was:
(a) Vesalius
(b) John Hunter
(c) Henry Trepaner
(d) William Morton

9. If Baby Heinie had analgesia, but not anesthesia, in his left ear, then he would:
(a) Experience a nearly constant state of ear pain
(b) Likely lose all feeling in the ear

(c) Perform a trepanation upon his grandmother after she had boxed his ear!
(d) Maintain all feeling in the ear, except for the sense of pain

10. Unlike general anesthesia, local anesthesia:
(a) Creates a false sense of security in many patients
(b) Involves the same factors as surgical anesthesia
(c) Requires no inhaling of ether-like substances
(d) Doesn't prepare the body for being biopsied

Memory Pillboxes for Chapter 2

Several key facts were tagged with numbered icons in the page margins of this chapter. Write a short summary of each of these key facts into a numbered cell or compartment within the appropriate type of *Memory Pillbox* that appears below.

Background and History **Pillboxes for Chapter 2:**

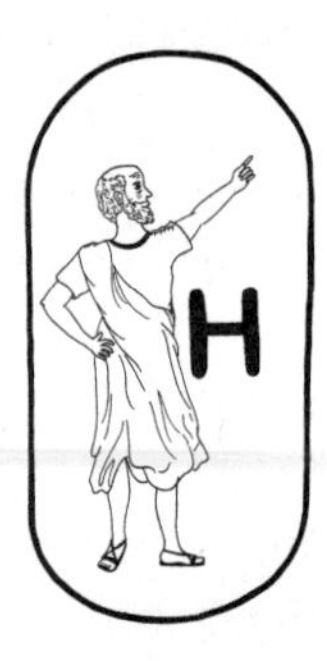

1	2

3	4

Anatomy **Pillboxes for Chapter 2:**

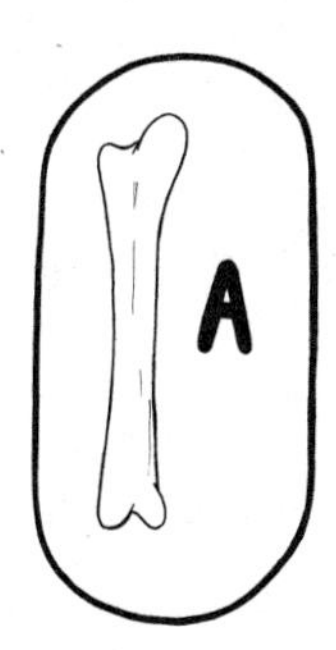

1

2	3

Disease/Injury **Pillboxes for Chapter 2:**

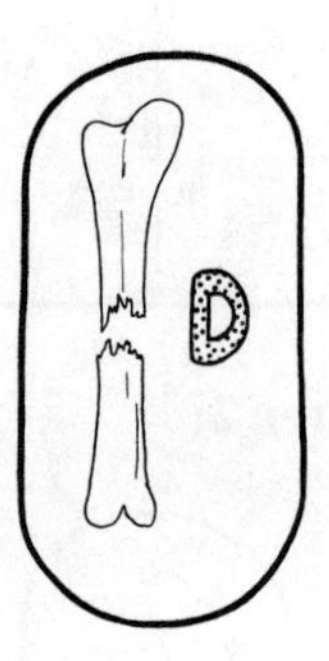

1	2

Therapy/Treatment **Pillboxes for Chapter 2:**

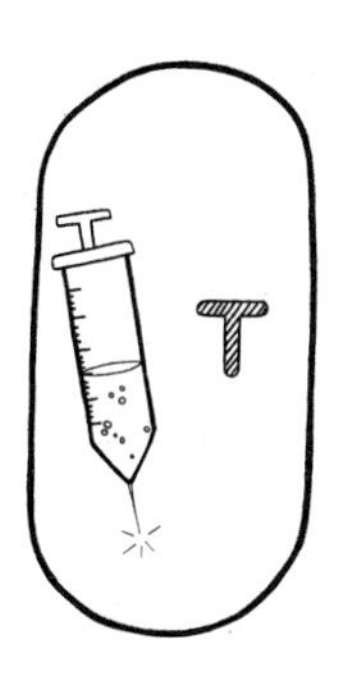

1	
2	3
4	5

6	7
8	9
10	11

Answers for Chapter 2 Summary Tables

FOR SUMMARY TABLE 2.1

1. "pertaining to work"
2. "pertaining to hand work"
3. "pertaining to the skull"
4. "the process of boring"
5. "one which is above"
6. "the process of quieting"
7. "pertaining to (something) before working"
8. "a condition without feeling"
9. "an abnormal condition of benumbing"
10. "pertaining to (something) after working"

FOR SUMMARY TABLE 2.2

1. "one which ties"
2. "the process of tying"
3. "pertaining to cutting (something) up or apart"
4. "one who specializes in cutting (something) up or apart"
5. "the process of seeing (for your) self"
6. "the process of seeing (something) living"
7. "the process of burning (something)"

FOR SUMMARY TABLE 2.3

1. "a condition without pain"
2. "pertaining to the lack of pain"
3. "pertaining to the lack of feelings or sensations"
4. "to cause to be without feelings or sensations"
5. "one who studies the lack of feelings or sensations"
6. "one who specializes in the lack of feelings or sensations"

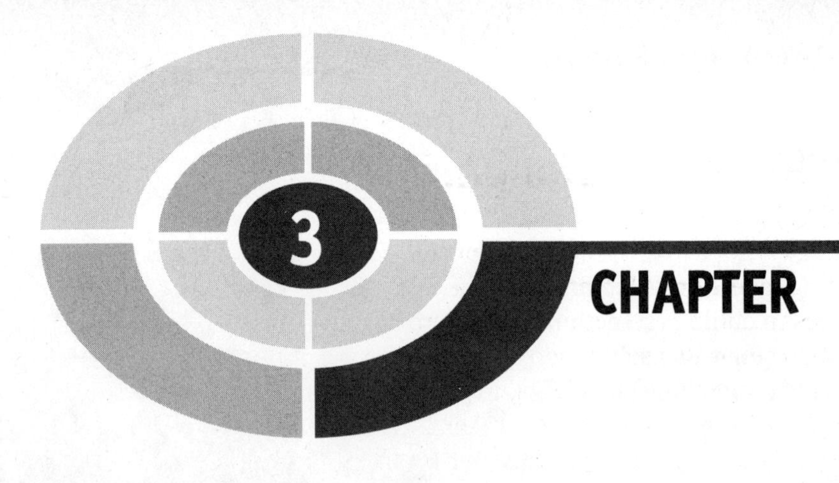

Terms of Microbiology and Infectious Diseases

For the most part, the terms we studied back in Chapter 2 focused upon the areas of anatomy, anesthesia, and surgery. Anatomy involves studying body structures, surgery involves cutting these body structures, and anesthesia involves numbing these body structures. Now, in Chapter 3, let's start *infecting* these body structures! The word *infection* ultimately comes from Latin and literally means "the process of" (*-ion*) "dipping into, corrupting, or invading" (*infect*). When we talk about *infectious* (in-**FEK**-shus) *diseases*, therefore, we are "referring to" (*-ious*) various types of body "invasions"!

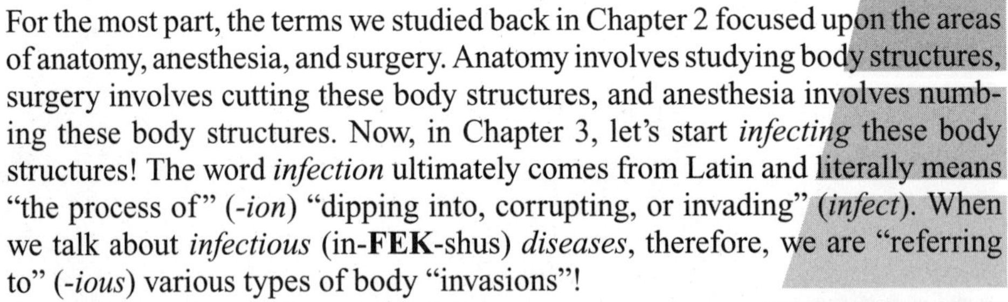

Hence, Chapter 3 will essentially give us access to a special kind of medical terminology: the terminology of infection—body invasion by alien (nonhuman) beings!

Background and History

We have already defined *infection* as "the process of invading." But this could be followed up by another question: "Infection is the process of invading *what*?" The answer is, invading an *organism* (**OR**-gah-**nizm**). An organism is literally a "condition of being" (*-ism*) a body having one or more "organs" (*organ*). Humans, all animals, and all plants, for instance, are classified as organisms. Organisms have living bodies with organs (such as the heart, which represents anatomy). And these organs carry out a variety of complex functions (such as the blood-pumping action of the heart, which represents physiology).

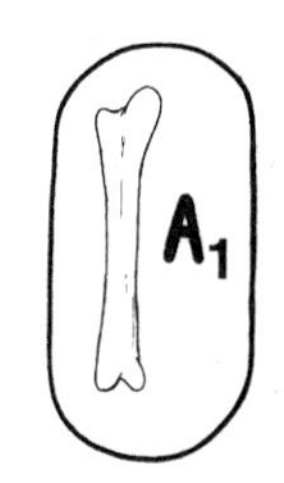

Because organisms are alive, they are considered part of *biology*, which is the "study of" (*-ology*) "life" (*bi*). Figure 3.1 shows some examples of both large and small living organisms, whose *biological* (buy-oh-**LAHJ**-ih-kal) characteristics "pertain to" (*-ical*) the "study of life."

There are two main ways that all types of organisms (humans, animals, or plants) are further categorized. These categories depend upon the relative size of the bodies of these organisms. *Macroscopic* (**MACK**-ruh-**SKAHP**-ik) or *gross* (**GROHS**) organisms are "large" (*macro-*) enough to be "examined" (*scop*) with

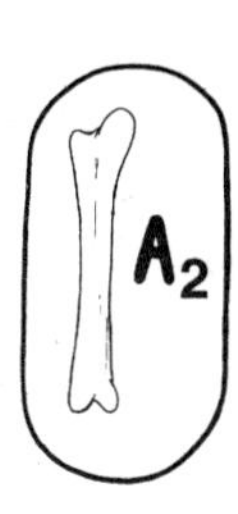

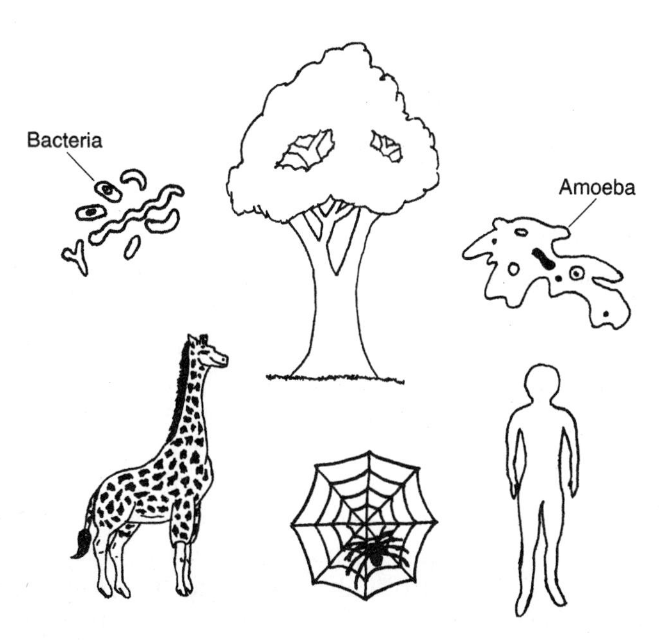

Fig. 3.1 Some large and small living organisms studied in biology.

the naked (unaided) eye. Such macroscopic (gross) organisms do, of course, include human beings!

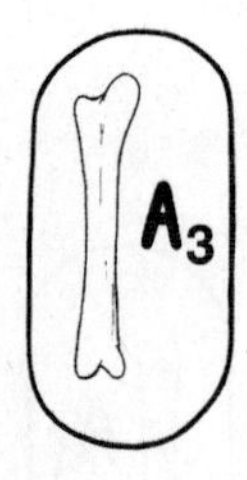

Microscopic (**my**-kroh-**SKAHP**-ik) *organisms*, in marked contrast, are so "tiny" (*micro-*) that they can only be "examined" (*scop*) using a special magnifying instrument: the *microscope*. In general, such microscopic organisms are called *microbes* (**MY**-krohbs). These are literally "tiny" (*micr*) "living" (*ob*) things that are "present" (*-e*) nearly everywhere on this planet! *Microbial* (my-**KROH**-be-al) life, in fact, may "pertain to" (*-al*) some of the most ancient "tiny living" (*microbi*) things!

In summary:

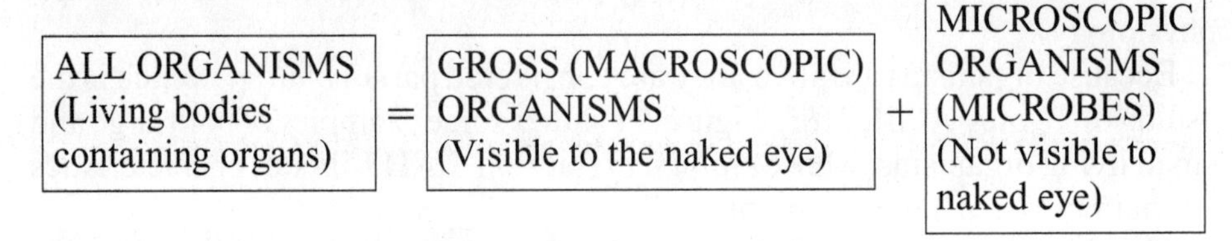

ALL ORGANISMS (Living bodies containing organs)	=	GROSS (MACROSCOPIC) ORGANISMS (Visible to the naked eye)	+	MICROSCOPIC ORGANISMS (MICROBES) (Not visible to naked eye)

[**Study suggestion:** Which of the living creatures shown in Figure 3.1 represent gross (macroscopic) organisms? Which are examples of microbes (microscopic organisms)?]

DEVELOPMENT OF THE MICROSCOPE: THE TINY BECOMES VISIBLE

To thoroughly understand the anatomy of microbes (microbial life or microscopic organisms), we must understand the development of the microscope. This is the tool that made such a tiny world visible to us in the first place! The science of *microscopy* (my-**KRAHS**-kuh-pea) is all about "the process of examining" (*-oscopy*) "tiny" (*micr*) things, both living and nonliving.

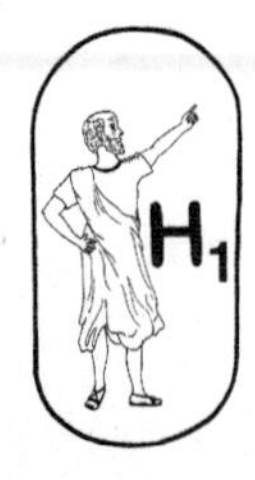

Let us talk about the very first *microscopist* (my-**KRAHS**-kuh-pist)—"one who specializes in" (*-ist*) "examining tiny" things. He is the Italian scientist, *Galileo* (**gal**-uh-**LEE**-oh). Galileo is most famous for his work with the telescope, but his experiments with glass lenses led him to develop the first microscope in the early 1500s. Although Galileo was probably the first microscopist, his intense interests in mathematics and astronomy soon led him far away from microscopy. Galileo did, however, create a lasting generalization about the connection between the mathematical subject of geometry and the study of all nature. "The Book of Nature is written in characters of Geometry," he wisely proclaimed. Because Galileo also studied medicine, he obviously would apply this statement to the study of the *internal environment*—the "inner space" of the body that lies deep under the surface of the skin. [**Study suggestion:** It is highly recommended that you follow up this idea with a careful reading of both *ANATOMY DEMYSTIFIED* and *PHYSIOLOGY DEMYSTIFIED*, which quite creatively carry out Galileo's geometric view of human body structure and function!]

Discovering "animalcules": A Dutchman creates the science of microbiology

About a century after Galileo, an uneducated Dutchman named *Anton van Leeuwenhoek* (**LOO**-en-**hohk**) began grinding glass lenses in his spare time. Leeuwenhoek earned his living as a *linen draper*. This is a person who uses linen from the stems of the flax plant (which has thin, threadlike parts) to sew cloth fabrics, such as drapes.

Leeuwenhoek probably began grinding his glass lenses to help him magnify and clearly see the intricate (and nearly microscopic) geometric patterns of crisscrossing linen threads in his fabrics. One common pattern of fabric studied by Leeuwenhoek is shown in Figure 3.2 (A). This intricate crisscrossing pattern creates a rectangle-shaped *matrix* (**MAY**-tricks) or "womb." The matrix (womb) is frequently used as a basic model for reproducing more complicated geometric designs. [**Thinking suggestion:** What is a possible connection between this matrix pattern of woven cloth fabrics and the rectangular "Memory Pillboxes" used to store key text facts at the end of each chapter in this book? Explain, and then discuss your insights with a friend!]

Like Galileo before him, Leeuwenhoek apparently concluded that, "The Book of Nature is written in characters of Geometry." He was referring, in particular, to the microscopic world of the rectangular thread matrix! Getting very excited about studying microscopic objects, he developed a keen interest in closely examining a wide variety of both living and nonliving things. In the early years, he used a cumbersome handheld device, but with later refinement, Leeuwenhoek developed the first stand-up microscope (Figure 3.2, B).

In one instance, he put a drop of greenish-looking pond water under the lenses of his microscope. Leeuwenhoek was amazed to see hundreds of what he called *animalcules* (**AN**-ih-mal-**kyools**), or "tiny" (*-cules*) greenish-yellow "animals," busily swimming around! In modern terminology, these animalcules are called the *protozoa* (**proh**-toh-**ZOH**-ah)—the "first or most primitive" (*proto-*) types of "animals" (*zoa*). These protozoa are living organisms, but they are extremely small, because in most cases their whole body is *unicellular*. This

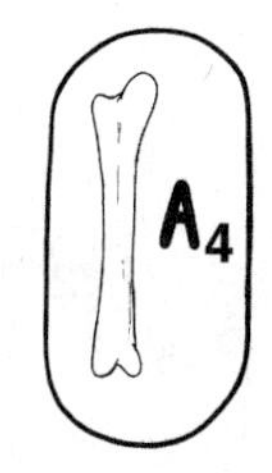

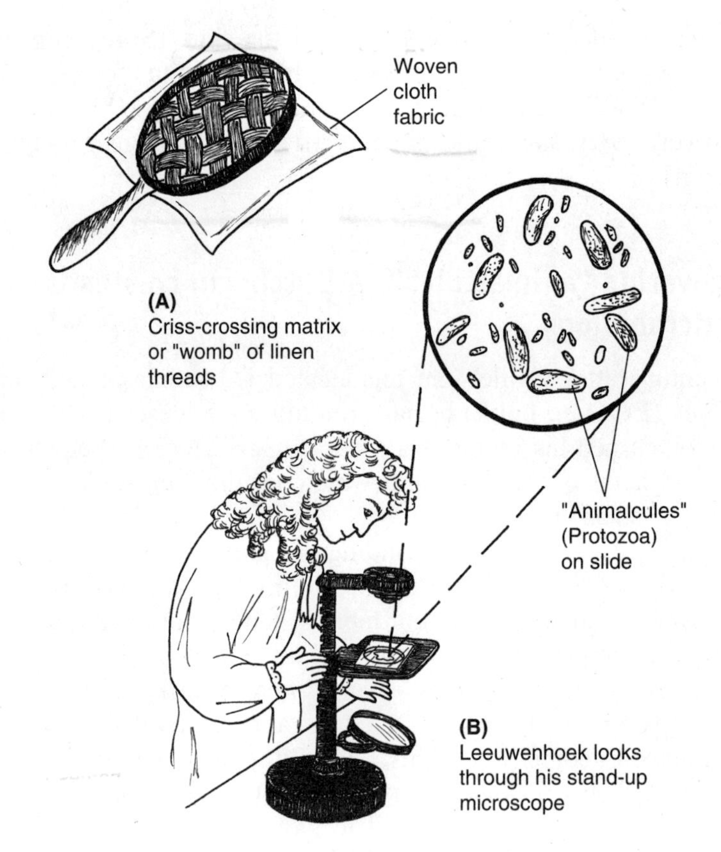

Fig. 3.2 Leeuwenhoek and his world of the microscope.

means that their body consists of just "one" (*uni-*) living "little cell" (*cellul*). [**Study suggestion:** Using your prior knowledge, try to build a single term that means "one who specializes in the study of the most primitive animals." Check your answer with the text that follows.]

Later, Leeuwenhoek also discovered *bacteria* in various places, such as in the scum covering the teeth in his own mouth! Therefore, we can call Leeuwenhoek the first *protozoologist* (**proh**-toh-zoh-**AHL**-uh-jist), because he studied "primitive animals." Likewise, Leeuwenhoek was the first *bacteriologist* (**bak**-teer-e-**AHL**-oh-jist). After all, he was a "specialist in studying" (*-ologist*) the "bacteria." The word, *bacteria* (**bak-TEER**-e-uh), literally translates to mean "little staffs, clubs, or rods" (*bacteri*) that are "present" (-a). Figure 3.3 provides an overview of the major types of bacteria. [**Study suggestion:** Name the major types of bacteria that you think look most like "little rods or clubs."]

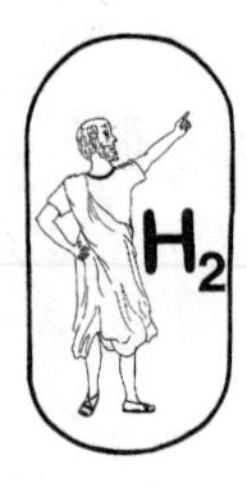

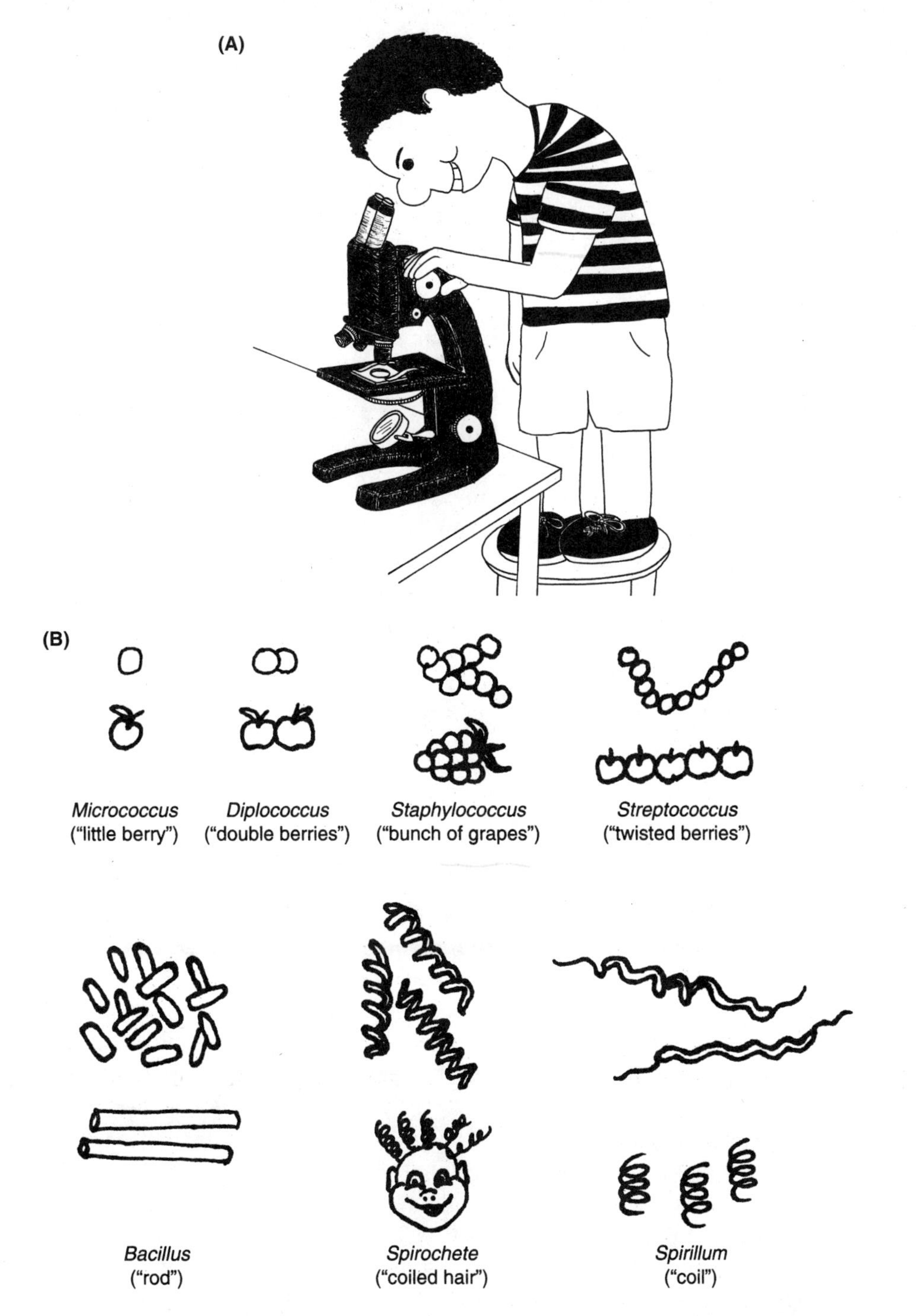

Fig. 3.3 The compound microscope used to view some major types of bacteria. (**A**) Baby Heinie gazing through a modern compound microscope (**B**) Some major types of bacteria that can be seen through a compound microscope.

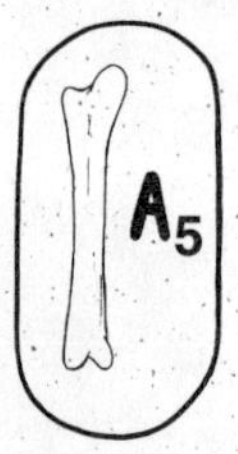

Each *bacterium* is just a single unicellular plant-like *microorganism* (**MY**-kroh-**OR**-gah-**nizm**) "present" (*-um*). As shown in Figure 3.3, the bacteria include these types: the *cocci* (**COCK**-see), which look like round "berries"; the *bacilli* (bah-**SIL**-ee), which resemble slender "rods"; the *spirochetes* (**SPY**-roh-keets), named for their likeness to tiny "coiled hairs"; and the *spirilla* (spy-**RIL**-uh), which look like tight "coils."

Observe from Figure 3.3 that Baby Heinie (a mischievous character who appears in both *ANATOMY DEMYSTIFIED* and *PHYSIOLOGY DEMYSTIFIED*) is standing upon a chair and looking at the different types of bacteria through a modern *compound microscope*. Unlike the very simple microscopes developed by Leeuwenhoek, the compound microscope has the magnification of the single lens in its main tube "compounded" or made better by additional lenses in the eyepieces. This compounded effect allows the modern microscopist (like mischievous little Baby Heinie) to view objects such as bacteria more readily. They can be magnified from about 100 to 1,000 times their actual size.

The electron microscope makes viruses visible

Some objects, such as *viruses*, are far too tiny to be viewed with a compound microscope. For examining these tiniest objects, which may have to be magnified 100,000 times, an *electron microscope* is required. As its name suggests, an electron microscope focuses a beam of *electrons* (tiny negatively charged particles) upon a specimen. Figure 3.4 (A) shows a *scanning electron microscope* being operated by none other than Professor Joe. (This studious fellow is the friendly host who guides readers through both our *ANATOMY DEMYSTIFIED* and *PHYSIOLOGY DEMYSTIFIED* books.)

Biologists (like Professor Joe) often use scanning electron microscopes to *scan* the surface of one or more cells that have been coated with metal. This metal coating stops the electron beam from passing through the cell, making it bounce off the cell so that its surface features may be seen. Figure 3.4 (B), for example, reveals the scanned surface of a *leukocyte* (**LOO**-koh-**sight**)—a "white" (*leuk*) blood "cell" (*cyt*). It is displayed as an image on a lit screen.

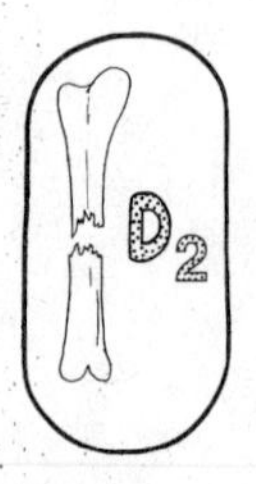

"What are those strange-looking objects dotting the surface of the leukocyte being scanned?" you might now be asking. These objects are an especially deadly type of virus known by its abbreviation, *HIV.* HIV stands for *human immunodeficiency* (ih-**MYEW**-noh-dee-**FIH**-shun-**see**) *virus*. This name reflects the fact that the virus causes a deficiency in the body's *immunity* (ih-**MYEW**-nih-**tee**), or protection from disease. Infection of leukocytes (and other human cells) with HIV may eventually result in the serious illness *AIDS* (*acquired immunodeficiency syndrome*).

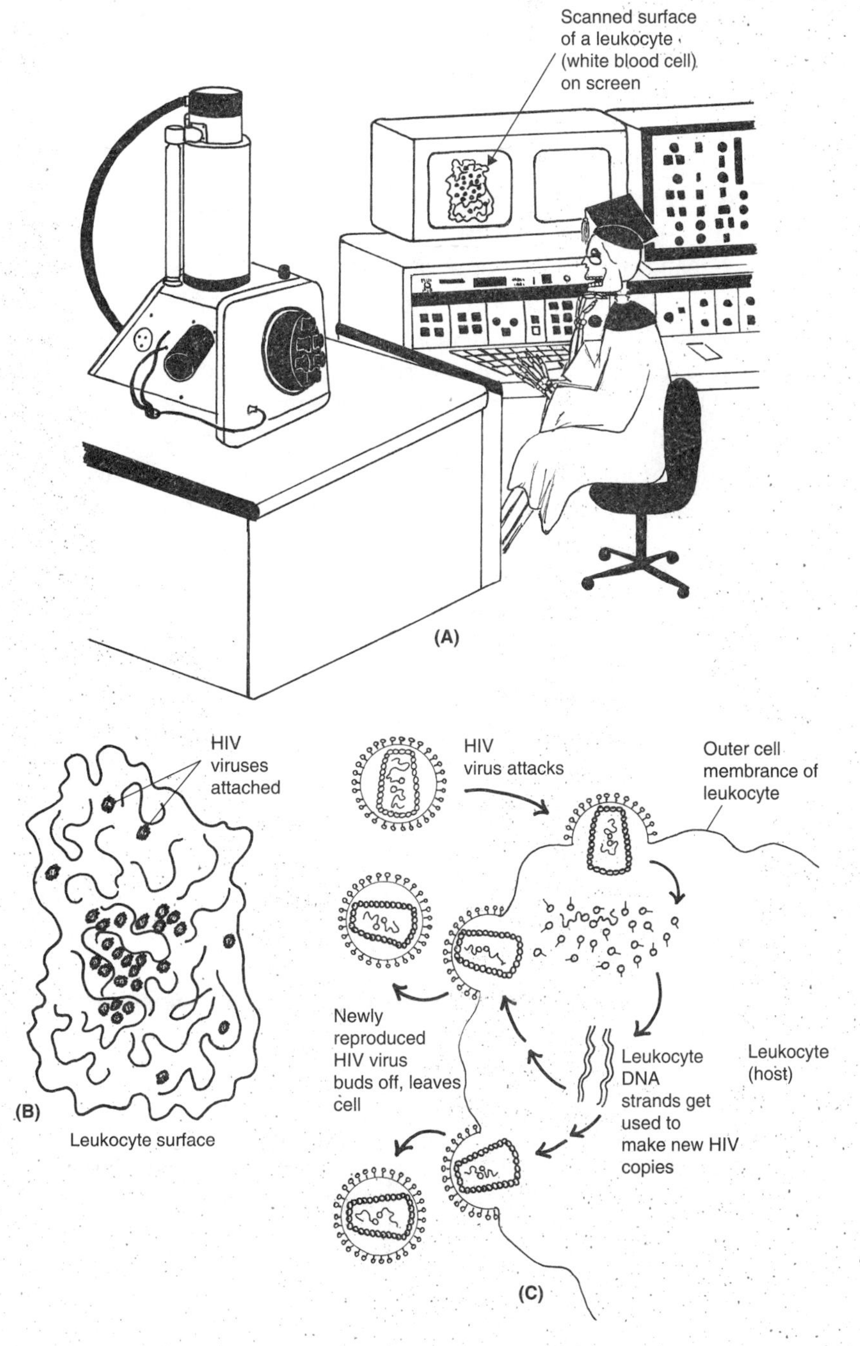

Fig. 3.4 The scanning electron microscope reveals the surface of a leukocyte being attacked by HIV viruses (**A**) Professor Joe (the Talking Skelton) operating a scanning electron microscope. (**B**) The scanned surface of a leukocyte (white blood cell) with HIV viruses (dark) studding its outer membrane (**C**) Detailed view showing how individual HIV viruses enter the leukocyte and use its DNA to reproduce and "bud off" from the cell's surface.

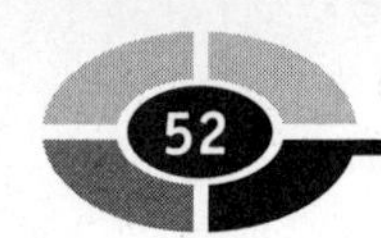

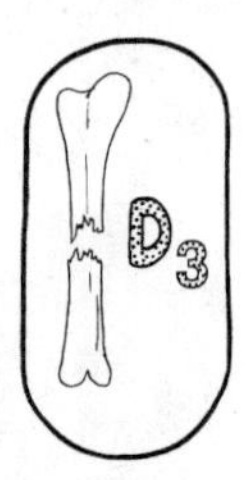

Like all viruses, HIV acts as a *parasite* (**PAIR**-uh-site) of living cells. A parasite is literally a creature that is an unwanted "guest" of some other organism, called the *host*. The *parasitic* (**pair**-uh-**SIT**-ik) "guest" in this case is the HIV, which enters the human leukocyte (white blood cell) host (Figure 3.4, C). Viruses are parasites because they need the *DNA* of other cells to reproduce themselves. (DNA is discussed in more detail in a later chapter.) As shown in Figure 3.4 (C), each HIV enters the leukocyte by fusing with its outer *cell membrane*. Chemical components of the fused HIV then enter the host leukocyte. Using strands of the host cell DNA, the virus makes several copies of itself. The reproduced HIV units then bud off from the host cell, eventually destroying it. Because so many thousands of leukocytes, a protective type of cell, are destroyed by these viruses, the person's immunity (ability to ward off disease) becomes greatly impaired.

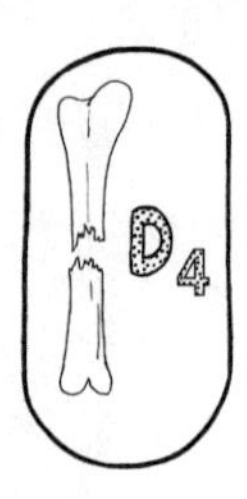

Summarizing all viruses, we can say that none of them is considered a living organism, because they cannot reproduce by themselves. Rather, viruses are nonliving superchemicals that act as parasites of living cells.

Overview of tiny objects seen through microscopes

Summary Table 3.1 provides an overview of the major classes of tiny objects that can be examined using various types of microscopes.

Summary Table 3.1 The Major Types of Tiny Object Viewed through Microscopes

Object Type	Chief Characteristics	Specific Example
Protozoon	A unicellular animal	An amoeba
Bacterium	A unicellular, plantlike microorganism	A staphylococcus
Virus	A nonliving superchemical that is a parasite of living cells	HIV (human immunodeficiency virus)

SUMMARY TABLE 3.2

Consult Summary Table 3.2 for a quick review of some important words and word parts.

Summary Table 3.2 Words and Word Parts

Write in the *exact* meaning (literal English translation) for up to 10 key terms selected from the preceding block of text. After you are done, check your word meanings with the correct answers given at the end of this chapter.

Key Terms	Prefixes	Roots	Suffixes	Exact Meanings
organism	(none)	organ "an organ"	-ism "condition of being"	1. ________
biological	(none)	bi "life"	-logical "pertaining to the study of"	2. ________
macroscopic	macr/macro- "large"	scop "examining"	-ic "referring to"	3. ________
microscopic	micr-/micro- "tiny"	scop "examining"	-ic "relating to"	4. ________
microscopy	micr-/micro- "tiny"	scop "examining"	-y "process of"	5. ________
microscopist	micr-/micro- "tiny"	scop "examining"	-ist "one who specializes in"	6. ________
unicellular	uni- "one"	cellul "little cell"	-ar "pertaining to"	7. ________
microorganism	micr-/micro- "tiny"	organ "organ"	-ism "condition of being"	8. ________
bacteriologist	(none)	bacteri "little staffs	-ologist "one who specializes in studying"	9. ________

PATHOGENIC MACROSCOPIC (GROSS) ORGANISMS

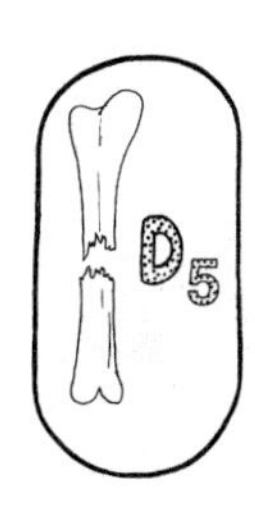

We have been discussing various types of microscopic organisms, especially those that may be *pathogenic* (**path**-oh-**JEN**-ik), that is, "disease" (*path*)

"producing" (*gen*). Many bacteria, for example, are *pathogens* (**PATH**-oh-jens) or "disease producers" in humans. Each bacterium, of course, is only a single cell—specifically, a unicellular organism. The pathogenic bacteria, therefore, that consist of just single cells (or relatively small groups of cells) are all microscopic.

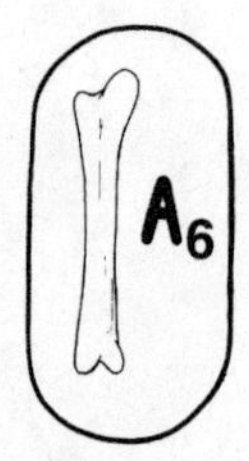

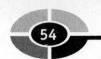

Most gross (macroscopic) organisms, in dramatic contrast, are *multicellular* (**mul**-tih-**SEL**-yew-ler) creatures. The human body is a well-known multicellular organism, because it consists of "many" (*multi-*) "little cells" (*cellul*). A great number of pathogenic organisms (pathogens) are also multicellular. Hence, they are visible to our naked eyes.

Consider the *nematodes* (**NEM**-uh-toads), a large group of roundworms that are named for the fact that their multicellular bodies are "shaped" (*-ode*) like long, slender "threads" (*nemat*). The common earthworm burrowing through the moist soil of your garden is a nematode familiar to most of us. [**Study suggestion:** Using the prefix *non-*, build a single term that means "not causing disease." Check your term with the one that follows in the text.]

The common earthworm is a *nonpathogenic* (**NAHN**-pah-thoh-**JEN**-ik) nematode, because it does "not" (*non-*) cause any human diseases. There are, however, a number of nematodes that *are* pathogenic to humans! These include the hookworm, technically known as *Ancylostoma* (**an**-suh-**LAHS**-tuh-muh). This name literally means "bent or crooked" (*Ancyl*) "mouth" (*stom*). When a person walks barefoot on feces-contaminated soil, the soil may contain hookworm *larvae* (**LAR**-vee), immature hookworms. These can burrow through the skin on the sole of the foot, causing "ground-itch." The larvae travel through the person's bloodstream and then migrate to the lungs. Above the lungs, they crawl up the person's windpipe and are eventually swallowed! After passing through the stomach, the larvae mature and attach to the lining of the person's small intestine. With their "bent," hook-like mouths, these parasitic worms eagerly suck the blood of their unwilling human host!

The medical term for this condition is *ancylostomiasis* (**an**-suh-**lahs**-tuh-**MY**-uh-sis). The suffix, *-iasis*, means "abnormal condition of." [**Study suggestion:** Using your knowledge, translate ancylostomiasis into its common English equivalent. Check your answer with the next sentence.] Technically speaking, ancylostomiasis is an "abnormal condition of hookworm" *infestation* (in-fes-**TAY**-shun). An infestation is an "attack" by macroscopic animal parasites, such as nematodes.

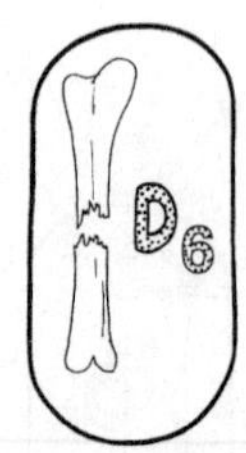

PATHOGENIC FUNGI: THEY'RE *NOT* ALL JUST *MUSHROOMS*!

Earlier, we learned about *infections*, which are caused by pathogenic unicellular *microbes* such as bacteria. And we have just learned about *infestations*, which are caused by pathogenic, multicellular, *macroscopic* organisms such as the hookworm. "What about the pathogenic *fungi* (**FUN**-jeye)?" the inquiring mind might well ask. "My doctor recently told me that I had a yeast *fungus* (**FUN**-gus) infection. But aren't mushrooms in the woods also fungi? Now, we can't see yeast cells with our naked eyes, but we can certainly go mushroom hunting! If parasitic fungi cause disease in our bodies, should these diseases be called *fungal* (**FUN**-gal) *infections*, or should they be called *fungal infestations*?"

Good question! But the answer is simply, "It depends." The fungi, you see, are a large group of plantlike, vegetable organisms that either live on decaying organic matter or are parasites of living plants or animals. The word *fungus* actually means "presence of" (*-us*) a "mushroom" (*fung*). But as Figure 3.5 shows, the *kingdom Fungi* consists of the unicellular yeasts, plus the multicellular molds and mushrooms.

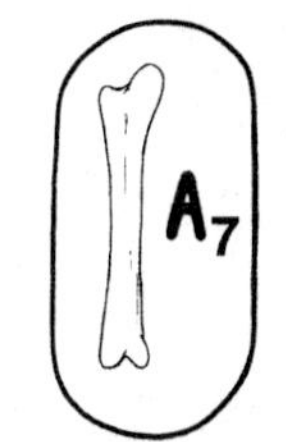

When a woman has many *vaginal* (**VAH**-jih-**nal**) *yeast cells*, for instance, this is a type of fungal *infection*, since the yeast cells are microscopic parasites. Attacks by other, larger, grossly visible multicellular fungi may result in a fungal *infestation* of the skin or other body organ. But whether the invading fungus is unicellular and microscopic, or multicellular and macroscopic, it still results in a *mycosis*—an "abnormal condition" (*-osis*) caused by a parasitic "fungus" (*myc*).

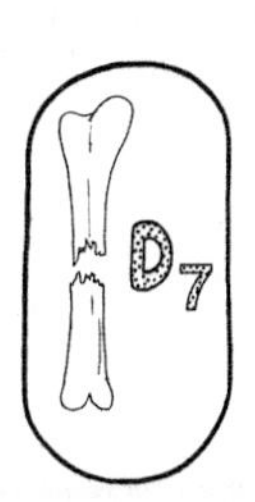

SUMMARY OVERVIEW OF INFECTIOUS DISEASES

Our discussion of ancylostomiasis (hookworm disease) revealed that some parasites can enter the human body without any help! Many parasites, however,

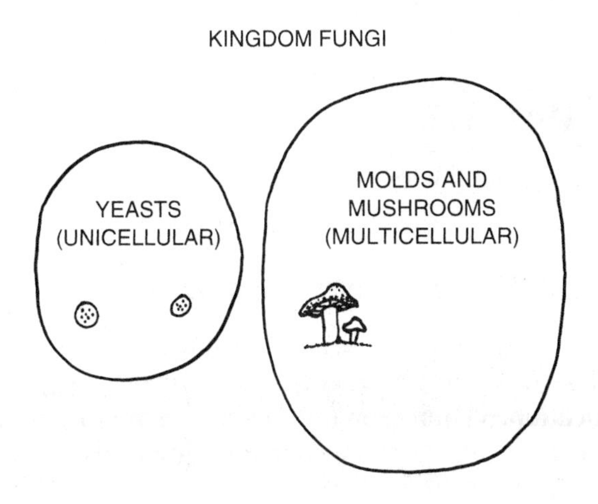

Fig. 3.5 The fungi, both unicellular and multicellular.

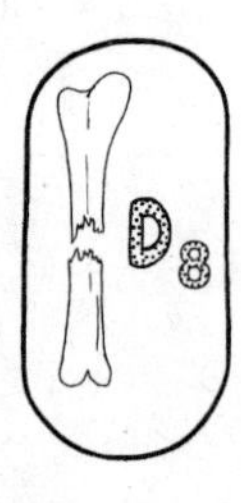

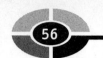

need the assistance of a *vector* (**VEK**-ter), which is the Latin word for "carrier." A biting wood tick, for example, can act as a vector (carrier) for Rocky Mountain spotted fever. Biting mosquitoes and the feces of infected birds often serve as vectors for dangerous protozoa or fungi that can create serious illness in the human host.

In general, vectors often play important roles in carrying both infections and infestations of human hosts.

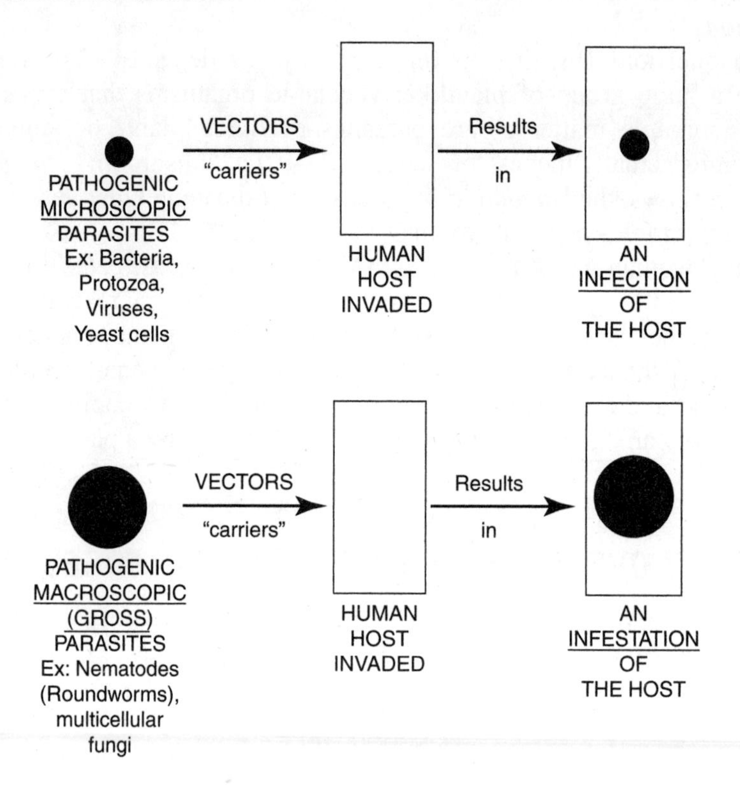

SUMMARY TABLE 3.3

Consult Summary Table 3.3 for a quick review of some important words and word parts.

Medical Case History: Histoplasmosis—It's from the Birds!

Now that we have completed the Background and History section for this chapter, we will examine a sample medical *case history* to provide a practical, real-world application of our growing medical terminology knowledge. Following the case history are a few short-answer questions.

Summary Table 3.3 Words and Word Parts

Write in the *exact* meaning (literal English translation) for up to 10 key terms selected from the preceding block of text. After you are done, check your word meanings with the correct answers given at the end of this chapter.

Key Terms	**Prefixes**	**Roots**	**Suffixes**	**Exact Meanings**
pathogenic	(none)	path "disease"; gen "producing"	-ic "pertaining to"	1. ___________
multicellular	multi- "many"	cellul "little cells"	-ar "referring to"	2. ___________
nonpathogenic	non- "not"	path "disease"; gen "producing"	-ic "relating to"	3. ___________
nematode	(none)	nemat "thread"	-ode "shaped"	4. ___________
ancylostomiasis	(none)	ancylostom "hookworm" ("bent mouth")	-iasis "abnormal condition of"	5. ___________

Mrs. Mortimer Tweet and seven members of her third-grade class at Lowland River Elementary were suddenly stricken with high fever, chills, coughing, and some difficulty in breathing. *Sputum* (**SPYOO**-tum) samples (samples of "spit") revealed the presence of a yeast-like organism called *Histoplasma* (**hiss**-toh-**PLAZ**-mah) *capsulatum* (**kap**-suh-**LAY**-tum). This is a parasitic fungus whose cells are surrounded by oval "capsules" or "little boxes." Questioning of the teacher and her students revealed the important fact that the class had been growing pea plants in small pots, which they left outside the classroom window every night. Several soil samples from these pots showed the presence of *spores* (*capsulat*) of the *Histoplasma capsulatum* fungus. Therefore, it was concluded that the teacher and students had inhaled the fungal spores from the potted soil, thereby causing the fungus to enter their lungs! The probable source of the spores was the droppings of many starlings, who nested in large flocks in trees overhanging the school. Fortunately, all cases of the disease were self-limiting, and the major *symptoms* disappeared after a few days. *Histoplasmin* (**hiss**-toh-**PLAZ**-min) skin tests were positive for all eight affected individuals. A variety of other lab tests confirmed a *diagnosis* (**die**-uhg-**NOH**-sis) of *primary acute* (ah-**KYOOT**) *histoplasmosis*. The disease of histoplasmosis gets its name from

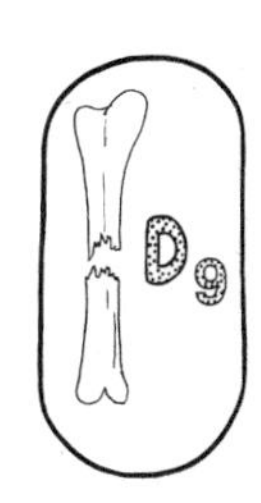

the fact that the fungus often forms a "webbing" (*hist*) of capsules ("little boxes") within the "matter" (*plasm*) of the lungs.

Probe of case history

(**A**) Was this medical case an example of an *infection* or an *infestation*? Briefly explain. (**B**) Name the probable *vector* of the disease in this case history. [Check your short answers with the key near the end of this chapter.]

Quiz

Refer to the text in this chapter if necessary. A good score is at least 8 correct answers out of these 10 questions. The answers are listed in the back of this book.

1. An *infestation* differs from an *infection* in that it:
   (a) Never hurts human beings
   (b) Involves macroscopic or gross pathogens
   (c) Can always be visualized using an electron microscope
   (d) Usually describes the death-causing actions of various microbes
2. "A virus *cannot* technically be classified as biological." This statement is true, because viruses:
   (a) Are closer to being dead animals, rather than living plants!
   (b) Must parasitize living cells to reproduce themselves
   (c) Have all the important characteristics of living organisms
   (d) Were once living unicellular organisms, but have dried up and died!
3. Probably the first protozoologist and the first bacteriologist:
   (a) George W. Bush
   (b) Galileo
   (c) Baby Heinie, Esquire
   (d) Anton van Leeuwenhoek
4. The _____ are a type of bacteria whose individual cells are named for their resemblance to "coiled hairs".
   (a) Spirochetes
   (b) Bacilli
   (c) Amoebae
   (d) Spirilla
5. The unwilling victim of a parasite is called a:
   (a) Microorganism
   (b) Vector

(c) Plasmodium
(d) Host

6. The entire Kingdom of unicellular animals:
(a) Fungi
(b) Mushrooms
(c) Protozoa
(d) Anopheles

7. Multicellular roundworms whose bodies are literally shaped like "threads":
(a) Liver flukes
(b) Nematodes
(c) Leukocytes
(d) Yeasts

8. The medical term for hookworm disease:
(a) Dermatitis
(b) Malaria
(c) Gastroenteritis
(d) Ancylostomiasis

9. Sputum is just a fancy term for:
(a) Urine
(b) Spit
(c) Blood
(d) Venom

10. You can get it by inhaling fungal spores deposited in the feces of infected birds!
(a) Wilm's tumor
(b) Malaria vivax
(c) Primary acute histoplasmosis
(d) Red blood cell rupture

Memory Pillboxes for Chapter 3

Several key facts were tagged with numbered icons in the page margins of this chapter. Write a short summary of each of these key facts into a numbered cell or compartment within the appropriate type of *Memory Pillbox* that appears below.

Background and History **Pillboxes for Chapter 3:**

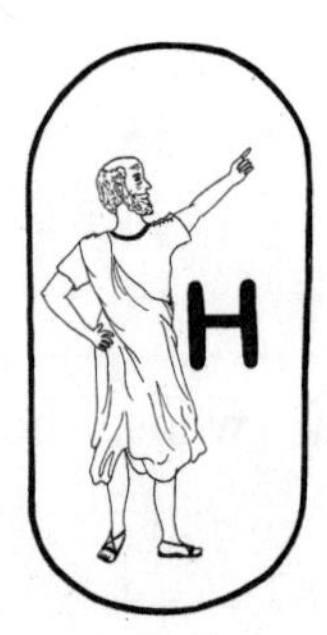

1	2

Anatomy **Pillboxes for Chapter 3:**

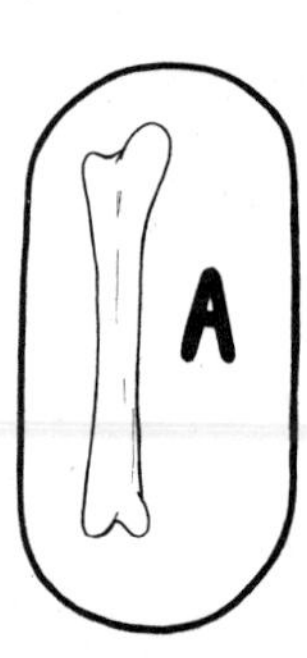

1	2

3	4

5	6

7

Disease/Injury **Pillboxes for Chapter 3:**

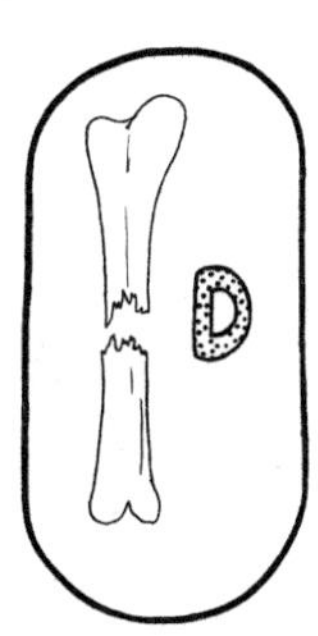

1

2	3
4	5
6	7
8	9

Answers for Chapter 3 Summary Tables

FOR SUMMARY TABLE 3.2

1. "condition of being an organ"
2. "pertaining to study of life"
3. "referring to examining (something) large"
4. "relating to examining (something) tiny"
5. "the process of examining (something) tiny"
6. "one who specializes in examining (something) tiny"
7. "pertaining to one little cell"
8. "condition of being a tiny organ"
9. "one who specializes in studying little staffs"

FOR SUMMARY TABLE 3.3

1. "pertaining to producing disease"
2. "referring to many little cells"
3. "relating to not producing disease"
4. "thread-shaped"
5. "abnormal condition of hookworm"

Answers to Probe of Case History

(**A**) An infection, because *Histoplasma* consists of yeast-like single cells that are microscopic. (**B**) The vector was probably the starlings.

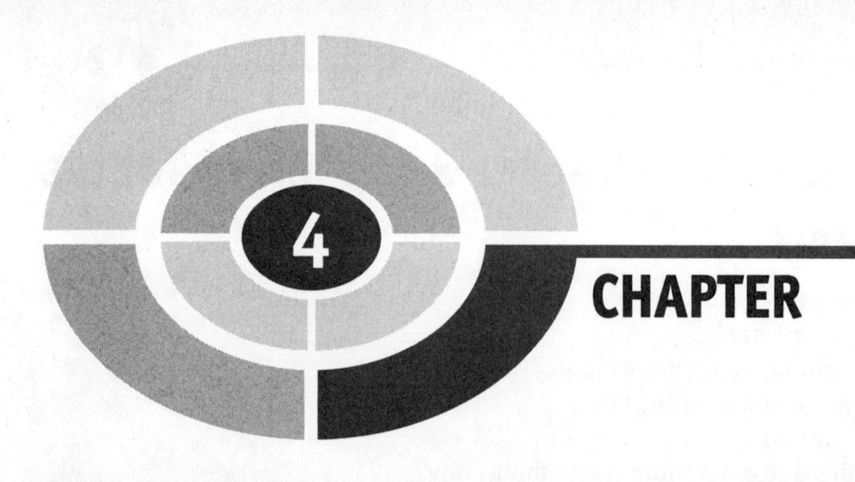

Terms of Therapy: Feeling Better!

When someone has a problem (of almost any sort, it seems), the common advice we give them is, "You need *therapy*!" In plain English, we are telling them that they need some kind of "treatment," which is represented by the medical word root *therap*.

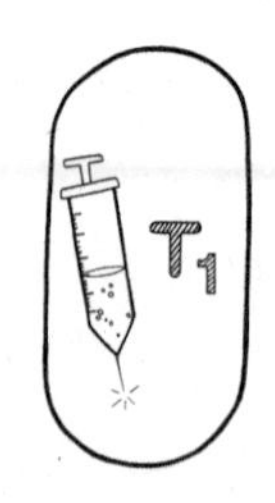

The main purpose of this chapter is to give you an overview of some of the chief *types* of therapy that medical specialists can give to patients. Along with these general types, some specific examples will be provided. This whole "operation" is supposed to make you feel a lot better, when we're finally through with it! We're "going into therapy," after all!

Background and History

Therapy, or the "process of" (*-y*) "treating" (*therap*), probably began very early in human history. There is evidence from cave paintings and other relics that *lesions* or "wounds" occurred quite frequently among groups of hunters

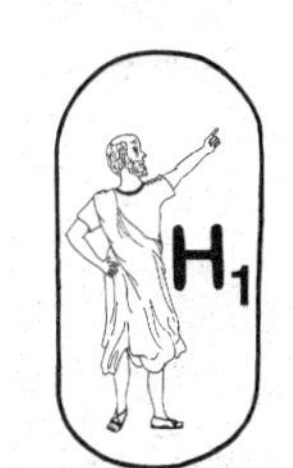

thousands of years ago. A spear could accidentally puncture the skin on a hunter's foot, for example, thereby creating a physical *trauma* (**TRAW**-muh) (in this case, a skin puncture). (The word *trauma,* like *lesion,* means "wound," but it is usually restricted to physical injuries or those involving the mind. Injuries involving say, a spot of cancer, in contrast, are usually called *lesions.*)

In this modern era, an entire discipline of medicine called *traumatology* (**traw**-mu-**TAHL**-uh-jee) has been developed. This discipline involves the "study of" (*-ology*) physical "wounds" (*traumat*), such as those that may be caused by automobile or firearm accidents.

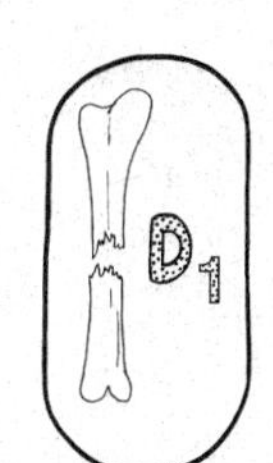

Closely related to traumatology is *pathology* (path-**AHL**-uh-jee). This is literally the "study of" (*-ology*) "disease and suffering" (*path*). A term for a "condition of" (*-ity*) "illness" (*morbid*) in general is *morbidity* (mor-**BID**-ih-tee). A person can have morbidity (illness), such as the common cold, but still not necessarily have visible body lesions.

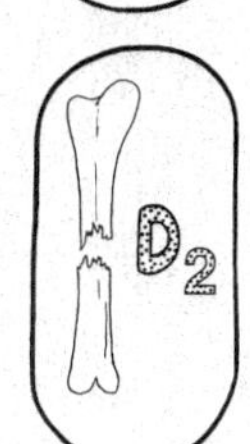

If morbidity becomes serious enough, then *mortality* (mor-**TAL**-ih-tee)—"a condition of" (*-ity*) "death" (*mortal*)—may result. A *pathologist* (path-**AHL**-uh-jist) may be called in to conduct a *postmortem* (post-**MORT**-em). The pathologist is "one who studies" (*-ologist*) "disease" (*path*) occurrence within the body tissues. He or she searches for evidence of the cause of mortality during the postmortem. The word *postmortem* literally means an examination of the body that takes place "after" (*post-*) "death" (*mortem*). [**Study suggestion:** A *synonym* for a particular word is another word that has a similar or identical meaning. Try to recall a synonym for postmortem that was on the word list in Chapter 2. Hint - - the word begins with the letter *a*.]

CARING HANDS OF NURSES BRING THERAPY

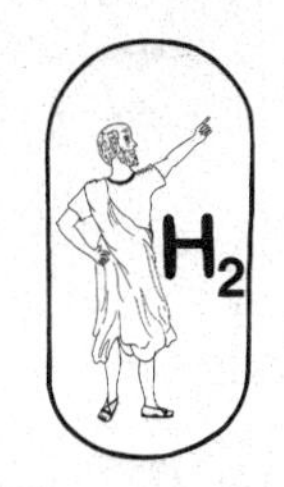

When *morbid* ("diseased") changes occur within our bodies, we naturally seek out comfort and therapy as a means to relieve or correct them. One of the important recent names in providing such comfort is *Florence Nightingale.* We can think of her as the Mother of Modern Nursing. Born in England in 1820, she became a nurse and eventually left to treat soldiers who had been injured in the Crimean (cry-**MEE**-an) War. She was known as the "Lady with the Lamp" by the soldiers who were receiving therapy in her military hospital (Figure 4.1). Nightingale noted that the wounded soldiers were kept in filthy rooms, shared the same beds, and were often still dressed in their uniforms, which she described as "stiff with dirt and gore." The high mortality rate in the hospital, originally attributed to gunshot wounds, was in fact a result of the widespread occurrence of bacterial diseases! Nightingale and her team of nurses cleaned the rooms and beds with strong chemicals, which served as good *disinfectants*

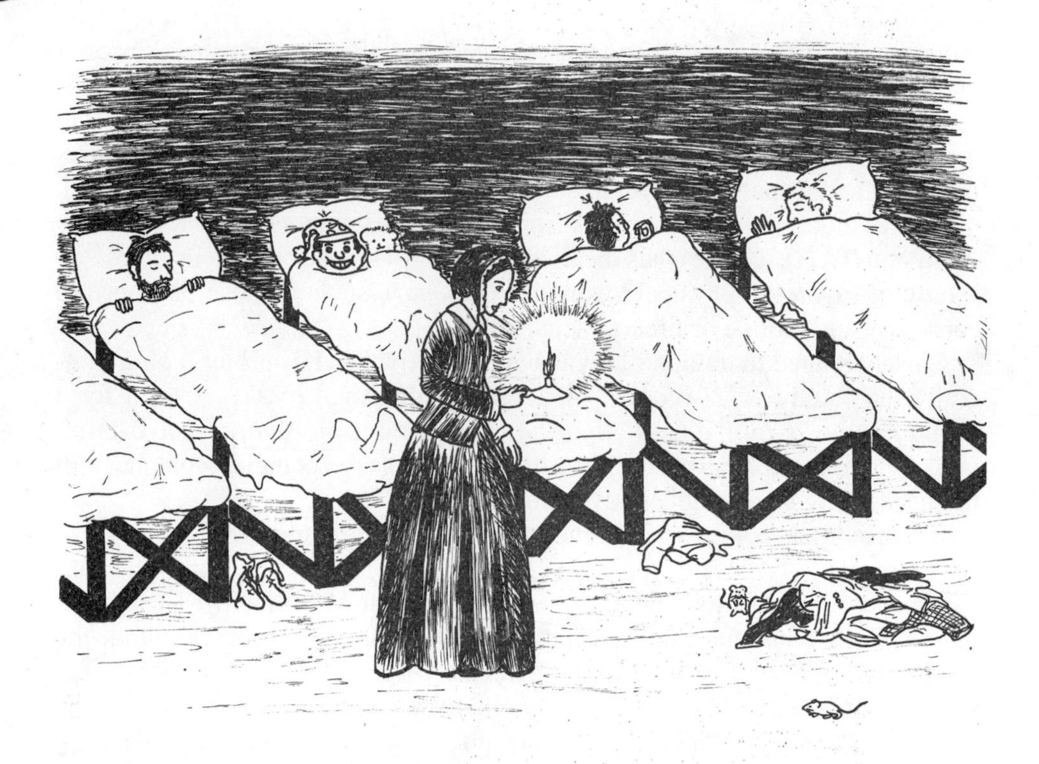

Fig. 4-1 Florence Nightingale, the Lady with the Lamp. The Mother of Nursing cares for injured soldiers ("*Wait!* What's *Baby Heinie* doing in that bed?")

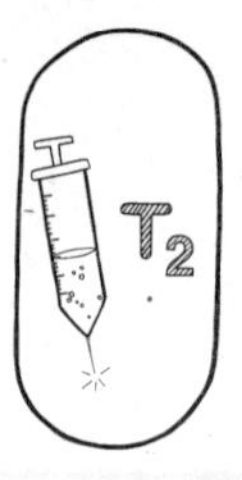

(**dis**-in-**FEK**-tunts)—"ones which" (*-ants*) take "away" (*dis-*) "infections" (*infect*). As a result, the number of bacterial pathogens in the hospital were greatly decreased, and the soldiers' previously high morbidity and mortality rates likewise declined.

SOME MAJOR TYPES OF THERAPY

Various specific techniques of therapy are now in existence. But there are two broad types: *physiatrics* (**fiz**-e-**AT**-riks) and *chemotherapy* (**keem**-oh-**THAIR**-uh-pea). Physiatrics involves medical "treatment" (*-iatrics*) and diagnosis using "natural" (*physi*), nonchemical agents. Physiatrics is a close synonym to *physiotherapy* (**FIH**-see-oh-**THAIR**-uh-pea), also called *physical therapy*.

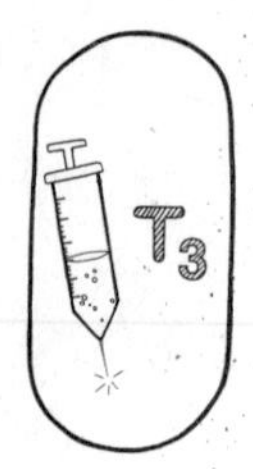

THERAPY = PHYSIATRICS (PHYSIOTHERAPY) + CHEMOTHERAPY

Physiatrics (physiotherapy or physical therapy) in turn consists of a collection of specific individual therapies. Each of these is involved with a specific force or characteristic in "nature" (*physi*). One of the more exotic is *electrotherapy* (e-**LEK**-troh-**THAIR**-uh-pea)—the use of "electrical current" (*electro*) as a "treatment" for mental illness and other clinical problems. *Diathermy* (**DIE**-uh-ther-mee) is the "process of" (*-y*) applying "heat" (*therm*) "through" (*dia-*) the body, as for easing the pain of sore muscles. Diathermy is a specific example of *thermotherapy* (**ther**-moh-**THAIR**-uh-pea). *Heliotherapy* (**HEE**-lee-oh-**THAIR**-uh-pea) involves use of the "sun" (*heli*) and its rays for healing purposes. Heliotherapy can help in cases of *rickets* (**RIK**-ets), a *pathological* (**path**-oh-**LAHJ**-ih-kal) condition of vitamin D deficiency in children in which the bones become abnormally soft, leading to easy deformity and fractures. By purposely exposing affected kids to the *ultraviolet* (**ul**-trah-**VEYE**-oh-let) *rays* in sunlight, heliotherapy stimulates their skin to greatly increase its rate of vitamin D production. This often helps cure or diminish the rickets.

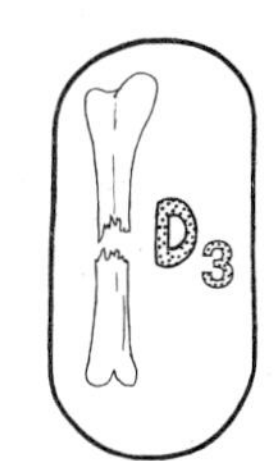

Cryotherapy (**cry**-oh-**THAIR**-uh-pea) is the exact opposite process of thermotherapy. **[Study suggestion:** See if *you* can provide the literal translation of cryotherapy, by writing it down. When done, check your answer with the sentence that follows.] Cryotherapy is the "process of" (*-y*) "treating" (*therap*) medical problems with the application of "cold" (*cry*). Placing a cold compress upon a bleeding wound in the skin and providing pressure, for instance, will tend to decrease the rate of bleeding and reduce tissue swelling.

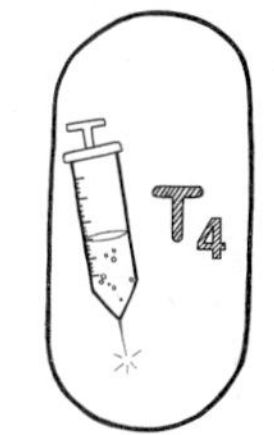

Radiotherapy (**ray**-dee-oh-**THAIR**-uh-pea) is "treatment" using "rays" (*radi*). In particular, we usually mean the *x-rays* that are released during *radiation* (**ray**-dee-**AY**-shun)—the "process of" (*-tion*) releasing "rays" (*radi*).

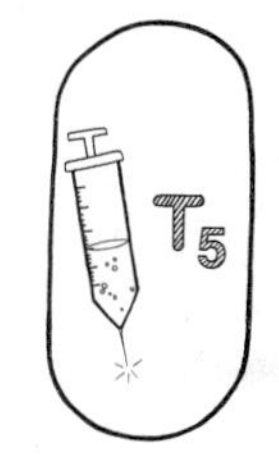

Physiotherapy sometimes involves helping a patient adapt to the replacement of lost body parts with *prostheses* (**prahs-THEE**-seez). A *prosthesis* (**prahs-THEE**-sis) is "an [artificial] addition" to the body, usually an artificial limb. In this modern computerized era, the primitive wooden arm or leg prostheses of earlier times are increasingly being replaced by sophisticated *robotic* (roh-**BAHT**-ic) limbs. The potential downside to an uncontrolled development of robotic prostheses—robot hands, arms, and legs—unfortunately, is that if we replace too many natural body parts with robotic ones, we will no longer be human! The resulting man-machine combination is technically called a *cyborg* (**SIGH**-borg), which is short for *cybernetic* (**sigh**-ber-**NET**-ik) *organism*. (Think about what happened to *Darth Vader* in the *Star Wars* movies!)

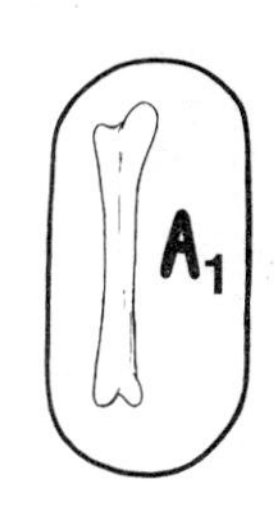

SUMMARY TABLE 4.1

Consult Summary Table 4.1 for a quick review of some important words and word parts.

Summary Table 4.1 Words and Word Parts

Write in the *exact* meaning (literal English translation) for up to 10 key terms selected from the preceding block of text. After you are done, check your word meanings with the correct answers, which are given at the end of this chapter.

Key Terms	Prefixes	Roots	Suffixes	Exact Meanings
therapy	(none)	therap "treating"	-y "process of"	1. ____________
traumatology	(none)	traumat "wounds"	-ology "the study of"	2. ____________
pathology	(none)	path "disease"	-ology "the study of"	3. ____________
morbidity	(none)	morbid "illness"	-ity "a condition of"	4. ____________
mortality	(none)	mortal "death"	-ity "a condition of"	5. ____________
pathologist	(none)	path "disease"	-ologist "one who studies"	6. ____________
postmortem	post- "after"	mortem "death"	(none)	7. ____________
disinfectant	dis- "away"	infect "infections"	-ant "one which"	8. ____________
physiatrics	(none)	physi "natural"	-iatrics "treatments"	9. ____________
diathermy	dia- "through"	therm "heating"	-y "process of"	10. ____________

THE SPECIAL WORLD OF CHEMOTHERAPY

Now that we have probed several aspects of physical therapy (physiotherapy or physiatrics), we are ready to explore the special world of chemotherapy. Quite obviously, chemotherapy involves "treating" morbid or *premorbid* (**PREE-mor-**bid) problems with the use of "chemicals" (*chem*).

Our current faith in the power of chemotherapy, and especially *medicinal* (meh-**DIH**-sih-nal) *drugs*, to solve all of our health defects has become far too strong! Consider, for instance, the common prescription of *placebos* by our physicians. Placebo means "I will please" in common English. This reflects the fact than a medical doctor may give a patient plain sugar pills or some other medically inactive tablet to satisfy an unreasonable demand for medicine!

The birth of chemotherapy

In Ancient China about 2000 BC, much of the early experimentation on the effects of drugs was carried out by *Shen Nung* (Figure 4.2). With the aid of his helpers, Shen Nung gathered many plants and herbs from the Chinese countryside. He then proceeded to grind up these plants and try them out on himself! Somehow, Shen Nung managed to survive without being poisoned to death, and he wrote the first classification of drugs. Therefore, Shen Nung is often called the Founder of Chinese *pharmacy* (**FAR**-muh-see)—the "preparation of drugs."

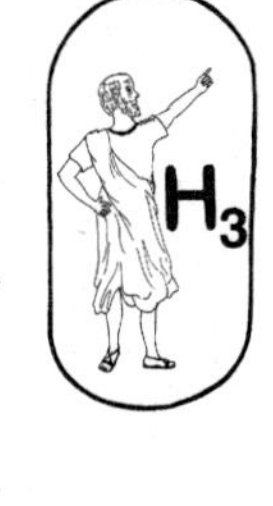

Shen Nung is also known as the Founder of *pharmacology* (**far**-muh-**KAHL**-uh-jee), which is literally "the study of" (*-ology*) "drugs" (*pharmac*). Shen Nung was a rather primitive *pharmacologist* (**far**-muh-**KAHL**-uh-jist) in that he was "one who studied" (*-ologist*) the effects of "drugs"—upon himself! For example, Shen Nung discovered the important *pharmacologic* (**far**-muh-kuh-**LAHJ**-ik) benefits of such naturally occurring Asian plants as *mandrake* (**MAN**-drayk) and *ginseng* (**JIN**-seng). *Mandrake* means "Man-dragon." That is, it looks somewhat like a weird man! (See Figure 4.3, A)

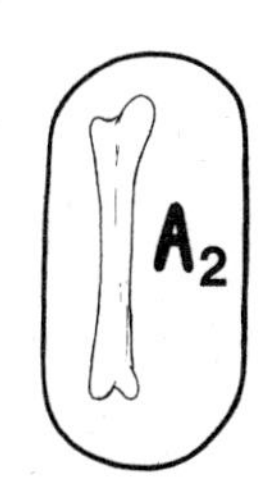

The mandrake plant has a very short stem (like the trunk of a human body) and a thick forked root (like two human legs). In Chinese legend, the mandrake

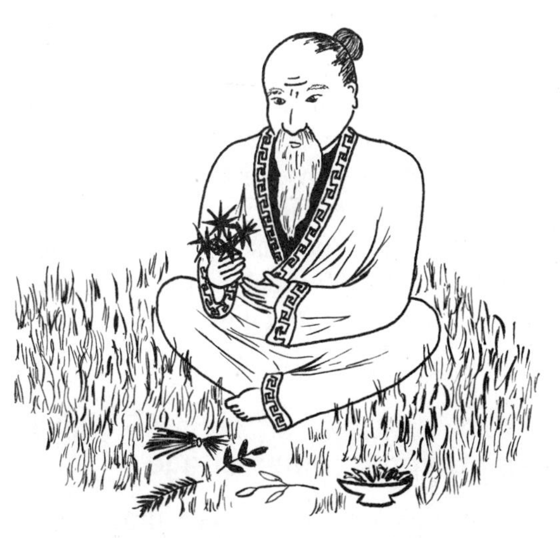

Fig. 4-2 Shen Nung, the Father of Pharmacy.

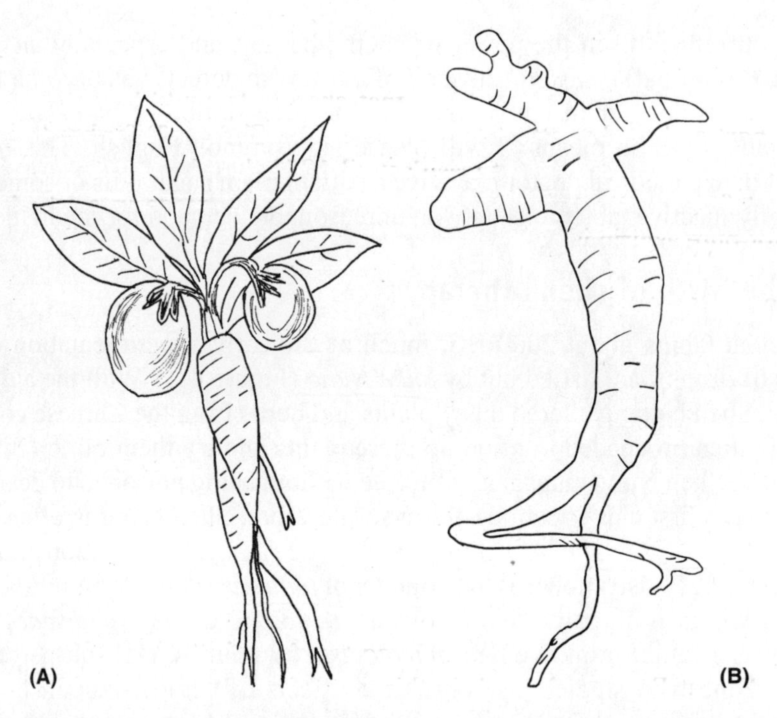

Fig. 4-3 Mandrake and ginseng: "man"-like roots! **(A)** Mandrake, the "Man-dragon." **(B)** Ginseng, the Chinese "Man."

root is said to cry out when it is pulled up from the ground! Shen Nung advocated use of the mandrake root as a medicine because it can induce *emesis* (**EM**-eh-sis) or "vomiting" when eaten and it has powerful narcotic (Chapter 2) properties. Nevertheless, mandrake root should not be consumed in large quantities, because it also contains powerful *toxins* ("poisons").

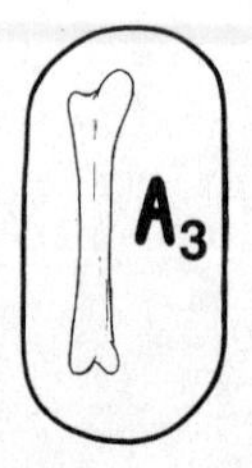

The word, *ginseng,* is Chinese for "man." Ginseng is a low-growing plant whose branched roots (like that of the mandrake) somewhat resemble the human form (Figure 4.3, B). Even today, the ginseng plant is a prized medicine in Chinese pharmacy. In general, ginseng is a powerful *stimulant* (**STIM**-you-lunt) that "goads or prods" the faster and stronger occurrence of many different body functions. Specifically, it is often used as a heart tonic and an *aphrodisiac* (**af**-roh-**DIZ**-e-ak), a stimulator of sexual desire. [**Thinking suggestion:** Considering the shape of the mandrake and ginseng plant roots, why do you think they might have powerful *placebo* effects? Speculate, and discuss your ideas with another person.]

Modern chemotherapy comes of age

When we think of chemotherapy in modern times, we usually don't have visions of man-shaped mandrake and ginseng roots swimming in our heads, do

we? Rather, we tend to imagine pills or capsules. These are the forms that most highly-purified modern drugs assume. Take common aspirin, for example. For many centuries, native people knew that chemicals could be extracted from *willow bark* and used as effective analgesics (see Chapter 2) for headaches and other painful problems. But it wasn't until 1852 that the important analgesic chemical found in willow bark, *aspirin,* was finally made in a lab. Another name for pure aspirin is *acetylsalicylic* (uh-**SEE**-til-**SAL**-ih-**SIL**-ik) *acid.*

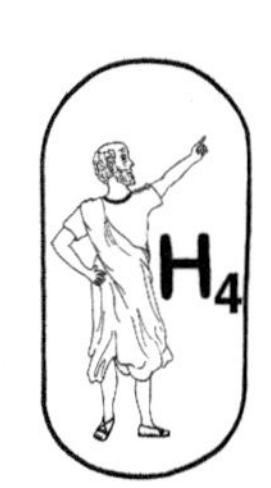

A French chemist, named *Ernest Fourneau* (foor-**NO**), who lived from 1872 to 1949, synthesized many other valuable drugs in their pure chemical forms. This included the forerunners to the modern *sulfa* (**SUL**-fah) drugs and the *antihistamines* (**an**-tih-**HISS**-tah-**meenz**). Such drugs act "against" (*anti-*) the natural substance called "histamine" (**HISS**-tah-**meen**). Now, histamine is released from injured cells during tissue *inflammation* (**in**-flah-**MAY**-shun)—a "condition of" (*-tion*) a "flame within" (*inflamm*). An inflammation of the skin, for example, such as sunburn or a mosquito bite, is accompanied by the four *symptoms* (**SIMP**-tums) of heat, redness, swelling, and pain. [**Thinking probe:** After which of these four symptoms do you think the word *inflammation* is named? Why?] Antihistamines, consequently, are drugs that operate to reduce the swelling and other symptoms caused by histamine release from inflamed tissues. Ernest Fourneau's work in this area was considered so important, in fact, that he has often been called the Father of Chemotherapy.

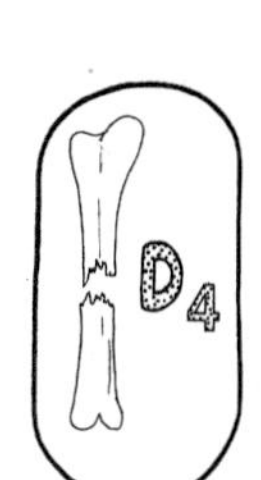

We have already mentioned that *pharmacology* involves the formal "study of" (*-ology*) "drugs" (*pharmac*). And a *pharmacologist* is "one who studies" these "drugs" and their various body actions. A *pharmacist* (**FAR**-muh-sist), in marked contrast, is "one who specializes in" (*-ist*) the preparation and dispensing of "drugs." [**Thinking probe:** Whom (a pharmacologist, or a pharmacist) would you expect to see behind the counter in your local drugstore? Whom would you expect to see working in a medical research lab? Why?]

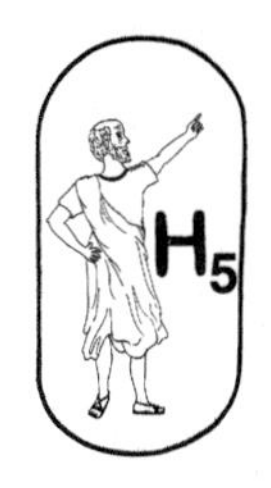

Main types of modern drugs

Having covered the key history of chemotherapy and pharmacology, let us now consider the twelve major types of drugs used for therapy. Many of the drug category names are based upon the kinds of effects they have upon the human body. [**Study suggestion:** As you read about each drug category, look over Figure 4.4 and enjoy the "intuitive" meanings of the little *icons* (picture-symbols) that represent each category.]

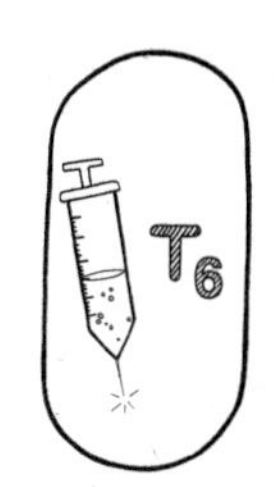

1. *Anti-inflammatory* (**an**-tih-in-**FLAM**-ah-toh-re) drugs literally act "against" (*anti-*) the symptoms of tissue "inflammation." One well-known specific type of anti-inflammatory drug, of course, is aspirin (acetylsalicylic acid).

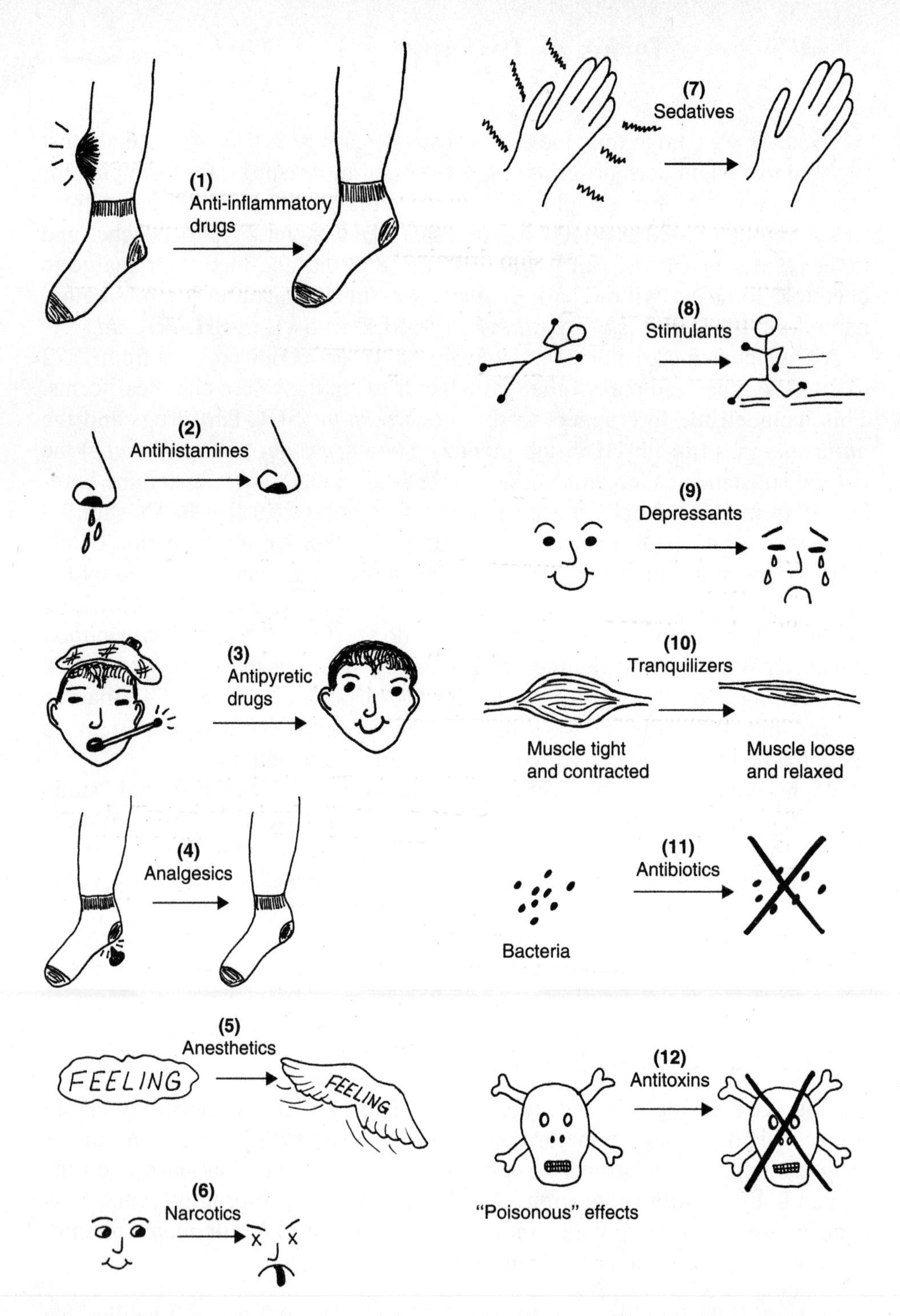

Fig. 4-4 The Great Mother diagram showing the twelve major categories of medicinal drugs.

2. *Antihistamines* we have previously mentioned as acting to counteract the tissue swelling caused by histamine after a tissue is injured. These antihistamines are often packaged in over-the-counter remedies that reduce swelling of the *nasal* (**NAY**-sal, "nose") *passages* during a common cold. They also help the nose stop dripping!
3. *Antipyretic* (**an**-tih-pie-**RET**-ik) drugs reduce or work "against" (*anti-*) the effects of a "fever" (*pyret*). Acetylsalicylic acid (the main ingredient in aspirin tablets) is a most-common antipyretic agent.
4. *Analgesics* (see Chapter 2) "take away" (*an-*) the sense of "pain" (*alges*).
5. *Anesthetics* (see Chapter 2) "take away" (*an-*) all body "feelings" (*esthet*).
6. *Narcotics* (see Chapter 2) create a powerful "benumbing" (*narc*) effect, as produced, for example, by injections of cocaine.
7. *Sedatives* (**SED**-ah-tivs) "pertain to" (*-ive*) "quieting down" (*sedat*) a patient, usually as a preop procedure carried out "before" surgery (Chapter 2). They usually act to decrease the level of a person's *consciousness* (**KAHN**-shus-ness) or "awareness," as well as reduce shaking.
8. *Stimulants* (**STIM**-you-lunts) "goad or excite" (*stimul*) the *central nervous system* (brain and spinal cord) or some other body system, causing an increase in their functions. *Caffeine* (kaf-**EEN**), for example, is the main stimulant chemical found in coffee, tea, and colas.
9. *Depressants* (de-**PRESS**-unts) literally "press down"—decrease—the functions of particular parts of the body. They include central nervous system depressants, *cardiac* (**KAR**-dee-**ak,** "referring to heart") *depressants*, and *respiratory* (**RES**-pir-ah-**tor**-ee) *depressants*, which inhibit us from "breathing again" (*respirat*).
10. *Tranquilizers* (**TRAN**-kwuh-**lie**-zers) "calm" anxious or agitated people, usually without decreasing their level of consciousness (awareness).
11. *Antibiotics* (**an**-tih-buy-**AHT**-iks) are chemicals extracted from mold or bacteria that function "against" or inhibit the "living" (*bi*) pathogenic microbes that cause infections. Good examples of antibiotic drugs are the *penicillins* (**pen**-ih-**SILL**-ins). They are extracted from the fungus, *Penicillium* (**pen**-ih-**SILL**-e-um), or are produced in the lab by pharmacologists.
12. *Antitoxins* (**an**-tih-**TAHK**-sins), as their name suggests, work "against" the body effects of *toxins* (**TAHK**-sins) or "poisons." Snake venom antitoxins, for instance, are drugs that counteract the sometimes deadly poisonous effects of various snake venoms.

SUMMARY TABLE 4.2

Consult Summary Table 4.2 for a quick review of some important words and word parts.

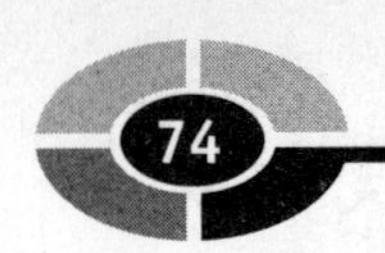

Summary Table 4.2 Words and Word Parts

Write in the *exact* meaning (literal English translation) for up to 10 key terms selected from the preceding block of text. After you are done, check your word meanings with the correct answers, which are given at the end of this chapter.

Key Terms	Prefixes	Roots	Suffixes	Exact Meanings
pharmacology	(none)	pharmac "drugs"	-ology "the study of"	1. ________
pharmacologist	(none)	pharmac "drugs"	-ologist "one who studies"	2. ________
inflammation	(none)	inflamm "flame within"	-tion "condition of"	3. ________
pharmacist	(none)	pharmac "drugs"	-ist "one who specializes in"	4. ________
anti-inflammatory	anti- "against"	inflammat "flame within"	-ory "pertaining to"	5. ________
antipyretic	anti- "against"	pyret "fever"	-ic "referring to"	6. ________
sedative	(none)	sedat "quieting down"	-ive "pertaining to"	7. ________
antibiotic	anti- "against"	biot "life"	-ic "relating to"	8. ________

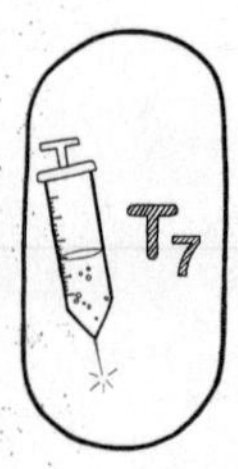

Medical Case History: Drug Addiction and Severe Accidental Overdose

Mrs. Claudia S. had been under treatment for severe clinical depression since early 1997. Previously, her former physician had prescribed a *barbiturate* (**bar-BITCH**-er-it)—a type of *CNS* (central nervous system) depressant. This drug was intended to help induce sleep and relieve the patient's overall high

state of tension and anxiety. The woman was instructed to take this medicine orally *t.i.d.* (*ter in die*, "three times a day"). Although the patient slept better, her state of depression worsened.

To help counteract these effects, a prescription of an *amphetamine* (am-**FET**-uh-**meen**)—a type of CNS stimulant—was used to help raise her mood. This was taken *b.i.d.* (*bis in die*, "two times a day"). The patient, however, soon gained a *tolerance* to these drugs. This is an adaptation to a particular dose level, with a loss of the drug's original effect. Without advice of her physician, the patient took higher and higher dosages to achieve a state of *euphoria* (you-**FOR**-e-uh)—an inappropriate feeling of "well-being." Eventually, Mrs. Claudia S. developed a severe amphetamine *addiction*. In general, an addiction is "a process of" (*-ion*) "giving over to" (*addict*) something, such as a drug. Technically speaking, a drug addiction involves a serious degree of *dependence* upon some drug to carry on in life. There are two main types of addiction (dependence): (1) *physical dependence* of normal body functions upon a drug, and (2) *psychic* (**SIGH**-kik) or "pertaining to" (*-ical*) "mind" (*psych*) *dependence* upon a drug.

DRUG ADDICTION = **Physical (body-affecting) drug dependence** + **Psychic (mind-affecting) drug dependence**

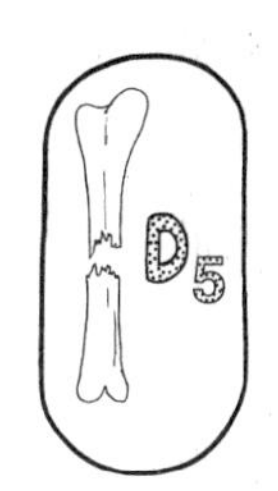

Mrs. Claudia S. began to take her prescribed amphetamine *q.i.d.* or *quater* (**KWAY**-ter) *in die* ("four times a day")—twice her recommended dosage! Even worse, she sought help from her teenage son, who was "doing" *marijuana* (**mahr**-ih-**WAH**-nah)! The kid took several thousand dollars from the family checking account and purchased *speed* from a local drug dealer. (Speed is an injectable liquid form of amphetamine that is sold illegally.) Junior learned from the drug dealer how to give a high dose of speed *intravenously* (**in**-trah-**VEE**-nus-lee), that is, "within" (*intra-*) a "vein" (*ven*). Such *IV*, that is, *intravenous* (**in**-truh-**VEE**-nus) doses, administered via a *syringe* (suh-**RINJ**) and needle into an arm vein, push a large amount of drug into the *addict's* (**AH**-dikts) bloodstream very quickly. This leads to a powerful euphoria.

Unfortunately, the teenage son gave his mom a huge IV injection of speed—about 400 milligrams (mg)! This represents 400 "thousandths" (*milli-*) of a gram. She quickly suffered *amphetamine poisoning*. This is the medical term for the *toxic* (**TAHK**-sik), "poisoning" effect of amphetamine *overdosage* (**OH**-ver-**doh**-suj). Mrs. S. became extremely overstimulated and her arms flailed about with severe *tremors* (**TREM**-ors), wild "shaking" motions. Loudly shrieking and running around the house, she suffered visual *hallucinations* (huh-**loo**-sih-**NAY**-shuns, "wanderings in the mind"). She thought she saw a red-eyed, green-skinned, lizard-like devil with a forked tongue (who closely resembled her former husband) breathing fire into her face! Her drug-induced *delirium*

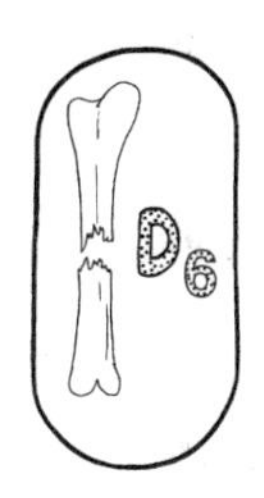

(dih-**LEER**-e-um) reflected the "presence of" (*-um*) extreme "raving" or "craziness" (*deliri*).

Mrs. S's pulse was racing, showing that the amphetamine overdose had created a state of *tachycardia* (**tak**-ih-**KAR**-dee-ah). In layman's language, her "heart" (*cardi*) was beating extremely "fast" (*tachy*). Her son was very alarmed by his mom's wild behavior, and he finally chased her down and grabbed her by both wrists. Mrs. S suddenly fell in a heap to the floor! Her body was wracked with severe *convulsions* (**kahn-VUL**-zhuns), which are also called *seizures*. These are "violent tearing or shaking" (*convuls*) contractions of the body limb muscles. When the son reached out to hold her, the mother went into *circulatory* (**SIR**-kyuh-lah-**tor**-ee) *collapse*. This means that there was a complete failure of the heart's pumping action and blood "circulation" (*circul*).

The kid called 911, and the ambulance immediately whisked her off to the nearest hospital *ER* (emergency room). The docs gave fluids IV to raise Mrs. S's *BP* (blood pressure), thereby correcting the circulatory collapse. A potent *tranquilizing* (**TRAN**-kwih-**lie**-zing) drug, *chlorpromazine* (**klor-PROH**-mah-zeen), was injected. The *IM* or *intramuscular* (**in**-truh-**MUS**-kyew-lar)—"within" (*intra-*) "muscle" (*muscul*)—route of injection was used. After a few hours, the patient's delirium and hallucinations completely subsided. Her pulse declined to normal, and she fell into a calm sleep.

Probe of case history

(**A**) In all three abbreviations indicating the frequency of drug taking—b.i.d., t.i.d., and q.i.d.—the same letter, *d*, is used to denote "die." What does *die* mean in common English? (**B**) If we said that the drug, chlorpromazine, has an *anti-amphetamine effect*, what precisely do we mean? [Check your short answers with the key near the end of this chapter.]

Quiz

Refer to the text in this chapter if necessary. A good score is at least 8 correct answers out of these 10 questions. The answers are listed in the back of this book.

1. By an addiction to some drug, we mean that the addicted person always has:
   (a) Just a mild case of the "blahs" whenever they can't get the drug
   (b) Only a physical dependence upon the drug
   (c) Both some physical and some psychic dependence upon the drug
   (d) Extreme depression whenever the drug is given

2. Morbidity differs from mortality in that:
   (a) Morbidity is always fatal
   (b) Some pathogens create mortality, with no morbidity involved
   (c) Morbidity literally means an "absence of feeling"
   (d) Mortality reflects death, while morbidity reflects illness
3. Florence Nightingale should be credited as:
   (a) A character in the Disney movie "Lady and the Tramp"
   (b) The Mother of Modern Medicine
   (c) The first person to state all the principles of chemotherapy
   (d) The Mother of Modern Nursing
4. Which of the following specialties is a subdivision of thermotherapy?
   (a) Diathermy
   (b) Heliotherapy
   (c) Physiatrics
   (d) Cryotherapy
5. This person discovered the potential medicinal value of many natural plants:
   (a) Abraham Lincoln
   (b) Shen Nung
   (c) W. K. Roentgen
   (d) Marie Curie
6. *Cyborg* is short for:
   (a) Cyanobiosis
   (b) Celluloborgitis
   (c) Cybernetic organism
   (d) Cell biology
7. *Prostheses* are best defined as:
   (a) Premorbid problems calling for *therapeutic* (**thair**-uh-**PYOO**-tik) interventions
   (b) Types of chemicals that aid in healing
   (c) Special applications of radiotherapy to the human body
   (d) Artificial additions (such as mechanical limbs) to the human body
8. One of the widely acknowledged "Fathers" of Modern Chemotherapy is:
   (a) W. K. Roentgen
   (b) Ernest Fourneau
   (c) Samuel Gompers
   (d) Mother Teresa

9. The four major symptoms of tissue inflammation:
   (a) Redness, cold, dehydration, and pain
   (b) Heat, convulsions, swelling, and tremors
   (c) Radiation emission, coldness, immunity, and swelling
   (d) Redness, heat, swelling, and pain
10. A placebo is usually given to a patient because:
   (a) It has hidden medicinal qualities not yet recognized by pharmacologists
   (b) Such a drug generally relieves the symptoms of chemical dependence
   (c) The psychic connection between always having to take a pill to get "healed" is deeply driven into many people's minds
   (d) Most placebos are narcotics, therefore providing a powerful calming effect

Memory Pillboxes for Chapter 4

Several key facts were tagged with numbered icons in the page margins of this chapter. Write a short summary of each of these key facts into a numbered cell or compartment within the appropriate type of *Memory Pillbox* that appears below.

Background and History **Pillboxes for Chapter 4:**

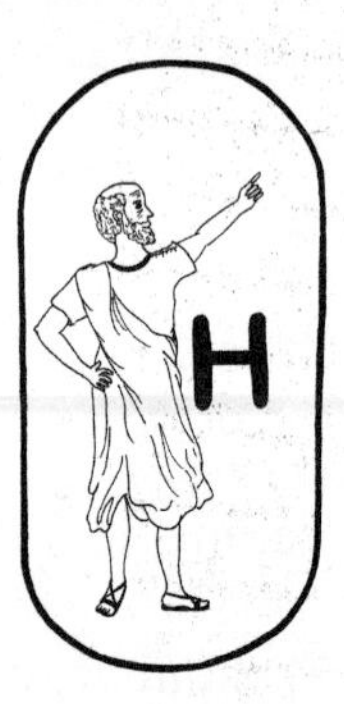

1

2	3
4	5

***Anatomy* Pillboxes for Chapter 4:**

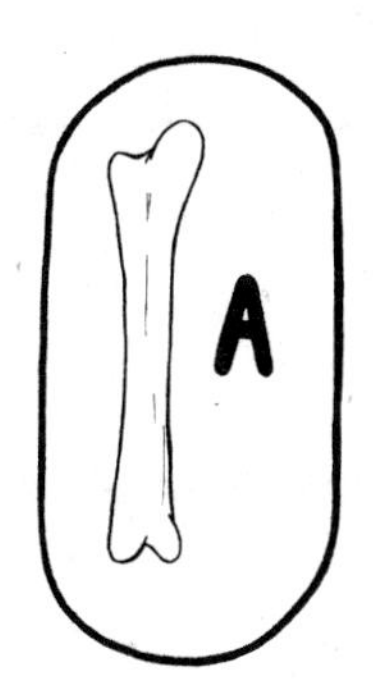

1

2	3

Disease/Injury **Pillboxes for Chapter 4:**

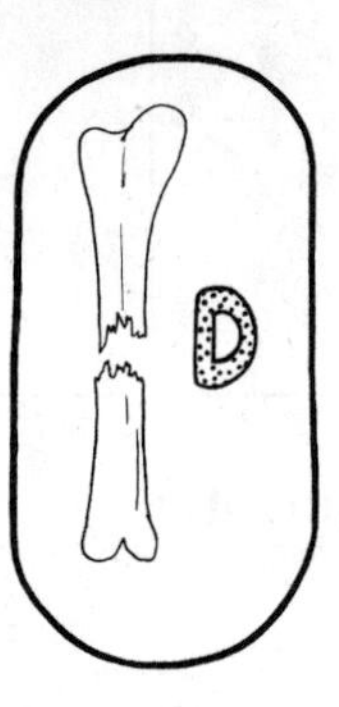

1	2

3	4

5	6

Treatment/Therapy **Pillboxes for Chapter 4:**

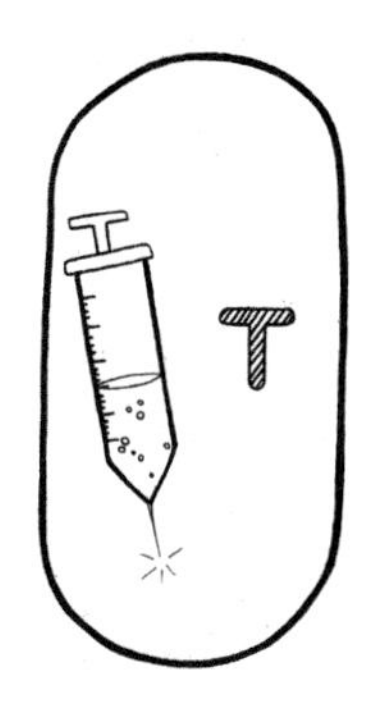

1	2

3	4

5	6

7

Answers for Chapter 4 Summary Tables

FOR SUMMARY TABLE 4.1

1. "process of treating"
2. "the study of wounds"
3. "the study of disease"
4. "a condition of illness"
5. "a condition of death"
6. "one who studies disease"
7. "after death"
8. "one which (takes) away infections"
9. "natural treatments"
10. "process of heating (something) through"

FOR SUMMARY TABLE 4.2

1. "the study of drugs"
2. "one who studies drugs"
3. "condition of a flame within"
4. "one who specializes in drugs"
5. "pertaining to (something) against a flame within"
6. "referring to (something) against fever"

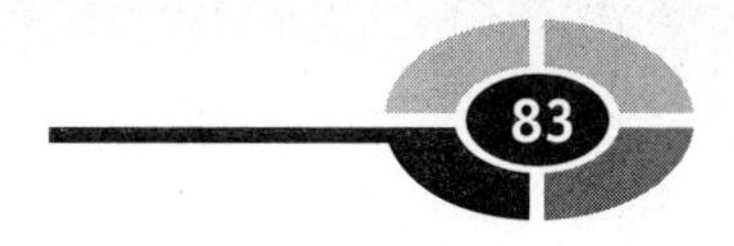

7. "pertaining to quieting down"
8. "relating to (something) against life"

Answers to Probe of Case History

(**A**) "day." (**B**) It exerts an action that is "against" or opposed to the stimulating body action of the amphetamines.

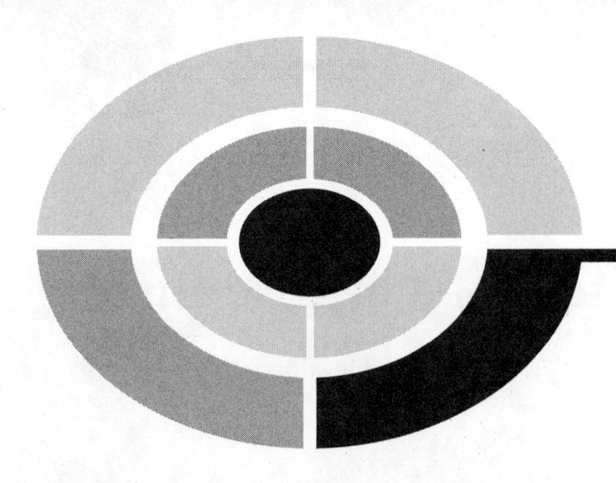

Test: Part 1

DO NOT REFER TO THE TEXT WHEN TAKING THIS TEST. A good score is at least 18 (out of 25 questions) correct. The answers are in the back of the book. It's best to have a friend check your score the first time so you won't memorize the answers if you want to take the test again.

1. The main idea or concept of a medical term is called its:
   (a) Suffix
   (b) Root
   (c) Prefix
   (d) Origin
   (e) Combining vowel
2. The suffix in the word, *premorbidity* (**pree**-mor-**BID**-ih-tee), is:
   (a) Pre-
   (b) Morbid
   (c) Post-
   (d) -ity
   (e) -idity

3. Pronouncing the word, *osteology* (**ahs**-tee-**AHL**-uh-jee), is considerably easier than pronouncing another word with the same meaning, *ostelogy* (**ahs**-tee-**LOH**- jee), because:
   (a) Ostelogy is based only upon Latin word parts
   (b) Osteology is created from both Greek and Latin word parts
   (c) Osteology contains a combining vowel
   (d) The word root in osteology is simpler than that in ostelogy
   (e) Ostelogy contains two suffixes
4. A word with the exact opposite meaning of *premorbidity* is:
   (a) *Postmortality* (**pohst**-mor-**TAL**-ih-tee)
   (b) *Morbiditis* (**mor**-bid-**EYE**-tis)
   (c) *Multimorbidity* (**mul**-tee-mor-**BID**-ih-tee)
   (d) *Postmorbidity* (**pohst**-mor-**BID**-ih-tee)
   (e) *Hypomortality* (**high**-poh-mor-**TAL**-ih-tee)
5. The prefix in *premorbidity* means ________ in regular English.
   (a) "Around"
   (b) "Before"
   (c) "Without"
   (d) "Removal of"
   (e) "After"
6. The plural of coccus is:
   (a) Cocci
   (b) Cockeyed
   (c) Coccidiosis
   (d) Coccusia
   (e) Coccusaces
7. Analgesia differs from anesthesia in that it:
   (a) Involves a removal of bony growths, not cartilage-containing ones
   (b) Points to a body inflammation
   (c) Entails the loss only of the sense of pain
   (d) Adds considerably more color to an otherwise dull day
   (e) Reflects a loss of essentially all types of body sensations
8. A surgical incision made superior and medial to the left eyebrow would probably cut through the:
   (a) Chin
   (b) Bridge of the nose
   (c) Middle of the forehead
   (d) Temple area of the head
   (e) Upper gumline

9. An "abnormal condition of benumbing":
   (a) Paresthesia
   (b) Anesthesia
   (c) Autopsy
   (d) Narcosis
   (e) Narcotic
10. When a surgeon says, "Nurse, please *ligate* that bleeding vessel!" he is telling the nurse to:
    (a) Perform a biopsy
    (b) Suture the vessel
    (c) Cut the vessel apart into two or more pieces
    (d) Pinch the vessel off using forceps
    (e) Tie a thread or wire tightly around the vessel
11. "Just *what* does that particular bone *do* in the human arm, Doc?" would be a question most appropriately asked of a:
    (a) Pharmacist
    (b) Pathologist
    (c) Anesthetist
    (d) Physiologist
    (e) Anatomist
12. Spending too much of your day sucking and chewing upon coca leaves would probably give you:
    (a) Sore lips
    (b) Preoperative anesthesia
    (c) Trephination
    (d) Postop tremors
    (e) Symptoms of extreme sleepiness
13. Excision of the tip of a patient's tongue would indicate that the tip was:
    (a) Turned inside-out
    (b) Reattached
    (c) Severely inflamed
    (d) Completely removed
    (e) Sutured onto the underside of the tongue
14. A hot branding iron can be effectively used for what medical purpose?
    (a) Administering cryotherapy
    (b) Cauterization
    (c) Inducing emesis
    (d) Studying gross anatomy
    (e) Providing sedation for an agitated patient

15. Infectious diseases literally “refer to” body:
    (a) “Infestations”
    (b) “Capitulation”
    (c) “Invasions”
    (d) “Rupture”
    (e) “Malaria”

16. One day, Professor Joe was bitten by an extremely aggressive gnat while walking through the jungle collecting medicinal plants! Two days later, the poor professor suddenly collapsed and was shown to have “jungle fever microorganisms” swarming within his bloodstream. We can logically conclude that the gnat was acting as a:
    (a) Protozoon
    (b) Parasite
    (c) Host
    (d) Vector
    (e) Bacterium

17. A toad’s entire eyeball probably couldn’t be photographed by a scanning electron microscope at once, owing to this reality:
    (a) The eyeball is far too squishy!
    (b) The scanning electron microscopy procedure is too costly to waste on a dumb toad
    (c) A toad’s forehead is more anterior than are the eyeballs, which are sunken back into their shiny skull sockets
    (d) The eyeball is far too shy to be photographed by any means!
    (e) The eye is macroscopic

18. Bacteria are classified as pathogenic if they:
    (a) Serve as food for humans
    (b) Produce helpful gases
    (c) Assist human cells in gaining nutrients
    (d) Cause cases of human illness
    (e) Aid in fermenting goat cheese

19. A little girl stricken with blue spots of mycosis all over her face would be suffering from an attack of what type of organism?
    (a) Rodent
    (b) Fungus
    (c) Bacterium
    (d) Virus
    (e) Bacillus

20. "Whewwww! I'm glad I wasn't bitten by an *Anopheles* mosquito!" expresses the relief of a man who just discovered:
    (a) His lazy dog had been kidnapped
    (b) He had a skin lesion that was completely nonpathogenic
    (c) Never again would he suffer the ill effects of parasitic nematodes
    (d) That his fever and chills probably weren't symptoms of malaria transmitted by a vector
    (e) A cure for cancer
21. Which of the items below is *not* a type of treatment?
    (a) Thermotherapy
    (b) Intravenous injections of healing drugs
    (c) Presentation of a placebo
    (d) Removal of excess body fluid
    (e) Plucking a thorn out of the sole of your crying grandmother's foot
22. A root for "drug":
    (a) Pharmac
    (b) Path
    (c) Mortal
    (d) Psych
    (e) Muscul
23. THERAPY = _______ + __________
    (a) HELIOTHERAPY + DIAGNOSTICS
    (b) PHYSICAL DEPENDENCE + DRUG ADDICTION
    (c) PHYSIOTHERAPY + CHEMOTHERAPY
    (d) RICKETS + DIATHERMY
    (e) DEFORMITY + FRACTURE
24. An *extramuscular* (**eks**-trah-**MUS**-kyoo-lar) *injection* would be given with a syringe whose needle was:
    (a) Stuck all the way through a muscle
    (b) Jabbed hard enough into a muscle to bend it
    (c) Completely blocked with slimy matter
    (d) Kept outside of the skin
    (e) Not penetrating a muscle surface
25. Are sometimes referred to as "uppers" because of their strongly stimulating physiological effect upon the Central Nervous System:
    (a) Amphetamines
    (b) Tranquilizers
    (c) Barbiturates
    (d) Sedatives
    (e) Antibiotics

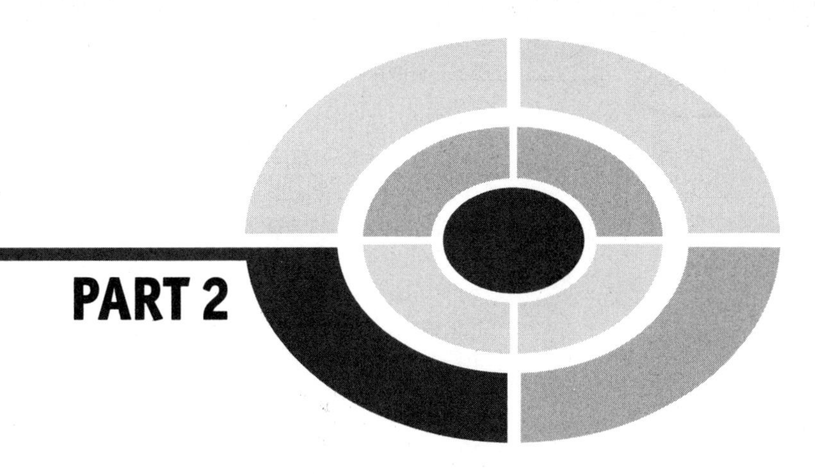

PART 2

Cells and Body Defense

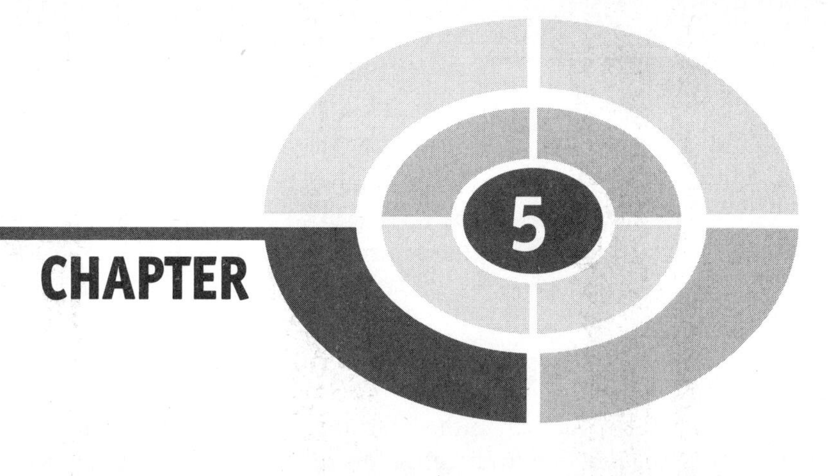

CHAPTER 5

Terms of Diagnosis, Immunity, and the Lymphatic System

In Part 1, we established the broad foundations for medical terminology. Topics such as the basic types of word parts, and the primary skills of terminology—word building, word dissection, and word translation—were all thoroughly examined. Now, in Part 2, we will begin to focus on the *cell level* of body organization, as well as the critical functions of *body defense*.

Background and History

Chapter 4 considered the main types of therapy or "treatments" for dealing with various kinds of body lesions ("wounds"), *pathologies* (**path**-**AHL**-oh-jees), and *morbidities* (**mor-BID**-ih-tees; "illnesses"). A lot of the terminology and related concepts in Chapter 5 now ask the important follow-up question, "Well, how come we're not always sick in the *first* place? What is it about normal body anatomy (structure) and physiology (function) that usually *keeps us* pretty healthy?"

AN OVERVIEW OF IMMUNITY

The answer to the first question posed above is, "We normally have a strong *immunity* to infection or infestation by the many kinds of pathogenic agents." [**Review suggestion:** Explain what is meant by the phrase *pathogenic agent.* Review Chapter 4 to find out, if necessary.] Immunity is literally a "condition of" (*-ity*) "not serving" (*immun*) disease.

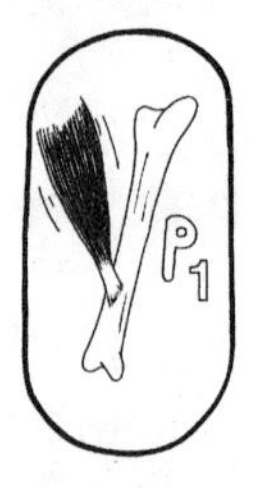

And the answer to the second question mentioned above is, "We have a strong immunity to disease because of the operation of the body's *lymphatic-immune* (**limpf-AT**-ik ih-**MYOON**) *system.*" The lymphatic-immune system is an *organ system* (collection of related *organs*) that function together to provide a broad *prophylaxis* or "guarding against" disease. The *prophylactic* (**prah**-fil-**AK**-tik) "guarding against" effect of the lymphatic-immune system is profiled in the summary equation below:

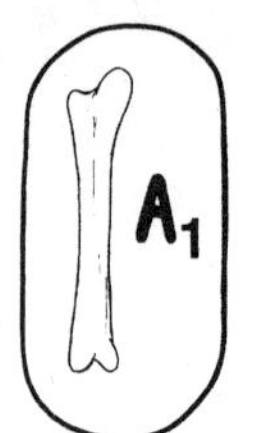

LYMPHATIC-IMMUNE SYSTEM	=	LYMPHATIC SYSTEM	+	IMMUNE SYSTEM
(provides broad immunity—prophylaxis or a prophylactic effect—from disease)		*(lymphatic vessels & organs containing lymph)*		*(antibodies and other protectors from disease)*

The lymph and lymphatic vessels

The human bloodstream is a *very* dirty place! "Why?" the inquiring reader might now ask. The answer is, "Because we always seem to be cutting ourselves, scraping and gouging and poking into our skin, popping blisters, and the like!" Therefore, we are frequently subject to the dangers of *bacteremia* (**bak**-ter-**E**-me-ah), which is a "blood condition of" (*-emia*) invading "bacteria" (*bacter*). In addition, *cancer cells* and *tumor cells* may be cast off into the bloodstream from various sites where they are growing, and then carried long distances throughout the body. Hence, doesn't there seem to be a dire need to have some kind of special blood filtration system—one that could filter out the dirt, debris, and cancer cells, and then return the cleansed blood back into circulation? [**Study suggestion:** Picture the oil filtration system of your car. How does it cleanse and purify the circulating oil? How is this somewhat like the situation for the *human* bloodstream?]

Figure 5.1 shows partly how the body achieves its blood-filtering functions. There is a *lymphatic circulation* with *lymphatic vessels* that closely shadow the *blood circulation* and its *blood vessels*. The tiniest vessels are called the *capillaries* (**CAP**-ih-**lahr**-eez). This is because they are extremely narrow and "have the nature of" (*-ary*) "tiny hairs" (*capill*). Therefore, the lymphatic capillaries shadow or run alongside the blood capillaries.

The *blood pressure* (BP), which pushes the blood through the blood capillaries, also pushes outward. This causes a net *filtration* (fil-**TRAY**-shun) or "process of filtering" of materials out of the bloodstream. When the *filtrate* (**FIL**-trayt)—filtration product—enters the nearby lymphatic capillaries, it then becomes the *lymph* (limpf). The lymph is named for its resemblance to "clear spring water." So, lymph is clear-looking and watery, rather than reddish (like

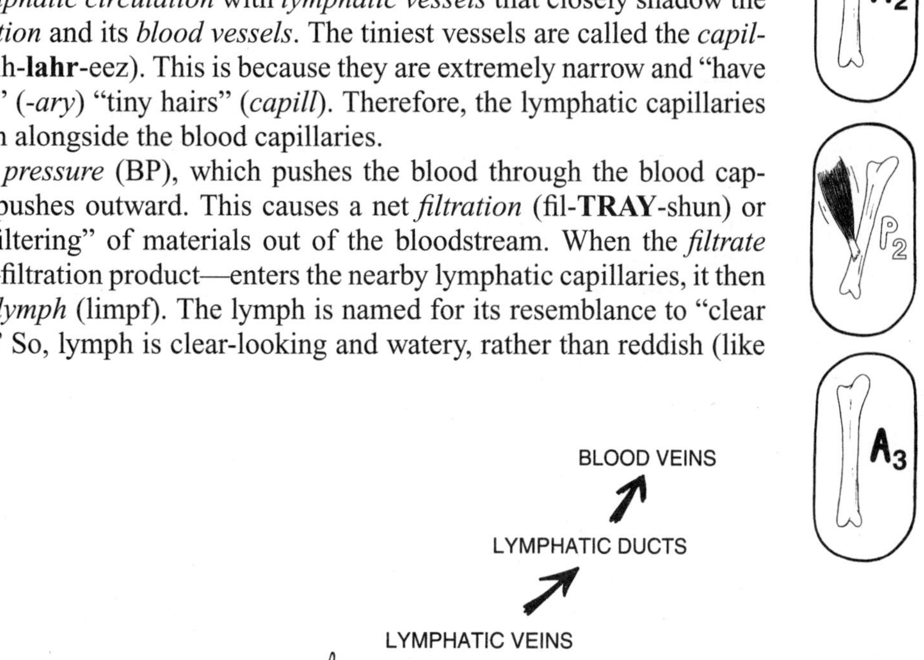

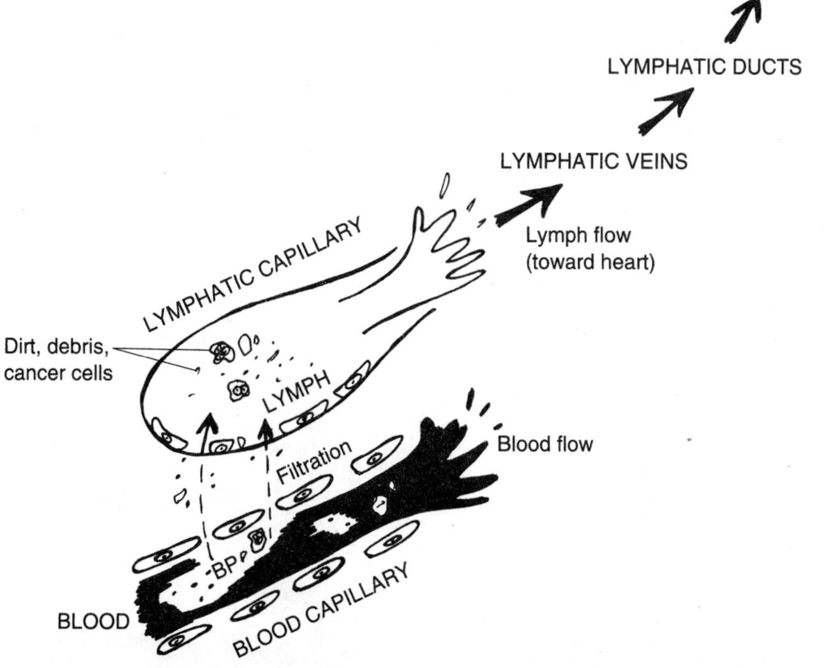

Fig. 5.1 "Dirty blood" in the blood capillaries becomes "dirty lymph" within the nearby lymphatic capillaries.

the blood). However, when the lymph is first formed by filtration of the blood, it is still quite *dirty*, because dirt, debris, bacteria, and cancer cells that were inside the bloodstream also get filtered into the lymph!

Tracing the lymph flow in Figure 5.1, you can see that the tiny lymphatic capillaries eventually flow into much larger *lymphatic veins*, then *lymphatic ducts*. Finally, the "cleansed" lymph returns back to the *blood veins*.

"Okay, but what *happens* to clean this dirty lymph along the way?" you might now be asking yourself. As you can see in Figure 5.2, it gets cleaned up by flowing through a number of different *lymphatic organs*.

A brief look at the immune response

Figure 5.2 shows the "dirty" lymph flowing into *lymph nodes* (nohds) at one end, and "clean" lymph flowing out, at the other. In between, we get the operation of the *immune response* (Figure 5.3). Foreign bacteria, cancer cells, and various other body invaders found in "dirty" lymph all have their surfaces tagged by *antigens*.

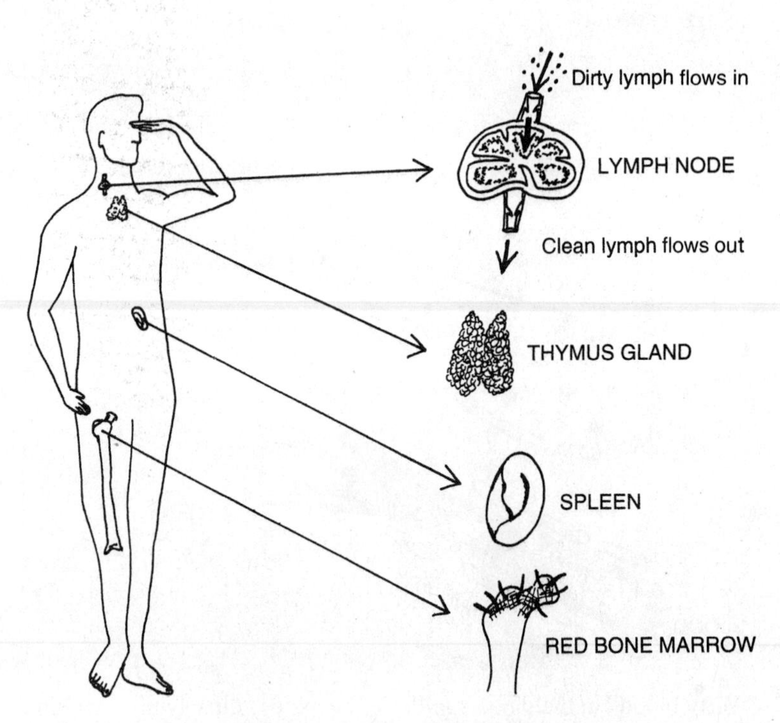

Fig. 5.2 The major lymphatic organs: Cleansers of dirty lymph.

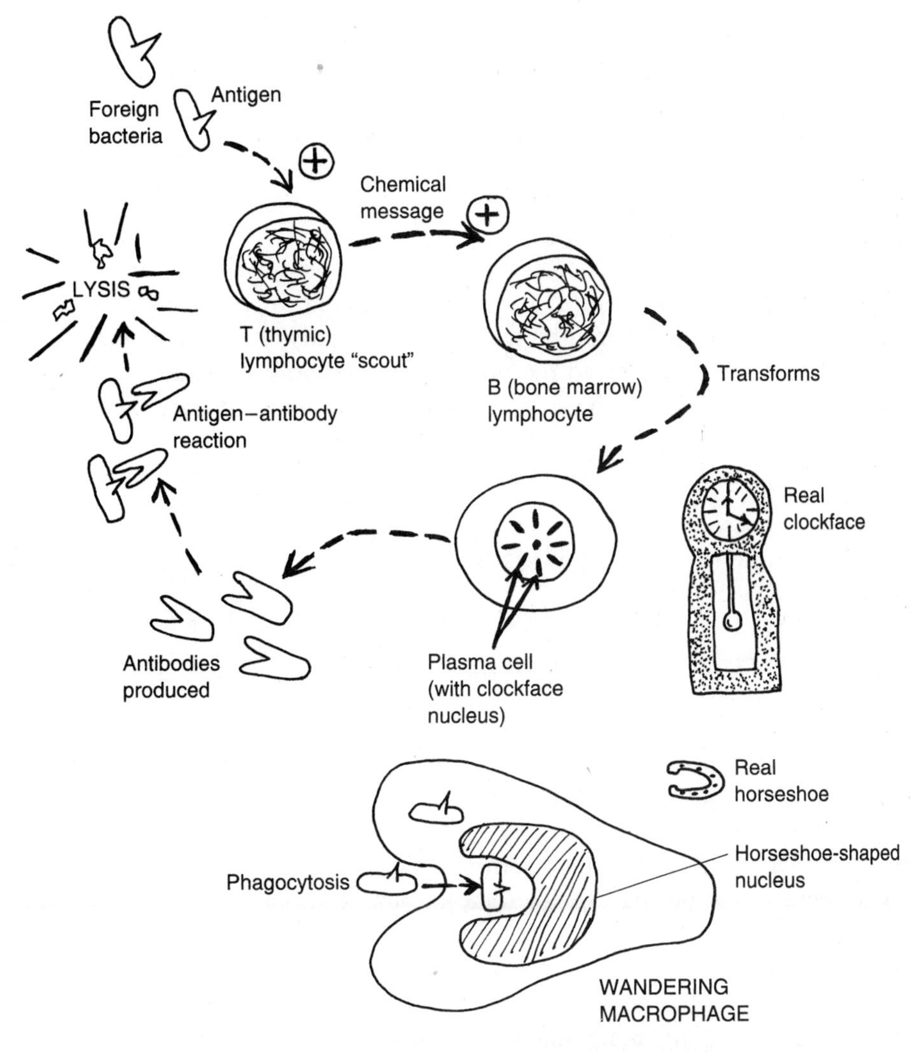

Fig. 5.3 A brief overview of the immune response.

The word *antigen* (**AN**-tih-**jen**) means "produced" (*-gen*) "against" (*anti-*). An antigen is a foreign *protein* (**PROH**-teen) or chemical marker that is present on the outer membrane surrounding an invading cell. (Figure 5.3 shows these invading cells as foreign bacteria.) Several types of *lymphocytes* (**LIMPF**-oh-**sights**)—literally "clear spring water" (*lymph*) "cells" (*cyt*)—are present within the lymph nodes. One type of lymphocyte acts as a scout, detecting the antigen (foreign protein marker) present on the invading bacterial

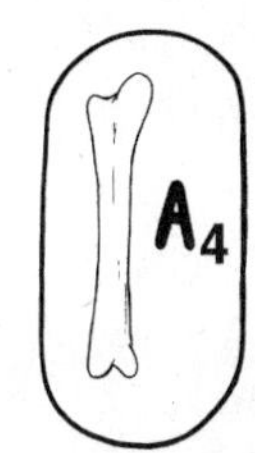

cells. It sends a stimulating message (indicated by the plus sign in Figure 5.3) to another type of lymphocyte. This second type of lymphocyte then transforms itself into an entirely different type of cell.

This new cell type is called a *plasma* (**PLAZ**-muh) *cell*. It is easily recognized under the compound microscope by the unique clock-face appearance of its *nucleus* (**NOO**-klee-**us**). (The nucleus is the small, rounded, "kernel" [*nucle*] "present" [*-us*] within most cells.)

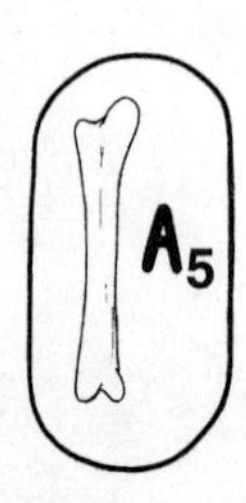

The plasma cell is unique because it is the main source of our *antibodies* (**AN**-tih-**bah**-dees). These antibodies are special types of proteins (Y-shaped *bodies*) that act "against" (*anti-*) foreign invaders. Specifically, the Y-shaped antibodies chemically attach and bind to the pointy antigens on the surfaces of the bacterial cells. (This is somewhat like two oppositely shaped puzzle pieces fitting together.)

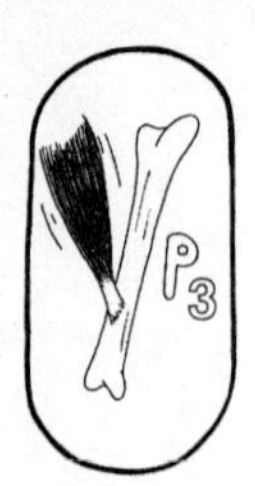

The result is called an *antigen-antibody reaction*:

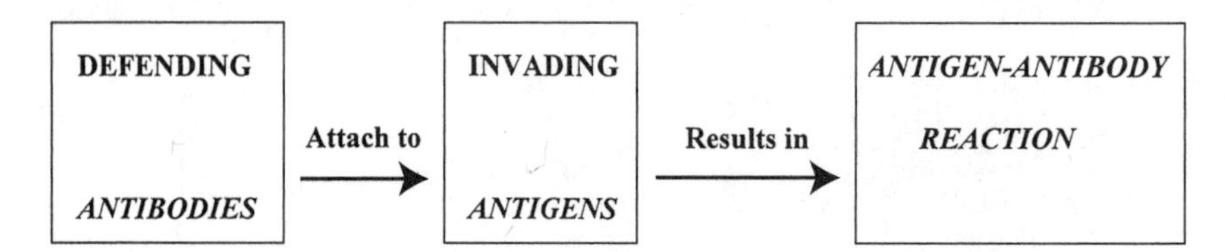

Following the antigen-antibody reaction (the combining of antibodies with antigens), the foreign bacteria cells undergo *lysis* (**LIE**-sis), a chemical explosion or "breakdown" (*lys*). This lysis ("process of breaking down"), of course, very effectively kills many thousands of the invading bacteria!

But there is another part of the total immune response we haven't yet mentioned. It is called *phagocytosis* (**fay**-go-sigh-**TOH**-sis)—a "process of" (*-osis*) "cell" (*cyt*) "eating" (*phag*). The bottom portion of Figure 5.3 shows a *wandering macrophage*, a "large" (*macr*) "eater" (*phag*) that is "present" (*—e*). Such macrophages, as their name suggests, wander throughout the vessels and organs of the lymphatic system. Whenever they encounter a foreign invader, they engulf or "eat" it.

Summary of the immune response

As we have seen, two major processes—antigen-antibody reactions and phagocytosis—make up our body's immune response. When they are both highly successful, we achieve a state of *clinical health.* By "clinical" health, we mean a lack of morbidity (illness), so that no visit to a medical *clinic* to receive treatment is necessary:

CLINICAL HEALTH	=	A SUCCESSFUL IMMUNE RESPONSE	=	ANTIGEN-ANTIBODY REACTIONS	+	PHAGOCYTOSIS
(lack of morbidity)		(state of immunity or prophylaxis from disease)		(within lymphatic organs; cause lysis of invading cells)		(eating of invaders by macrophages that wander throughout the lymph)

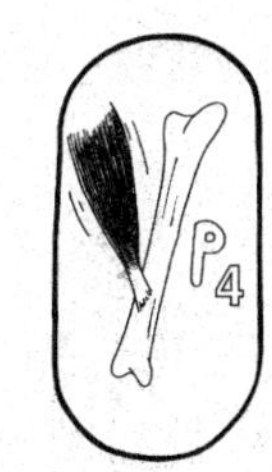

[**Study suggestion:** You may want to explore the subject of the lymphatic system and immunity in further detail within two of our very helpful companion volumes: *ANATOMY DEMYSTIFIED* and its separate partner, *PHYSIOLOGY DEMYSTIFIED*.]

SUMMARY TABLE 5.1

Consult Summary Table 5.1 for a quick review of some important words and word parts.

Summary Table 5.1 Words and Word Parts
Write in the *exact* meaning (literal English translation) for up to 10 key terms selected from the preceding block of text. After you are done, check your word meanings with the correct answers, which are given at the end of this chapter.

Key Terms	**Prefixes**	**Roots**	**Suffixes**	**Exact Meanings**
immunity	(none)	immun "not serving"	-ity "condition of"	1. ________
prophylactic	(none)	prophylact "guarding against"	-ic "pertaining to"	2. ________
lymphocyte	(none)	lymph "clear spring water"; cyt "cell"	-e "presence of"	3. ________
phagocytosis	(none)	phag "eating"; cyt "cell"	-osis "process of"	4. ________
lymphatic	(none)	lymphat "clear spring water"	-ic "referring to"	5. ________

THE WORLD OF DIAGNOSIS: TAKING STOCK WHEN IMMUNITY FAILS

In reality, of course, the immune response isn't always perfect, so that humans sicken and die. There is a whole World of Clinical Diagnosis, therefore, that has been developed over the centuries to describe this morbid reality.

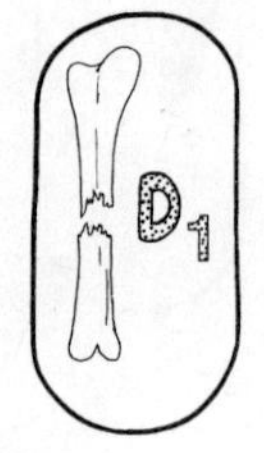

The word, *diagnosis* (**die**-uh-**NOH**-sis), literally means "a condition of" (*-is*) "knowledge" (*gnos*) "through" (*dia-*). Although its literal meaning is rather clumsy, diagnosis does represent the physician's "knowledge" about what a person has wrong with them at the present time. In other words, it is knowledge about what the person is now going "through." Say, for instance, that your family caregiver makes a diagnosis of *acute coryza* (**kor-EE**-zah). The word, *acute*, can be subdivided with a single slash mark as acut/e. The root, *acut*, means "sudden." **[Thinking probe:** What is the suffix in *acute*? What does it mean in Common English? Hint: The suffix is the same as that in *macrophage.* Check your thinking with the next sentence.] In plain layman's language, acute means the "presence of" (-e) something "sudden" (*acut*). An acute problem, therefore, is one that has a sudden onset and usually lasts for only a relatively short time.

The other word in the preceding diagnosis, *coryza*, derives from the Greek for "runny nose." An alternative term with almost the same meaning is *rhinitis* (**rye-NEYE**-tis)—an "inflammation of" (*-itis*) the lining of the "nose" (*rhin*). Hence, a person who is *diagnosed* (**die**-ahg-**NOHSD**) with acute coryza or rhinitis is suffering, essentially, from the effects of a sudden head cold.

There are several characteristic *symptoms* or "happenings" that are detected by the patient. Certainly, the coryza (runny nose) associated with a head cold would be a symptom perceived by the patient. Quite frequently, in fact, it is one or more symptoms that bother the patient enough to seek medical help in the first place!

Another self-observed symptom of a cold is an *edema* or "swelling" of the membranes lining the *nasal* (**NAY**-sal) *passages*. The word, *nasal*, literally "pertains to" (*-al*) the "nose" (nas). It is an edema (swelling) that causes nasal *congestion* (**kahn-JES**-shun). This is a "process of" (*-ion*) one's nasal passages becoming "stuffed up" (*congest*).

Along with such *clinical symptoms* reported by the patient, however, the examining caregiver will also base his or her *diagnostic* (**die**-ug-**NAHS**-tik) findings upon a certain number of *clinical signs*. In general, a sign is "a mark" of some illness or disease that is detected by a doctor or other examiner—*not* by the patient. If an assisting nurse places an *oral thermometer* into a patient's "mouth" (*or*), for example, she may report the clinical *sign* of an oral temperature of 101 degrees *F* (*Fahrenheit*). "You are somewhat *febrile*," the nurse informs you. "What does *that* mean?" you (the patient) nervously ask. "Oh, it just means that you have (*-ile*) a moderate fever (*febr*)," she casually replies. "Gosh,

my face *does* seem to feel rather hot!" you say, confirming this clinical finding. [**Thinking probe:** Is the nurse's conclusion that you have a fever based upon a clinical symptom or a clinical sign? How about your self-report that your face has been feeling hot? Is this a clinical symptom or a clinical sign? Why?]

When we put all of the above clinical info "together" (*syn-*), we get a *syndrome*. The word *syndrome* comes from the Greek and means "a running together." A *clinical syndrome* (**SIN**-drohm), consequently, is a whole group of clinical symptoms and signs that more or less "run together" in a particular patient at the same time. The doctor making a diagnosis of acute coryza or rhinitis would base this decision upon a *cold syndrome*. Such a syndrome includes a characteristic set of *cold symptoms* and *cold signs* "running together" in a patient.

Summarizing, we obtain the following handy word-equation:

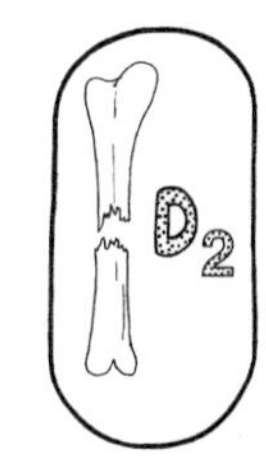

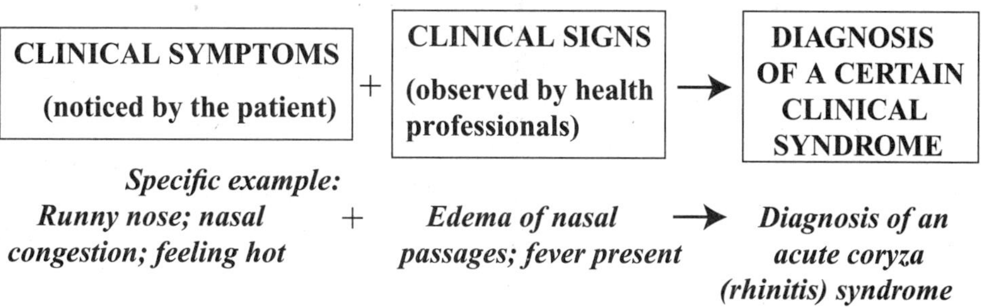

"Okay, but how do you *know* that you're getting a cold *before* the disease actually happens?" the careful student may further probe. The physician may say you have a particular *prodrome* (**PROH**-drohm)—literally "a running" (*drome*) "before" (*pro-*). A prodrome, then, involves the symptoms that occur *before* a full-blown disease syndrome. In our example, there would be a case of the sniffles. This might also include *malaise* (mah-**LAYZ**)—a vague feeling of body weakness or "discomfort." Both sniffles and malaise, then, are often part of the PRODROME leading up to a full-blown SYNDROME of acute coryza/rhinitis.

Remember:

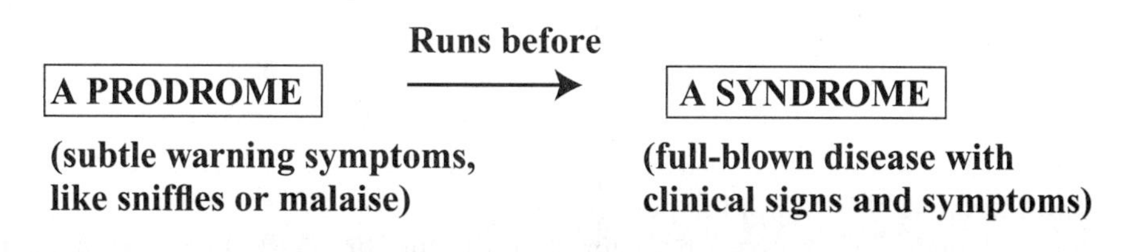

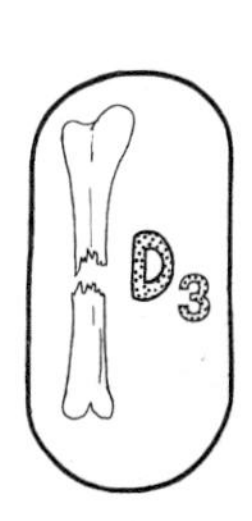

"I understand," the motivated learner may now exclaim. "But can you tell me what happens *after* a diagnosis of a disease syndrome is made? What happens *next*?"

Once a disease is diagnosed, it is only natural for the patient (who is often worried) to ask the caregiver, "How is this thing going to work out?" Speaking medically, the patient is asking the doctor to make a *prognosis* (prahg-**NOH**-sis). This word literally means "a condition of" (*-is*) "knowledge" (*gnos*) "before" (*pro-*). Prognosis, then, is a condition of foreknowledge. It is a situation in which the knowledgeable caregiver makes a prediction concerning the outcome of a particular disease the patient has, including the chances for full recovery. "You have 3 months to live!" is definitely *not* the prognosis any of us would like to hear! Hopefully, we will hear our caregiver make a much more optimistic prediction, such as, "Your head cold should disappear in just a few more days. But I have prescribed a *nasal decongestant* [**dee**-kahn-**JES**-tant] that will help you breathe easier in the meantime." [**Thinking probe:** From your recent study of the word, *congestion,* what do you think that the word, *decongestant*, literally means?]

In overview, remember:

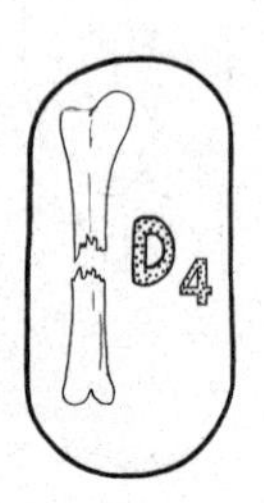

A *DIAGNOSIS*	but	A *PROGNOSIS*
(summarizes what you are going "through" [*dia-*] during a disease)		(predicts the future outcome of a disease "before" [*pro-*] it actually happens)

IMPORTANT TOOLS AND TECHNIQUES USED IN MAKING DIAGNOSES

We have now discussed various concepts involved in making *diagnoses* (**die**-uhg-**NOH**-seez; statements of present disease conditions). And we have contrasted this with *prognoses* (predictions about future disease outcomes). It is now appropriate for us to discuss some of the major tools and techniques that are used to make such knowledgeable statements.

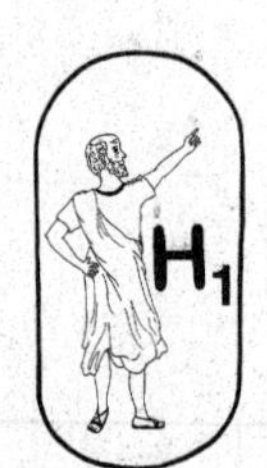

Even as far back as Hippocrates (Chapter 1), healers made diagnoses by *palpation* (**pal-PAY**-shun). The earliest physicians *palpated* (**PAL**-pay-ted) or "touched" (*palpat*) the bodies of their patients in numerous places. They used only their sensitive fingertips as diagnostic tools. By palpation (a "process of touching") the abdomen, for example, Hippocrates was able to diagnose an enlarged liver right through his patient's skin!

Closely related to palpation is another diagnostic skill, *percussion* (per-**KUSH**-un)—"a process of" (*-ion*) "striking" (*percuss*). Percussion is used in physical examination by tapping (striking) the body surface fairly hard with the fingertips. Such tapping helps the *clinician* (clin-**ISH**-un) working in a "clinic" to evaluate the size, borders, and consistency of underlying *viscera* (internal organs). Percussion can also help reveal the relative amount of fluid accumulated within a body cavity.

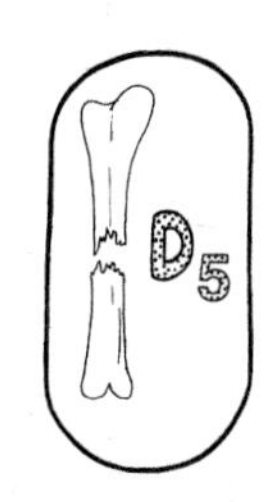

Often following percussion is *auscultation* (**aws**-kul-**TAY**-shun)—"a process of" (*-ion*) "listening" (*auscult*). (The combined sequence is often called *percussion and auscultation*, abbreviated as *P & A*.) For many centuries, auscultation was performed by simply placing an ear tightly against a body surface, such as the back or chest. This permitted the hearing of internal body sounds, like the beating of the heart and movement of air into and out of the lungs.

Laennec invents the stethoscope

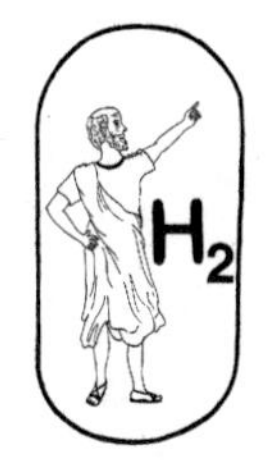

One of the most vital improvements in the quality of auscultation (internal body listening) came with the inventive mind of a Frenchman named *Rene Laennec* (**LAY**-uh-**nek**), who lived in Europe from 1781 to 1826. Dr. Laennec was walking home one day, and he noticed two young boys playing. One boy was holding a thick stick up to his ear, while the other was scratching a long pin over the other end. This simple trick gave Laennec a brilliant insight. "Why not try that with my patients?" he must have said to himself. As a result, Laennec set to work and invented the first *stethoscope* (Figure 5.4). Laennec originally developed it as an "instrument used to examine" (*scope*) the sounds of the "chest" (*steth*). Basically, it was a hollow wooden cylinder over which Laennec pressed one of his ears. The resulting *amplification* (**am**-plih-fih-**KAY**-shun) or "enlargement (boosting)" of chest sounds made auscultation of the thorax much more accurate and efficient. Today, of course, the basic stethoscope design consists of Y-shaped rubber tubing connecting two earpieces to a single bell that is held against the body.

Ultrasound goes far "beyond"

Traditional auscultation using a stethoscope, of course, depends upon the existence of *audible* (**AW**-dih-**bl**) sound waves—those that are "capable" (*-ible*) of being "heard" (*aud*). Around 1957, a whole new science called *ultrasonics* (**ul**-trah-**SAHN**-iks) was developed. This name translates to mean "pertaining to" (*-ic*) vibrations that are far "beyond" (*ultra-*) the range of audible "sound" (*son*).

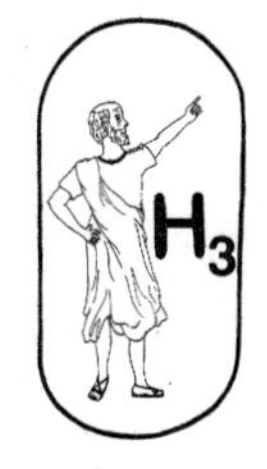

Ultrasound (**UL**-trah-**sound**) *technology* for medicine was developed largely by a British physician named Ian Donald. During World War II, *ultrasonics* was first used to bounce sound waves of very high frequency off the hulls of enemy submarines. Later, it detected cracks, flaws, and bubbles in the metal of machine parts. But Ian Donald altered this technology to create *medical ultrasonography*

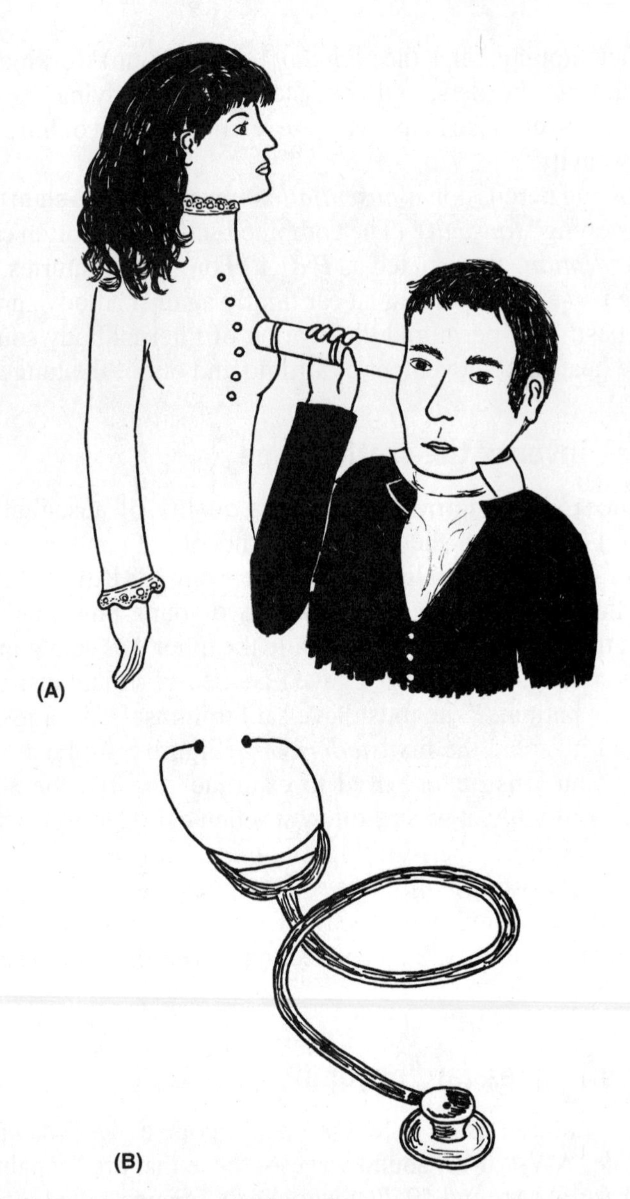

Fig. 5.4 Laennec invents the stethoscope for auscultation. **(A)** Laennec using a hollow wooden cylinder as his primitive stethoscope for auscultation of the chest. **(B)** A modern stethoscope with Y-shaped tubing.

(**ul**-trah-son-**AHG**-rah-fee). This new field involves the "process of recording" (*-graphy*) extremely high-frequency sound waves reflected off internal body structures.

Sound waves of very high frequency can easily and harmlessly pass through human flesh. They are reflected or bounced off tissues with different degrees of density. These reflected high-frequency waves then make a visible tracing on an electronic screen. The visible tracing is called a *sonogram* (**SOH**-noh-gram) or "sound record." Because the high-frequency rays are harmless, they are especially helpful in creating ultrasound pictures (sonograms) of the human *fetus* (**FEE**-tus). A fetus is technically the unborn "offspring" (*fet*) during the later stages of pregnancy. This technique enables physicians to diagnose many *prenatal* (**pree-NAY**-tal) problems—those that occur "before" (*pre-*) "birth" (*nat*).

X-rays come out from the "unknown"

A third major diagnostic technology is *radiography* (**ray**-dee-**AHG**-rah-fee)—the "process of recording" (*-graphy*) x-"rays" (*radi*). The interesting story behind x-rays involves a German *physicist* (**FIZZ**-ih-**sist**) named *W. K. Roentgen* (**RENT**-gun). In 1895, Roentgen was experimenting with a new device called a *vacuum tube*. This is a sealed glass tube that encloses a vacuum (space completely "empty" of air). The tube contains a *cathode* (**KAY**-thohd) or filament that gives off *electrons* (negatively charged particles) when heated. Roentgen was surprised to find that something very different (in addition to a stream of electrons) was coming out of his heated vacuum tube. There were also mysterious, invisible rays of unknown origin, which he called *x-rays*. These rays were able to pass right through softer, less dense body tissues, such as the skin and muscle tissue of his wife's hand. (See Figure 5.5, A.) However, the rays bounced off the harder, denser body tissues, such as bone and *cartilage* (**KAR**-tih-**lahj**). The result was the very first *radiogram* (**RAY**-dee-oh-**gram**) "x-ray" (*radi*) "record" (*gram*)—of the human body. [**Thinking probe:** Please observe that the radiogram of the hand of Roentgen's wife has the bones clearly standing out as a black image upon a white background of the softer skin and muscle tissue. Now, think about the modern radiograms you have seen of people's bones. Do the x-rayed bones show up black, as they did in Roentgen's day?]

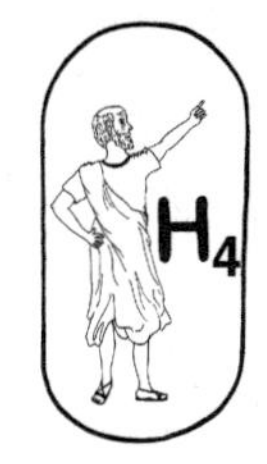

Because of his pioneering work, W. K. Roentgen can be given credit as the Father of Radiology, which is "the study of" (*-ology*) "rays" (*radi*). Therefore, he was also the first *radiologist*, because he was "one who studied" (*-ologist*) these mysterious "rays."

Soon after Roentgen's discovery, early *fluoroscopes* (**FLOOR**-oh-**skohps**) were developed. These are technically "instruments that examine" (*-scopes*) the interior of the body by casting x-ray "shadows" (*fluor*) of them. In 1896,

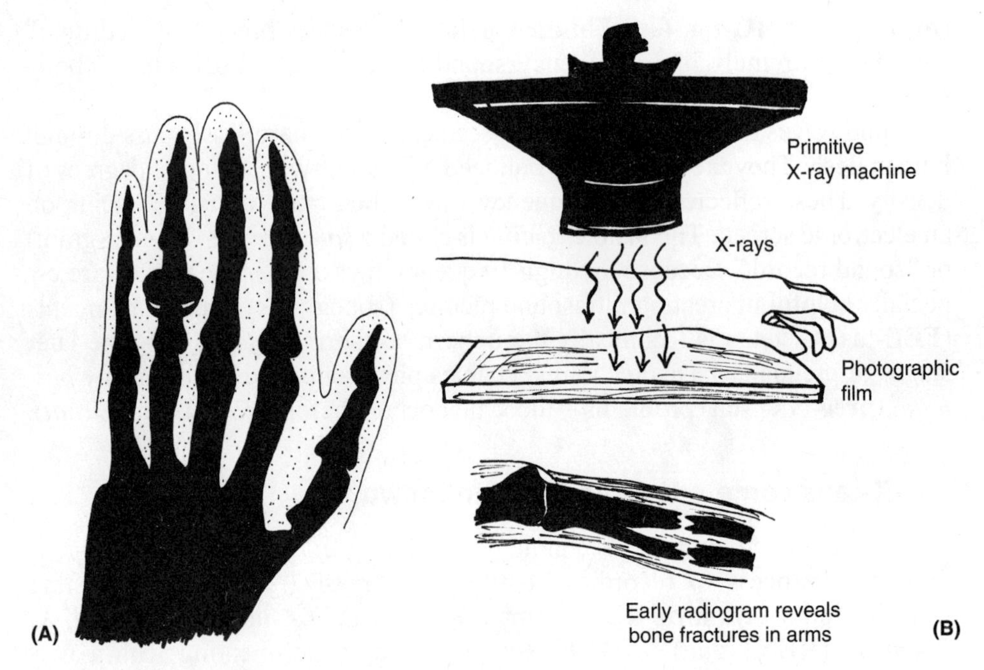

Fig. 5.5 Some of the earliest radiograms of the human body. **(A)** A Sketch of the radiogram Roentgen took of his wife's hand. Observe that her large finger ring was also recorded. **(B)** A primitive fluoroscope records the fractured bones in the lower arm of Eddie McCarthy.

such a primitive fluoroscope made a radiogram of the broken bones in the forearm of a man named Eddie McCarthy (Figure 5.5, B). This radiogram was the very first one used to help set the broken bones of a patient!

Today, highly advanced *radiologic* (**ray**-dee-oh-**LAHJ**-ik) techniques are available. Among the most impressive of these is the making of *CAT scans*. CAT is an abbreviation for *computed axial* (**AKS**-ee-ul) *tomography* (**toh-MAH**-grah-fee). An alternate name is *CT* (an abbreviation for the shorter version, *computed tomography*.) Now, recall that the word root, *tom* (as in *anatomy*), means "cut." Hence, a *tomogram* is an x-ray "record" (*-gram*) of only a particular "cut or slice" (*tom*) through the body, not an entire part of the body! *Tomography* is the "process of recording" (*-graphy*) such thin body cuts or slices. Computed axial tomography, then, is just a very efficient and modern type of tomography (making x-ray records of thin body slices or tomograms). This CAT (CT) procedure is illustrated in Figure 5.6. A large fluoroscope is rotated on an axis around the patient, such that a thin *cross-section* all the way through the body can be viewed. An attached computer generates the actual image.

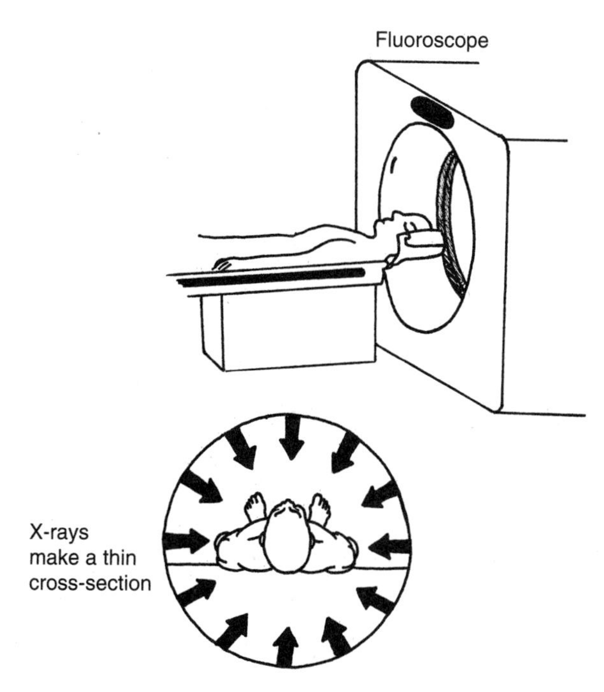

Fig. 5.6 A CAT scanner in operation.

THE ULTIMATE CHALLENGE: FINDING THE "CAUSE"

With all its powerful diagnostic procedures, modern medicine still faces this key question asked by suffering patients: "What is *causing* my medical problem, Doctor?" The answers to such questions involve *etiology* (e-tee-**AHL**-uh-jee)—the "study of" (*-ology*) disease "causes" (*eti*).

D6

While the doctor may be able to give you a proper diagnosis, such as, "You have an acute coryza syndrome," finding its specific cause or etiology often involves some extra detective work. "With whom have you recently come into contact? Did they have a common cold? Do you wash your hands frequently?" The preceding are all some relevant *etiological* (**ee**-tee-oh-**LAHJ**-ih-kal) or "cause-related" questions the clinician might ask you.

D7

Many times, of course, the exact cause of a person's morbidity is *never* found. In such cases, the caregiver may say that your disease is *essential* or *idiopathic* (**id**-e-oh-**PATH**-ik). In Common English, this means that it appears to be your "own" (*idio*) private "disease" (*path*)!

SUMMARY TABLE 5.2

Consult Summary Table 5.2 for a quick review of some important words and word parts.

Summary Table 5.2 Words and Word Parts

Write in the *exact* meaning (literal English translation) for up to 10 key terms selected from the preceding block of text. After you are done, check your word meanings with the correct answers, which are given at the end of this chapter.

Key Terms	Prefixes	Roots	Suffixes	Exact Meanings
diagnosis	dia- "through"	gnos "knowledge"	-is "a condition of"	1. ________
acute	(none)	acut "sudden"	-e "presence of"	2. ________
rhinitis	(none)	rhin "nose"	-itis "inflammation of"	3. ________
prodrome	pro- "before"	drom "running"	-e "presence of"	4. ________
prognosis	pro- "before"	gnos "knowledge"	-is "condition of"	5. ________
percussion	(none)	percuss "striking"	-ion "a process of"	6. ________
auscultation	(none)	auscult "listening"	-tion "a process of"	7. ________
stethoscope	(none)	steth "chest"	-scope "instrument used to examine"	8. ________
ultrasonography	ultra- "beyond"	son "sounds"	-graphy "process of recording"	9. ________
etiology	(none)	eti "causes"	-ology "study of"	10. ________

***Medical Case History:* Suddenly Stricken with Tonsillitis**

Andrew M. L., age 21, was working at his summer job cleaning out dorm rooms on his college campus. This job was quite dirty, because Andrew had to flip over old mattresses and shake them out. (We all know that college students in dorms collect a lot of debris under their sheets!) As a result, Andy inhaled lots of house dust, which was heavily laden with pathogenic bacteria.

Quite obviously, poor Andy had a dire need for assistance from his lymphatic-immune system! Now, in addition to our full-blown lymphatic organs, there are some smaller masses of lymphatic tissue scattered here and there throughout the body. Very familiar to most of us are the *tonsils*. [**Thinking and discovery suggestion:** Get up right now and go to the bathroom. Look straight into the bathroom mirror, and open your mouth nice and wide! Do you see the pair of whitish-colored tonsils located on either side of the entrance to your throat, at the back of your tongue? We will name these specific tonsils in a moment.]

Because of their oval shape and whitish color, the tonsils are literally "almonds" of lymphatic tissue located in the back of the throat (Figure 5.7). There are five tonsils in all. Perhaps the most noticeable of these (when you look into a wide-open mouth) are the two *palatine* (**PAL**-ah-**tyn**) *tonsils*. The word, *palatine*, actually "refers to" (*-ine*) the "roof of the mouth" (*palat*). The palatine tonsils lie just inferior to the *palate* (**PAL**-aht)—roof of the mouth. They are two almond-shaped masses on either side of the back of the throat, flanking the root of the tongue.

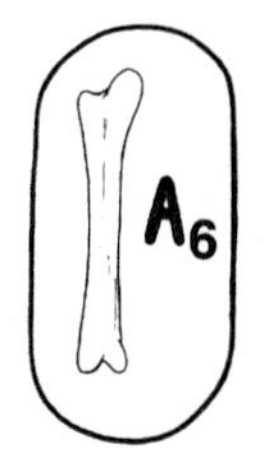

The term, *lingual* (**LING**-gwal), "relates to" (*-al*) the "tongue" (*lingu*). The two *lingual tonsils*, therefore, sit on the far posterior (rear) end of the tongue. And as you can see from Figure 5.7, behind the palate (roof of the mouth) lies the *pharynx* (**FAIR**-inks). The pharynx is the correct anatomic term for the "throat." There is a single, large *pharyngeal* (fah-**RIN**-jee-al) *tonsil* attached to the back of the upper pharynx (throat). The word *pharyngeal* "relates to" (*-al*) the "throat" (*pharynge*), so you can see how the pharyngeal tonsil gets its name.

An alternate name for the pharyngeal tonsil is the *adenoids* (**AD**-uh-**noyds**). *Aden* (**AH**-den) is a root for "gland," while *-oids* (**oyds**) means "resemblers." Hence, *adenoids* translates to mean "______________." [**Study suggestion:** *You* go ahead and fill in this blank with the complete anatomical term.] This alternate name reflects that fact that the pharyngeal tonsil or adenoids consists of several rounded, lumpy, gland-like masses pushed close together.

A bad case of tonsillitis

Returning to Andy, we can speculate that the lymphocytes and macrophages within his tonsils were not able to fight off the huge number of pathogenic

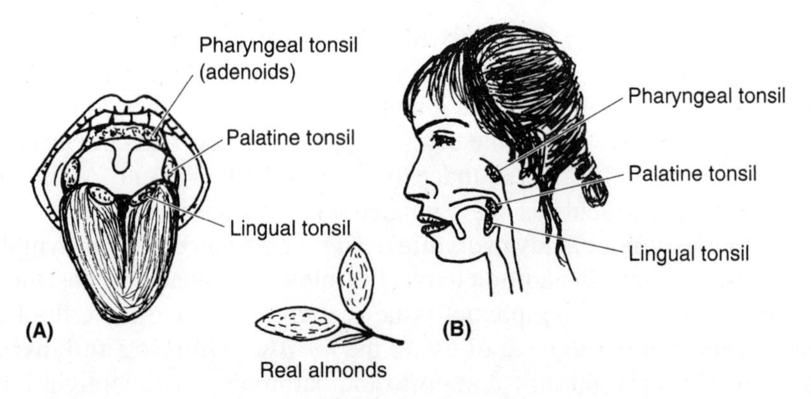

Fig. 5.7 The tonsils: "Little almonds" tucked away in our throats.

bacteria he inhaled into his throat during bed cleaning. As a result, he came down with a bad case of *tonsillitis* (**tahn**-sil-**EYE**-tis)—an "inflammation of the tonsils." Secondarily, this general tonsillitis included a severe ________ or "inflammation of the adenoids." [**Study suggestion:** Why don't *you* try to build this term, and write it into the preceding blank. You'll get feedback about your answer, very soon!]

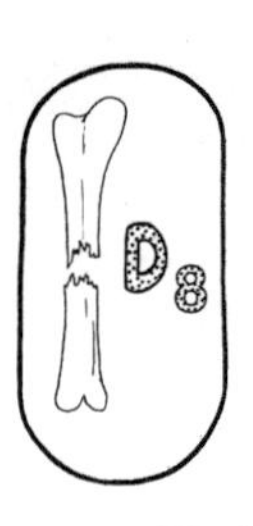

The *adenoiditis* (inflammation of the adenoids) was so severe that it was accompanied by *adenoid hypertrophy* (**high-PER**-truh-fee). Hypertrophy, broadly speaking, is "a process of" (*–y*) "excessive" (*hyper-*) "stimulation or nourishment" (*troph*). When a body structure (such as the adenoids) is excessively stimulated, it often responds by enlarging—that is, undergoing hypertrophy. In Andy's case, his adenoids were overstimulated as they tried to fight off the invading bacteria he had inhaled, so that they underwent a dramatic enlargement (hypertrophy).

His visit to the college campus health center resulted in a diagnosis of *chronic inflammation of both palatine tonsils and the pharyngeal tonsil* (*adenoids*). A *throat culture* (swab of the throat to collect infecting organisms) revealed that the pathogenic bacteria were *streptococci* (**STREHP**-toh-**kahk**-sigh). These bacteria are of the coccus type (see Chapter 3). The individual bacterial cells are attached to one another like a "curved" (*strept*) chain of little "berries" (*cocci*).

The news that this infection was chronic was bad, because it suggested that it had been present for a long "time" (*chron*). Careful interviewing with Andrew indicated that he had probably suffered repeated bouts of *acute* (short-term) *tonsillitis* many times before. He had an extremely sore *edematous* (eh-**DEM**-ah-tus) or "swollen" throat. Fever, chills, and *cephalalgia* (**sef**-al-**AL**-juh) were present. Cephalalgia is literally an "ache or pain condition" (*-algia*) located within the "head" (*cephal*). The palatine tonsils and adenoids showed a bright *rubor* (**ROO**-bor) or "redness." The *cervical* (**SIR**-vih-**kal**) *lymph nodes* in

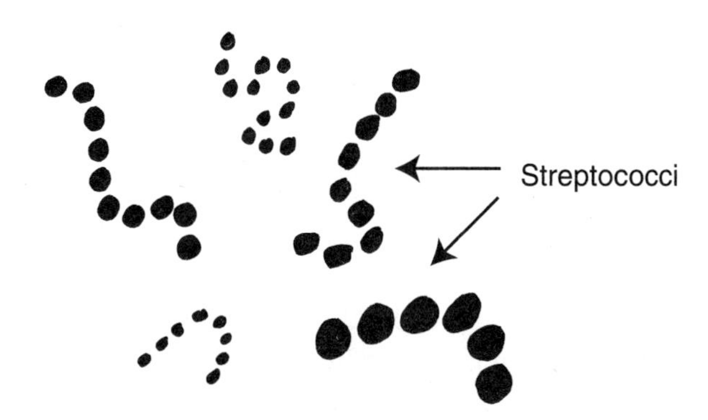

the "collar" (*cervic*) area of the neck were also *hypertrophied* (**high-PER**-truh-feed). Specifically, they were enlarged.

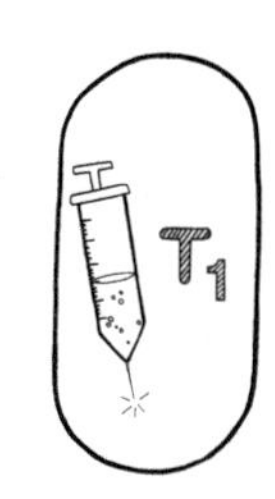

The patient's malaise prevented him from talking freely, and his adenoids were so big that he was having difficulty breathing. Because he was so *febrile* (**FEB**-ril) or "feverish," however, surgery to remove the tonsils and adenoids was *contraindicated* at this time. (*Contraindicated* means that the indications were "against" [*contra-*], or not in favor of, surgery.) It was determined that the infectious streptococci were the true *etiologic* (**ee**-tee-oh-**LAHJ**-ik) or "causative" agents of this recurring problem.

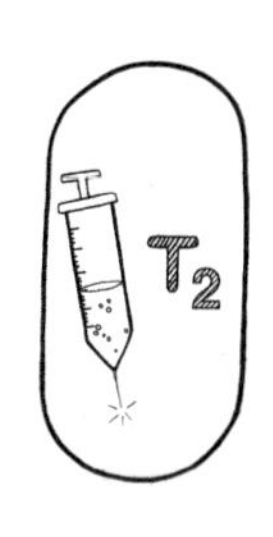

Antibiotics were given t.i.d. for 5 days. After the acute infection had temporarily stopped and the fever was reduced, a combined *tonsillectomy and adenoidectomy* was performed. This *T & A* involved the surgical "removal of" (*-ectomy*) both the palatine tonsils and the adenoids (pharyngeal tonsil).

Probe of case history

(A) The patient, Andy L., was said to suffer from a *chronic* case of tonsillitis, rather than just an *acute* one. How are the words *chronic* and *acute* exactly opposite in meaning to one another? (B) Andrew had a bad case of cephalalgia. What if he also had a case of *cephalitis* (**sef**-al-EYE-tis)? Translate this medical term into its common English equivalent. [Check your short answers with the key near the end of this chapter.]

Quiz

Refer to the text in this chapter if necessary. A good score is at least 8 correct answers out of these 10 questions. The answers are listed in the back of this book.

1. The lymph is most closely related to:
   (a) Burning rubber

(b) Reddish blood
(c) Clear, salty water
(d) Creamy white toothpaste

2. If we say that taking Vitamin C on a regular basis tends to have a *prophylactic* effect, we mean that it:
(a) Tends to provide a protective influence from disease
(b) Promotes edematous changes
(c) Adds cancer cells to the bloodstream
(d) Inhibits the normal processes of digestion

3. The immune response equals:
(a) Brain + spinal cord
(b) Lymphocytes + plasma cells
(c) Lymphatic system minus the spleen
(d) Antigen-antibody reactions + phagocytosis of foreign invaders

4. If a doctor tells you that "You have 6 months to live!," then she is making a:
(a) Syndrome
(b) Diagnosis
(c) Prognosis
(d) False and biased accusation

5. Sniffles can be considered part of the _____ for acute coryza.
(a) Prodrome
(b) Postdrome
(c) Palindrome
(d) Mortality

6. "Doc, I came here because of my aching back!" reflects the expression of a:
(a) Morbid preoccupation
(b) Clinical sign
(c) Clinical symptom
(d) Severe congestion

7. Palpation of your forehead involves:
(a) Kissing it lightly
(b) Pinching it between your toes
(c) Digging out some flesh with a scalpel
(d) Touching it with your fingertips

8. Invented the stethoscope:
   (a) Albert Schweitzer
   (b) Friedrich von Helmholtz
   (c) Rene Laennec
   (d) Beatrice Arthur
9. If "a prenatal diagnosis was obtained via ultrasonography":
   (a) A pregnant lady had her abdomen examined by high-frequency sound waves
   (b) Disturbed memory of a senile patient was cured by auscultation
   (c) Severe morbidity in an unborn child was identified by careful fluoroscopic probing of the *uterus* (**YOU**-ter-**us**) or "womb"
   (d) The patient had a severely depressed functioning of her lymphatic organs
10. An x-ray taken of just a thin section or slice through the body is most appropriately called a:
    (a) Sonogram
    (b) Radiography
    (c) Roentgenogram
    (d) CAT scan

Memory Pillboxes for Chapter 5

Several key facts were tagged with numbered icons in the page margins of this chapter. Write a short summary of each of these key facts into a numbered cell or compartment within the appropriate type of *Memory Pillbox* that appears below.

***Background and History* Pillboxes for Chapter 5:**

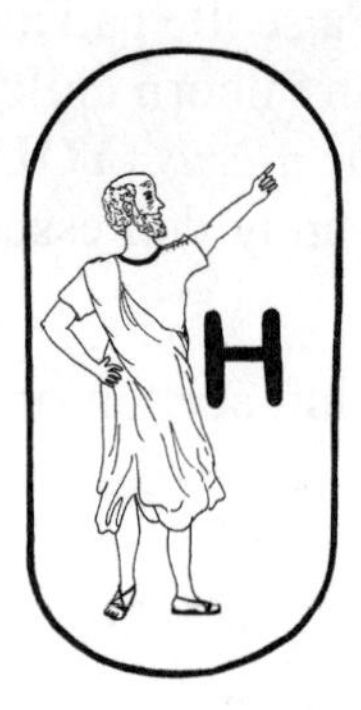

1	2
3	4

***Anatomy* Pillboxes for Chapter 5:**

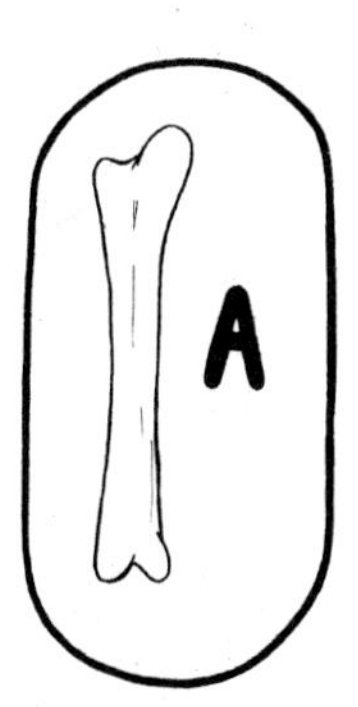

1	
2	3
4	5
6	

***Physiology* Pillboxes for Chapter 5:**

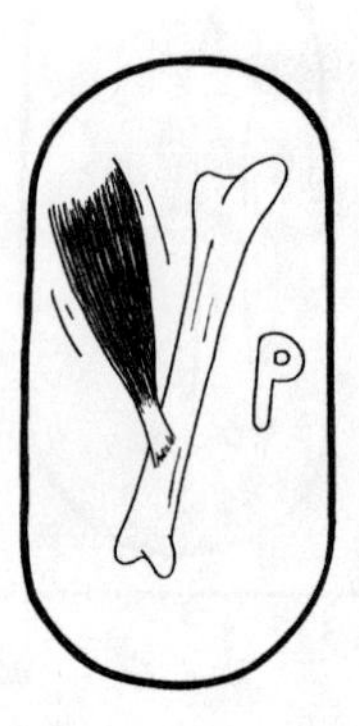

1	2
3	4

Disease/Injury **Pillboxes for Chapter 5:**

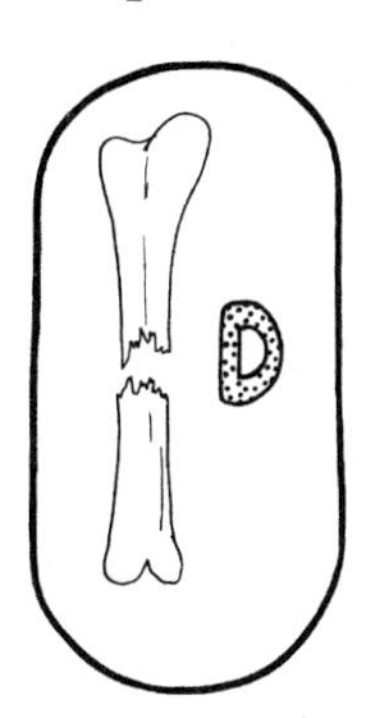

1	2
3	4
5	6

7	8

***Treatment/Therapy* Pillboxes for Chapter 5:**

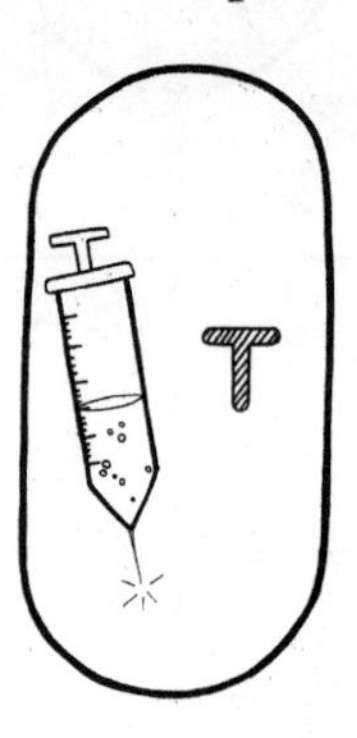

1	2

Answers for Chapter 5 Summary Tables

FOR SUMMARY TABLE 5.1

1. "condition of not serving"
2. "pertaining to guarding against"
3. "presence of a clear spring water cell"
4. "process of cell eating"
5. "referring to clear spring water"

FOR SUMMARY TABLE 5.2

1. "a condition of knowledge through"
2. "presence of (something) sudden"
3. "inflammation of the nose"
4. "presence of a running before"
5. "condition of knowledge before"
6. "a process of striking"
7. "a process of listening"
8. "an instrument used to examine the chest"
9. "a process of recording sounds beyond"
10. "study of causes"

Answers to Probe of Case History

(**A**) *Chronic* refers to disease of long duration, while *acute* refers to one of short duration. (**B**) *Cephalitis* means "inflammation of the head."

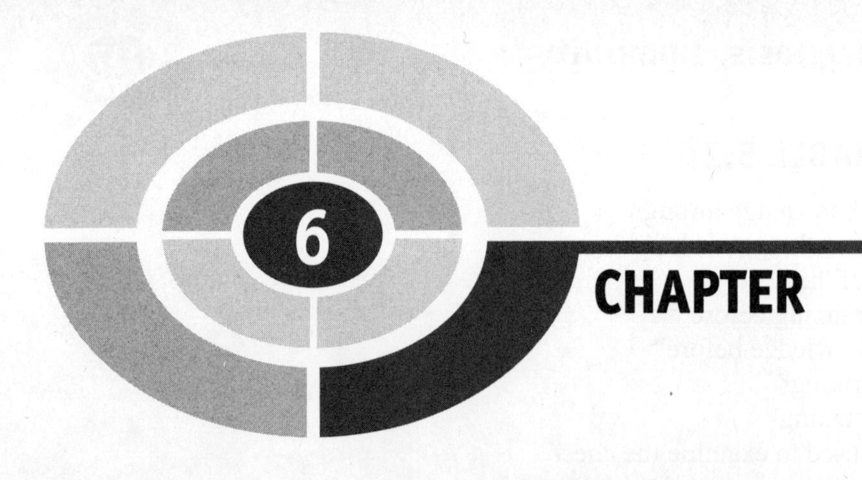

Terms Related to Disorders of the Cells and Body Tissues

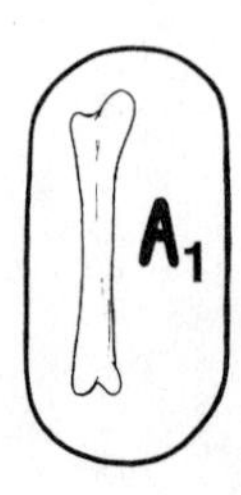

Two very similar words—*cell* and *cellular* (**SELL**-you-lar)—are used to identify the tiny "chambers" or "little boxes" that represent the lowest *living* level of body organization. *ANATOMY DEMYSTIFIED* brought in the concept of the ancient Egyptian pyramid (see Page 119) as an organizing superstructure to help us frame the various levels of anatomy (body structure).

Back in Chapter 5, several specific examples of living body cells were mentioned. You may recall that these were the lymphocytes, plasma cells, and macrophages. Now, in Chapter 6, we will begin dissecting the *cell level of body organization* (anatomy) in much greater depth. Rising above it, we shall also analyze the *tissue level*. And we will employ the majestic *Great Body Pyramid*, composed of stacked horizontal levels, as our organizing frame of reference.

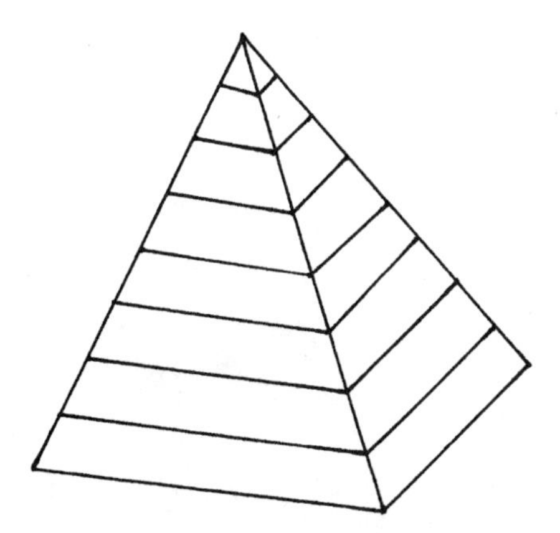

Background and History

Figure 6.1 (A) shows that nine different levels (I to IX) of body organization subdivide the total study of anatomy. At the broad base of the Great Body Pyramid lie the smaller and simpler levels. As we proceed toward the top, the various types of body structures contained within these horizontal levels become increasingly larger and more complex.

Figure 6.1 (B) reveals the idea that each horizontal level of body organization is like a grid containing a series of square fact-cells. (In this book, we have visualized each level as a pillbox that holds a number of Memory Pills representing key text facts.)

Figure 6.2 provides the names for each of these nine different levels of body organization. Starting at the broad base of the Great Body Pyramid, we have *subatomic* (**sub**-ah-**TAH**-mik) *particles*, which exist "below" (*sub-*) the level of the individual *atom*. And rising above the atoms are the *molecules* (**MAH**-leh-**kyools**), then the *organelles* (**or**-gah-**NELS**), and above them the *cells*. Figure 6.2 calls this cell level the *Life-line*.

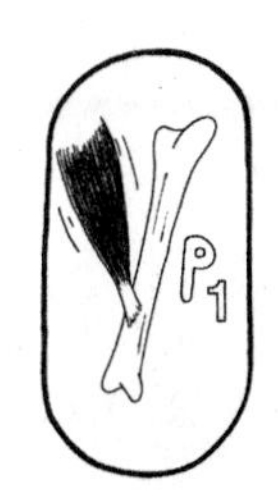

The Pyramid rises above the cell to include the *tissues*, *organs*, *organ systems*, and finally, the *organism*—our entire human body!

THE TWO SIZE-WORLDS OF ANATOMY

Perhaps you remember (from Chapter 3) that the broad discipline of anatomy (body structure) can be subdivided into two main sections. These are *microscopic anatomy* on the one hand, and *macroscopic* or *gross anatomy* on the other:

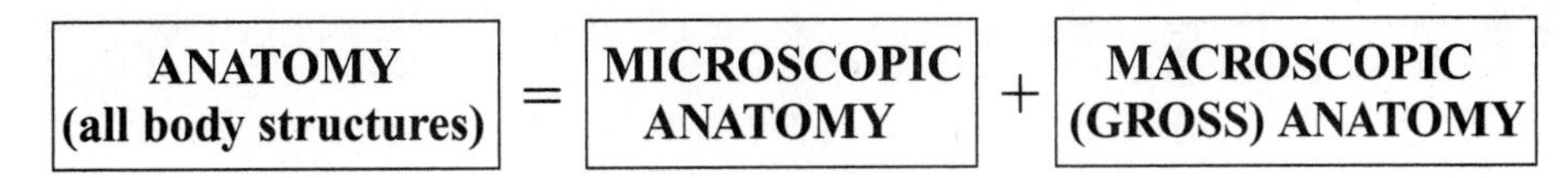

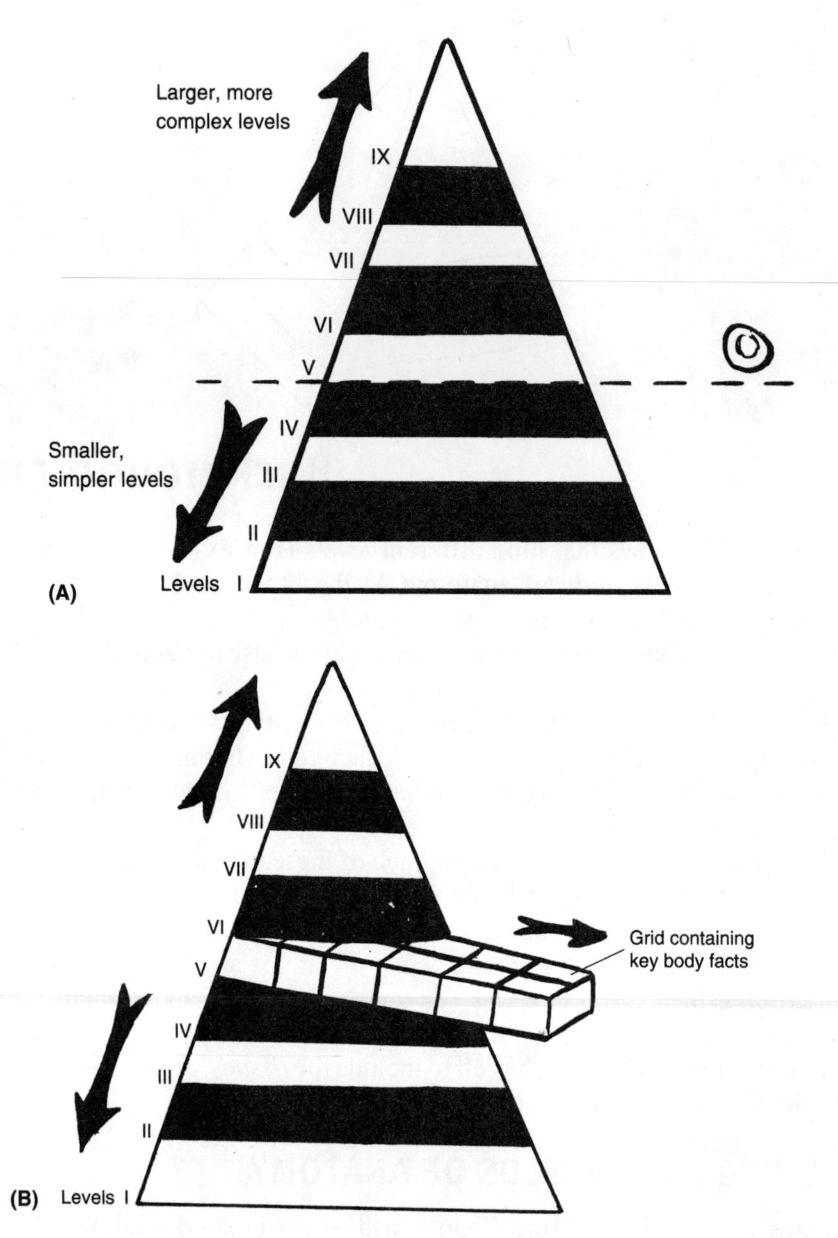

Fig. 6.1 An introduction to the Great Body Pyramid.

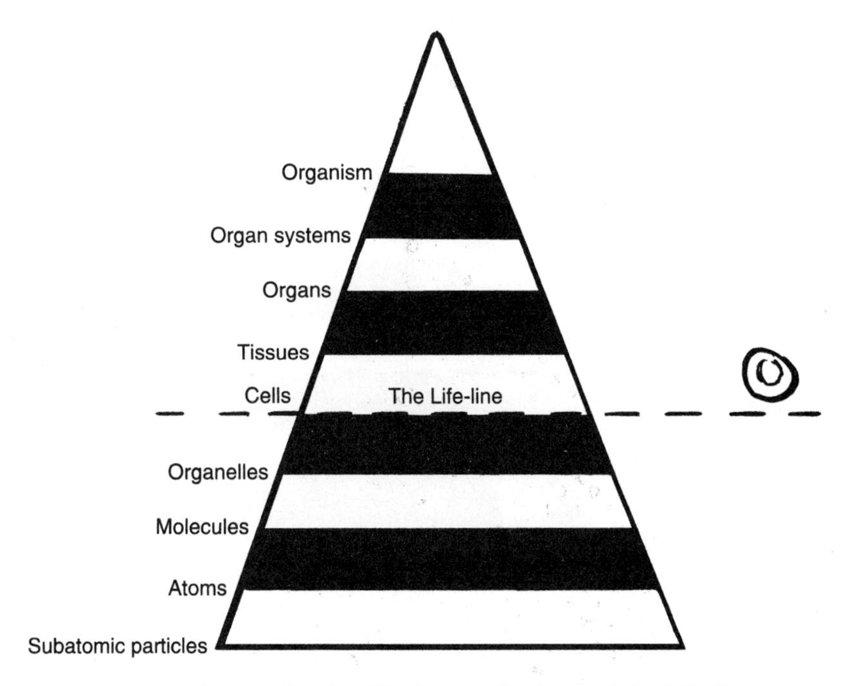

Fig. 6.2 The nine levels of body organization and the Life-line.

Each of these two broad subdivisions is, in effect, its own "size-world"! Microscopic anatomy is the world of the "________" (*micr*), while macroscopic or gross anatomy is the world of the "________" (*macr*). [**Memory probe:** Using your memory of word parts presented in Chapter 3, try to fill in the blanks within the preceding sentence, writing their common English translations. Answers will directly follow! By the way: How is your memory doing? Do you need to take more "pills"?]

Chapter 3 talked about various types of creatures whose name includes the root for "tiny" (*micr*). Specifically, these were microbes or microorganisms. (A related book, *BIOLOGY DEMYSTIFIED*, fleshes out this "tiny world." This helps us understand a great variety of *nonhuman* microorganisms studied in microbiology.) In *MEDICAL TERMINOLOGY DEMYSTIFIED*, of course, our focus is on the levels of *microanatomy* (**MY**-kroh-ah-**NAT**-oh-**mee**) that are contained within the *human* organism.

The tiny world is *unicellular* (**you**-nee-**SEL**-you-lar)—"single-celled." Thus, microscopic anatomy (microanatomy) must be examined with the aid of a microscope (or some other type of special instrument). This fact is reinforced by Figure 6.3. To summarize:

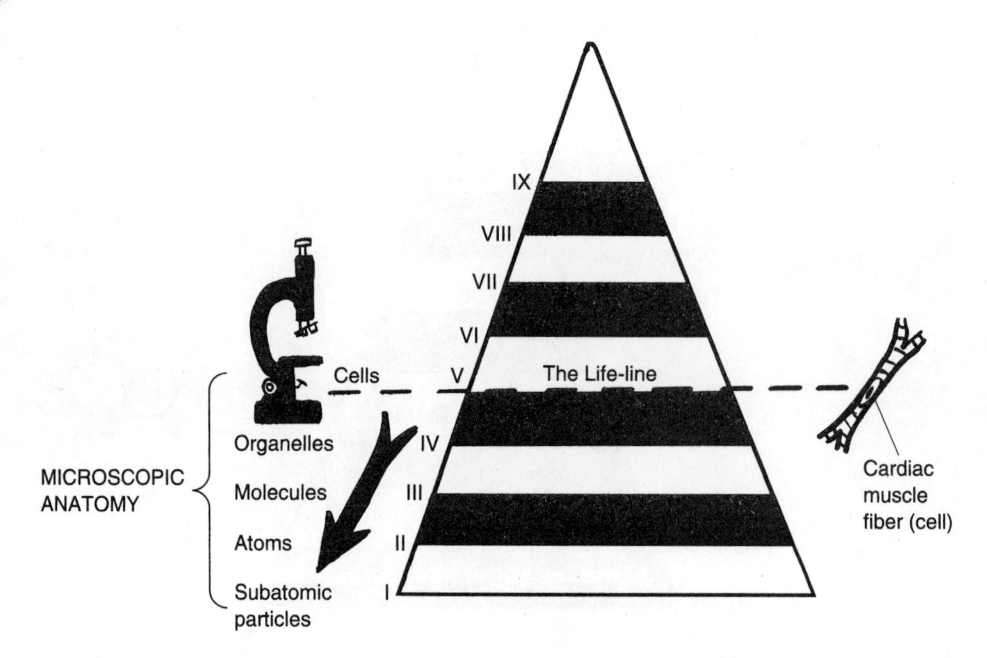

Fig. 6.3 Microscopic levels of the Great Body Pyramid.

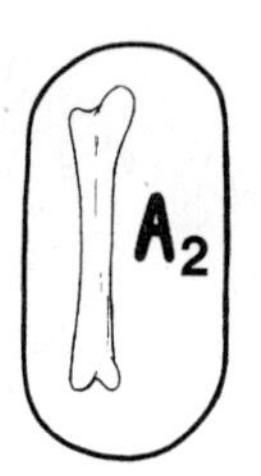

MICROSCOPIC ANATOMY (micro-anatomy)	= **levels of "tiny" body structures that must be studied with a microscope (or some other type of instrument)**
	= **subatomic particles + atoms + molecules + organelles + cells**

Note that the Life-line (cell level) within Figure 6.3 is tagged with a specific example—a *cardiac* (**KAR**-dee-ak)—or "referring to" (*-ac*) the "heart" (*cardi*)—*muscle fiber*. (This is actually a long, slender, cardiac muscle *cell* that has a *fiber* shape.)

Above the cell level, in dramatic contrast, lies the "big" (*Macr*) world of macroscopic or gross anatomy (Figure 6.4). Observe that this big world starts with the *tissue level*. It then proceeds on up, until the *organism* (entire human body) *level* at the very pointy tip of the Great Body Pyramid is finally reached. The big world is multicellular ("many-celled"). Hence, gross anatomy is visible to the naked eye. To summarize:

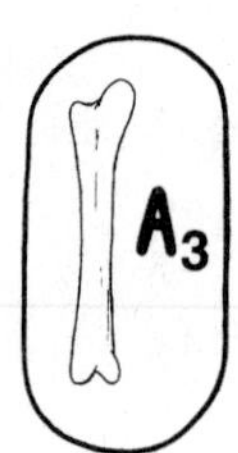

MACROSCOPIC (GROSS) ANATOMY	= **multicellular levels of "big" body structures visible to the naked eye**
	= **tissues + organs + organ systems + organism**

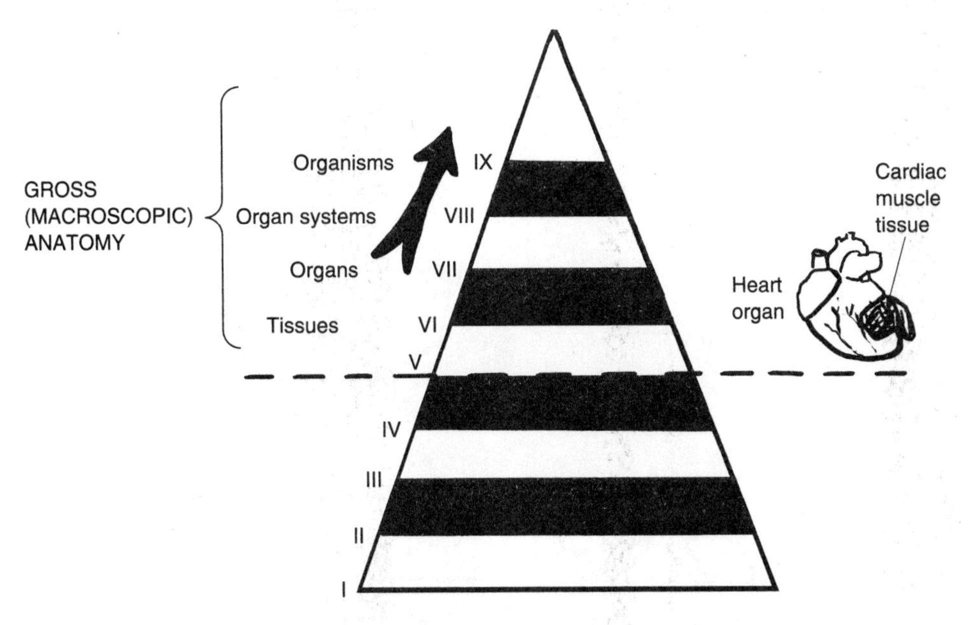

Fig. 6.4 Macroscopic levels of the Great Body Pyramid.

BIOLOGICAL ORDER AND CLINICAL HEALTH

"Good Hippocrates!" you may now be saying to yourself. "I thought this book was all about demystifying *medical* terminology! So, why is it that we are spending so much time discussing the levels of *normal* anatomy?" Good question! The reason is that, in general, normal anatomy (body structure) and normal physiology (body function) are examples of *biological order*. And biological order, in turn, usually results in a state of *clinical health* (no observed disease). Now:

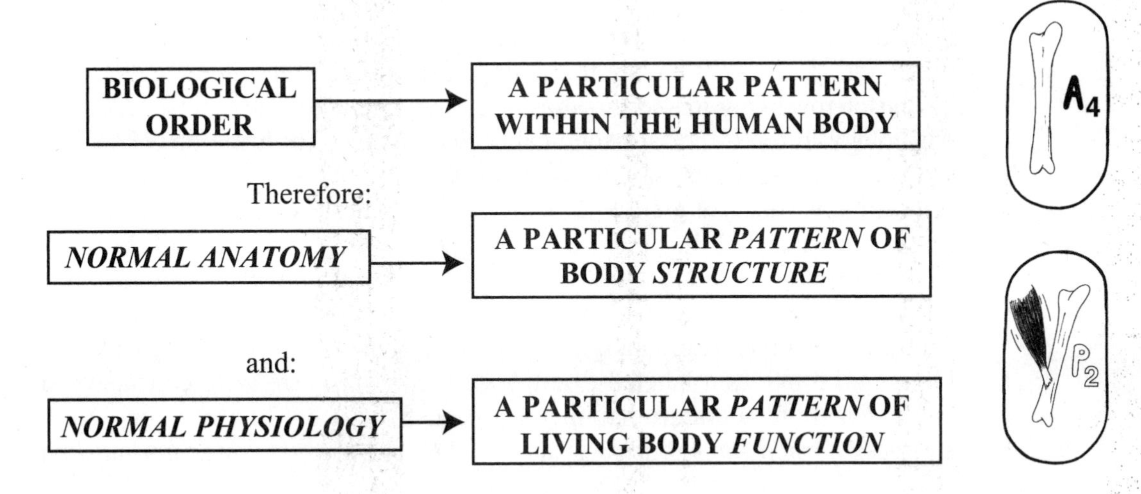

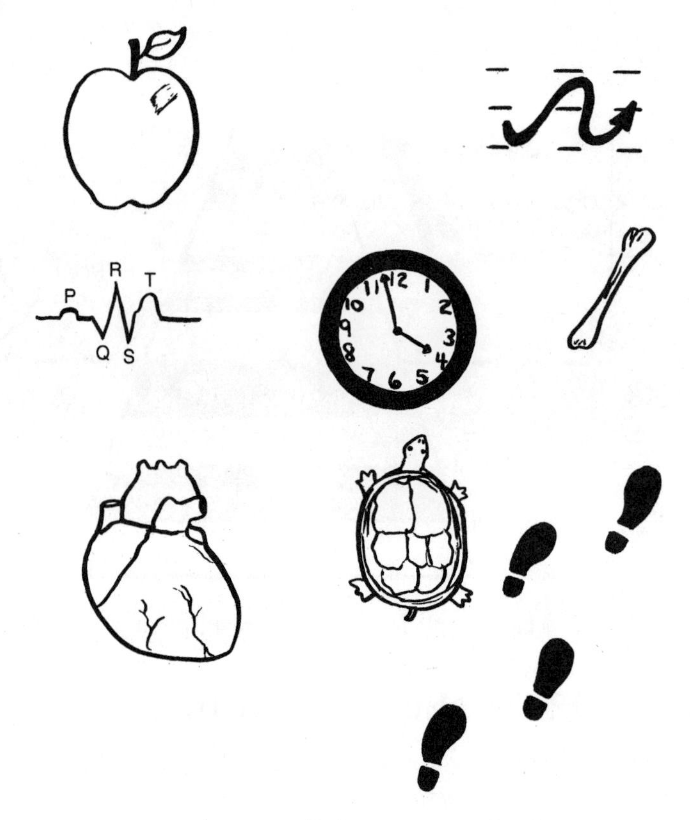

Fig. 6.5 Some distinct patterns of order.

So normal A&P (anatomy and physiology) is mainly about intact patterns of body structure and function. Figure 6.5 provides some examples of intact patterns of order. [**Thinking probe:** What examples of normal *anatomy* are provided in Figure 6.5? What are the examples of normal *physiology*?]

The top row in Figure 6.5 shows a dark, wavy line. This line represents normal physiology in the important state called *homeostasis* (**hoh**-me-oh-**STAY**-sis). The root, *homeo*, means "sameness," while the suffix *-stasis* denotes "control of." Hence, homeostasis is literally a "control of sameness" or a *relative constancy* of various aspects of the body's *internal environment*.

Suppose, for instance, that we are considering *oral body temperature*, which is often measured in units of *degrees Fahrenheit* (°*F*). We can call oral body temperature in degrees Fahrenheit a *physiological parameter* (pah-**RAM**-uh-**ter**). Figure 6.6 provides a labeled example of homeostasis (relative constancy) of the oral body temperature parameter. Because the wavy line rises only up to an *upper normal limit* of 99.6°F and falls down only to a *lower normal limit*

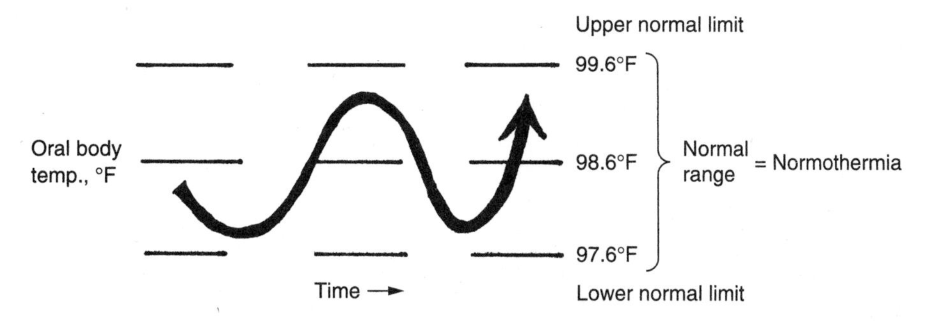

Fig. 6.6 Normothermia and homeostasis of body temperature.

of 97.6°F, we say that it is being tightly controlled within its *normal range*. In this case, since body "heat" (*therm*) or temperature is being followed, we call this state *normothermia* (**nor**-moh-**THERM**-ee-ah). Normothermia is a "condition of" (*-ia*) "normal" (*normo-*) "heat or temperature" (*therm*). Therefore, normothermia (homeostasis of oral body temperature within its normal range) is a good example of a state of clinical health. It is also an elegant example of strict biological order being maintained for body temperature over time. Many other body parameters in addition to oral temperature are also maintained in such a normal range (condition of homeostasis, clinical health, and biological order) over time. Starting with the cell level, various physiological parameters are maintained in a state of homeostasis (relative constancy) within all the organ systems. [**Reference suggestion:** To learn much more about the fascinating topics of physiology, biological order, body parameters, and homeostasis, you are highly advised to read *PHYSIOLOGY DEMYSTIFIED.*]

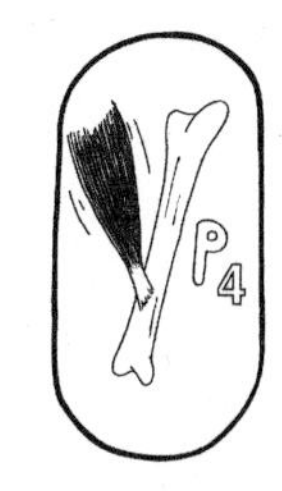

Summary of biological order

We can bring together these ideas about biological order, homeostasis, and clinical health by using a handy word equation:

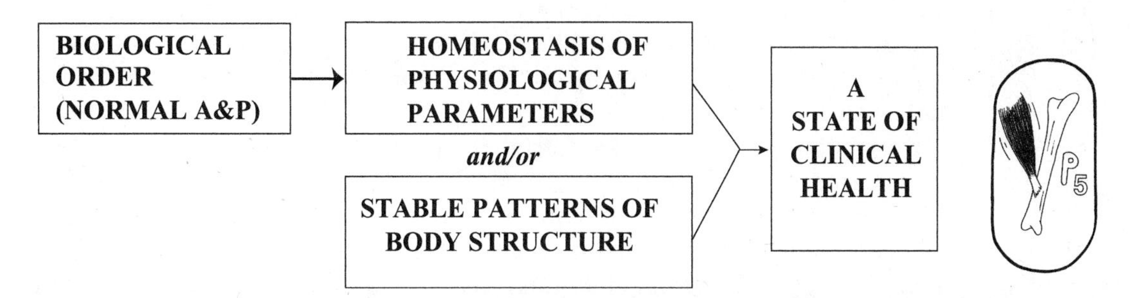

From the above summary, we can see that biological order of normal anatomy and physiology tends to result in a state of clinical health. And although clinical health means there is no morbidity (disease or injury) present, it is still important to learn some of this basic Latin-Greek terminology. Why? The reason is that medical terminology students need a solid *frame of reference*—a collection of physiological parameters in states of homeostasis, plus body structures with stable patterns—to make intelligent decisions about identifying disease when it is present. In short, the student needs to refer back to the normal A&P associated with the various levels of the *Great Pyramid of Structure-Function Order*. Figure 6.7 colorfully portrays this Great Pyramid, being pointed to by our kind teacher in both *ANATOMY DEMYSTIFIED* and *PHYSIOLOGY DEMYSTIFIED*: Professor Joe, the Talking Skeleton!

We are making a big deal about normal A&P here in Chapter 6, because it is at the cell level of body organization where both life and physiology first appear! Below this level (as you can see in Figure 6.7), we have *normal plain body functions*, rather than physiology.

NORMAL A&P OF THE HUMAN CELL

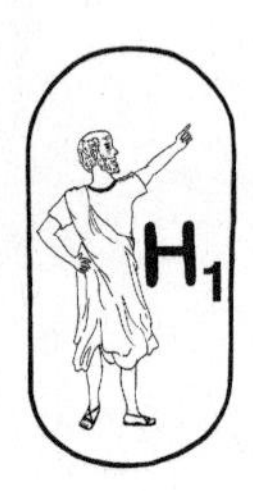

The cell, as we have already pointed out, is crucially important because it is the lowest *living* level of body organization. This critical importance has been quite evident ever since the year 1838, when two German scientists, *Matthias Schleiden* and *Theodor Schwann,* proposed the *modern cell theory*. This theory states that the cell is the basic unit of all living things. Therefore, the discipline of medical terminology, which talks about diseases and healing, really does have its own roots at the cellular level of body organization!

The cell organelles

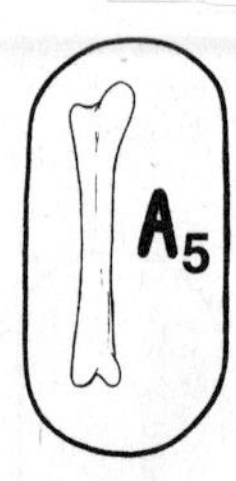

As soon as we begin talking about cell A&P, we start referring to the *organelles* (**or**-gah-**NELS**). These are the "tiny" (*-elle*) "organ"-like structures that carry out specific functions within the cell. For our purpose, we will only look at some of the most prominent organelles. Figure 6.8 shows, for instance, that the cell is surrounded by a very thin *plasma* (**PLAZ**-mah) *membrane*. It is the soft covering that creates the outer "form" (*plasma*) of the cell.

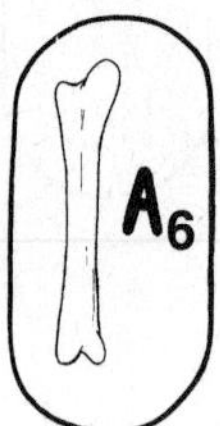

The most prominent organelle is the *nucleus,* which is a fairly oval "kernel" (*nucle*)-shaped structure in the middle of the cell. The nucleus of each adult human cell (except for *sperm* and *egg cells*) contains 46 *chromosomes* (**KROH**-moh-**sohms**). These chromosomes are dark, worm-like, "colored" (*chrom*) "bodies" (*somes*). They contain the basic *genetic* or hereditary material. The chromosomes mainly consist of a double-stranded molecule of *DNA*—short for the tongue-twisting full name: *deoxyribonucleic*

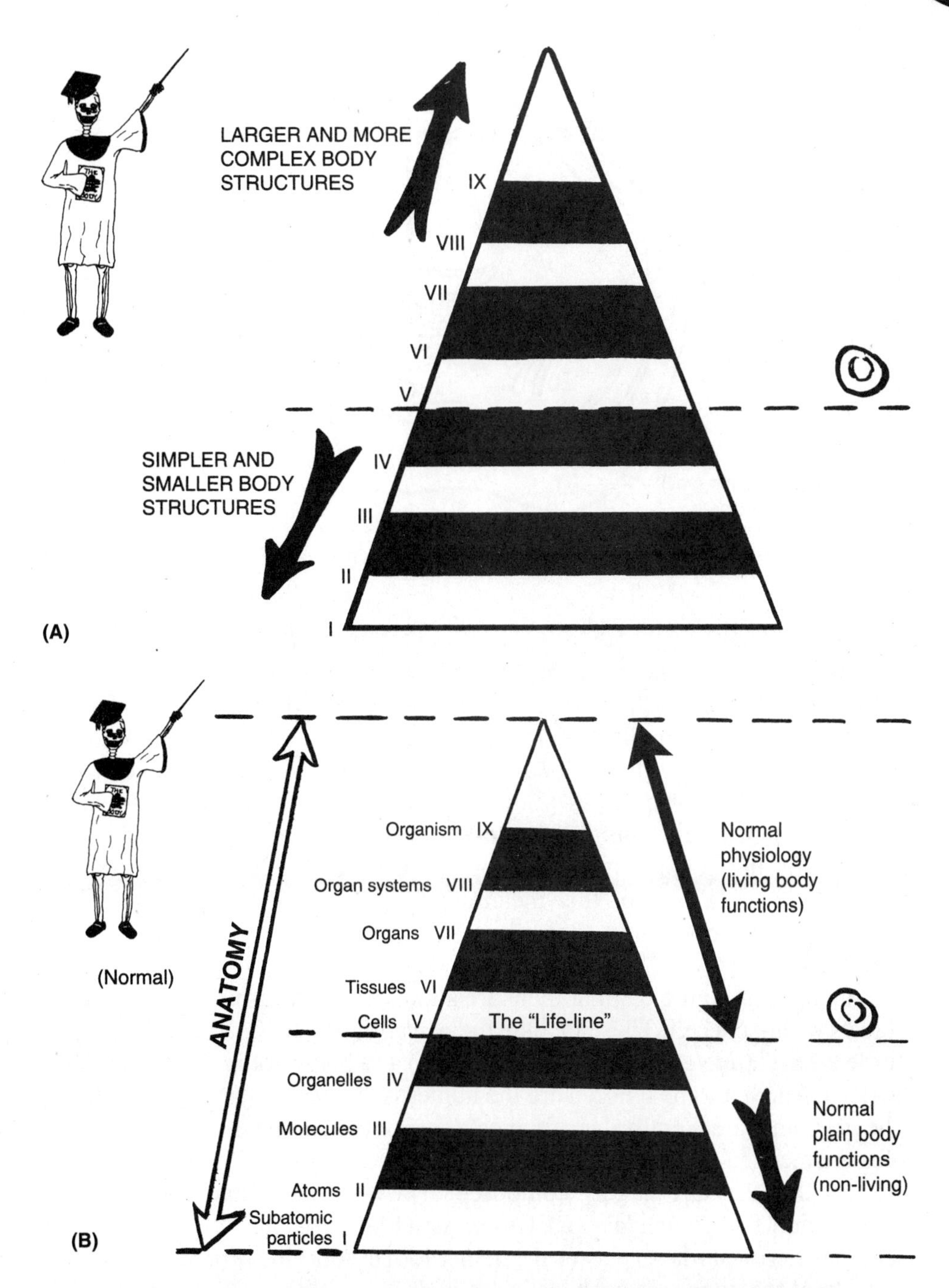

Fig. 6.7 Normal A&P and the Great Pyramid of Structure-Function Order.

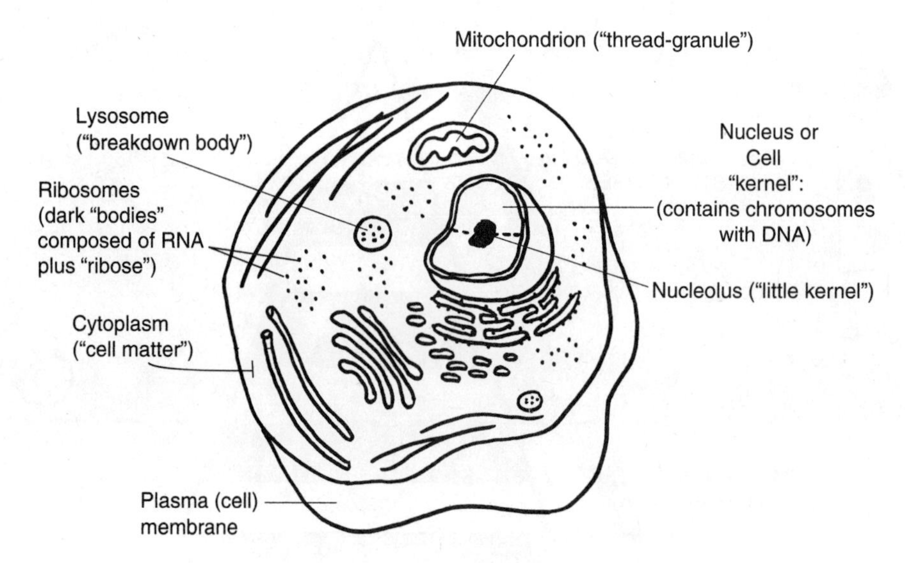

Fig. 6.8 Some of the organelles within a cell.

(dee-**ox**-ee-**RYE**-boh-new-**klee**-ik) *acid.* Each DNA molecule, in turn, consists of many short sections called *genes* (**JEANS**). It is the genes that are our basic units of heredity. Whether you have blue, green, or brown eyes, for instance, is largely determined by the particular sequence of genes found within the DNA molecules of your chromosomes. You may have heard the recent news that scientists have unraveled the *genome* (**JEE**-nohm). What is meant by the genome is the "group" (*-ome*) of "producers" (*gen*) within a cell. In layman's lingo, this means that the genome is the total collection of chromosomes and their genes, which act to produce many body *proteins*.

Note back in Figure 6.8 that there are a number of darkish-colored, rounded objects within the cell. These include the *nucleolus* (new-**KLEE**-uh-lus). It is a "little kernel" (*nucleol*) that is "present" (*-us*) as a black dot in the center of the nucleus. And not to be ignored are the numerus *ribosomes* (**RYE**-boh-**sohms**). The ribosomes are literally dark "bodies" (*somes*) containing the important sugar substance called ribose. Both the nucleolus and ribosomes have in common the fact that they are largely composed of *RNA*. These three letters are the abbreviation for *ribonucleic* (**RYE**-boh-new-**klee**-ik) *acid.* RNA (ribonucleic acid) has a critical role to play as the helper for DNA during *protein synthesis*—creation of the important proteins in the body.

Another sphere-shaped cell organelle is called the *lysosome* (**LIE**-soh-**zohm**). This word exactly translates to mean "breakdown" (*lys*) "body" (*som*) that is "present" (*-e*). The lysosomes are really tiny bags of *digestive* (die-**JES**-tiv)

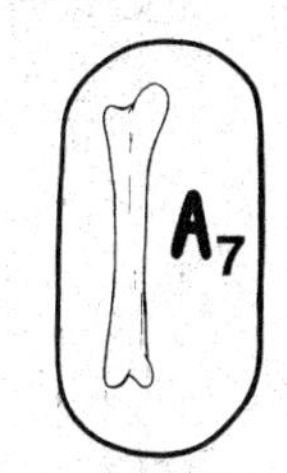

enzymes (**EN**-zighms), surrounded and contained with a thin membrane. Let's say that a particular cell, such as a leukocyte, carries out an extensive phagocytosis (Chapter 5) of bacteria. One or more lysosomes move toward the ingested bacteria and rupture. Their digestive enzymes are released and chemically dissolve the bacterium. The resulting *nutrients* (**NOO**-tree-**unts**)—"ones that" (*-ents*) "nourish" (*nutri*)—are then used by the cell for its *metabolism*. By *metabolism* we mean a "state of" (*-ism*) "change" (*metab*). The breakdown of various nutrients provides the *free energy* required to carry out cell metabolism. These involve the various body "changes" (such as cell division, protein synthesis, and movement) necessary for life.

Finally, we will consider a distinct organelle with a very unusual personality of its own: the *mitochondrion* (**my**-toh-**KAHN**-dree-un)! A careful look at Figure 6.9 makes known the underlying *etymology* (**et**-uh-**MAHL**-uh-jee)—"study of" (*-ology*) the "original meaning of a word" (*etym*). The etymology (original Latin-Greek meaning) of mitochondrion is "presence of" (*-ion*) a "thread" (*mito*) "granule" (*chondr*). The mitochondrion assumes two differing shapes. In some cases it is long and slender, much like a thread (*mito*). In other instances it is rather rounded and oval, much like a granule (*chondr*).

Observe that the internal anatomy of the two *mitochondria* (**my**-toh-**KAHN**-dree-ah) pictured in Figure 6.9 includes thin "crests" or "ridges" called *cristae* (**KRISS**-tee). These cristae resemble the teeth of a comb.

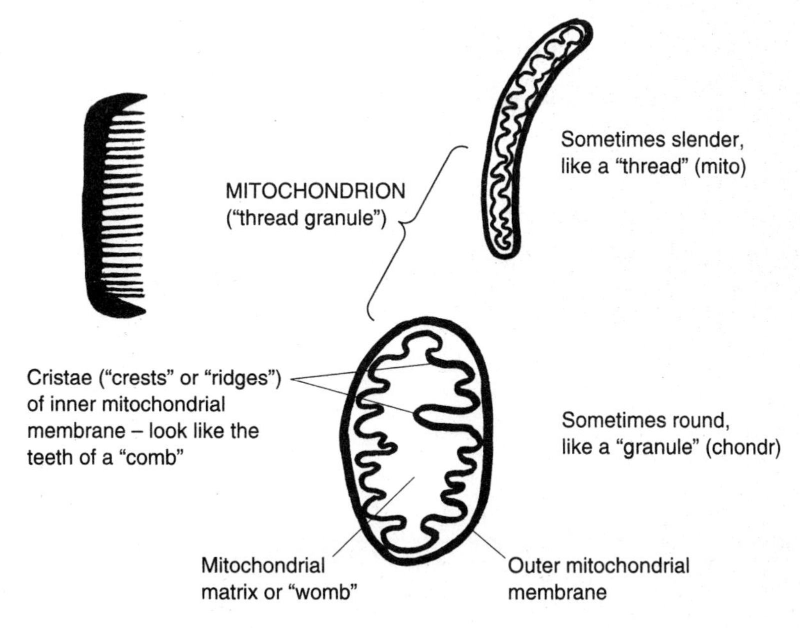

Fig. 6.9 The internal anatomy of a mitochondrion.

Aerobic cell metabolism and ATP

The mitochondrion is frequently nicknamed the Powerhouse of the Cell. The reason is that the *mitochondrial* (**my**-toh-**KAHN**-dree-al) cristae are the main sites for *aerobic* (air-**OH**-bik) *metabolism* within human cells. By *aerobic* we mean "pertaining to" (*-ic*) something that "lives" (*ob*) in "oxygen or air" (*aer*). The mitochondria take in both oxygen and *glucose* (**GLOO**-kohs) from the surrounding *cytoplasm* (**SIGH**-toh-**plazm**). The cytoplasm is the fluid "matter" (*plasm*) in the "cell" (*cyt*). (Review Figure 6.8.)

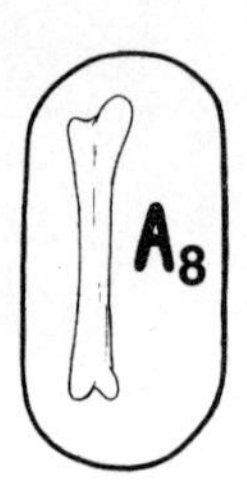

Glucose is the most important sugar or "sweet" molecule used for fuel within our body's cells. Glucose is a ring-shaped *molecule* or "little mass" composed of six *carbon* (C) atoms and a number of oxygen (O) and *hydrogen* (H) atoms. (View Figure 6.10.) These C, O, and H atoms are all linked to another by means of *chemical bonds*. The *molecular* (muh-**LEK**-you-ler) or "pertaining to little mass" *formula* of glucose is $C_6H_{12}O_6$, or $C_6(H_2O)_6$. When written as $C_6(H_2O)_6$, the nature of glucose as a type of *carbohydrate* (**kar**-boh-**HIGH**-drayt) molecule is revealed. Specifically, glucose is a "carbon" (*carbo*) and "water" (*hydr*) molecule—a molecule whose formula can be written as an equal number of carbon atoms and water molecules (in this case, six of each). (The molecular formula for water, of course, is H_2O.)

Glucose is the key type of carbohydrate (carbon-water molecule) broken down for energy during metabolism. Glucose is broken down within each mitochondrion under aerobic (oxygen-living) conditions, yielding a molecule called *ATP* as its end product. And ATP, in turn, is the final chemical broken down by cell metabolism that releases free energy to do body work. The technical name for this metabolic process is *glycolysis* (gleye-**KAHL**-ih-sis)—the "breaking down" (*lys*) of a "glucose" or "sweet" (*glyc*) carbohydrate molecule. (Look over Figure 6.11.)

[**Further study suggestion:** Two of our related books, *BIOLOGY DEMYSTIFIED* and *PHYSIOLOGY DEMYSTIFIED,* include much more extensive discussion about the vital subject of aerobic metabolism and cell energy production using ATP.]

To summarize:

AEROBIC METABOLISM (occurs within mitochondria) —Uses O_2, Glucose→ **ATP MOLECULES PRODUCED** (broken down by cells for energy)

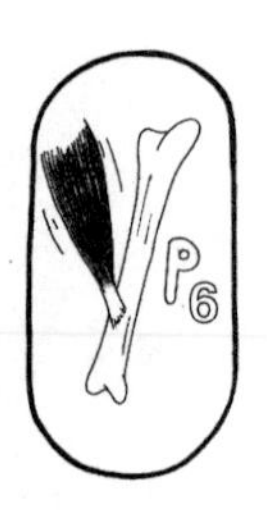

NORMAL A&P OF THE BODY TISSUES

A quick glance back at some of our earlier sketches of the Great Body Pyramid (such as Figure 6.2) reveals the *tissue level* of body organization. A *tissue* is a

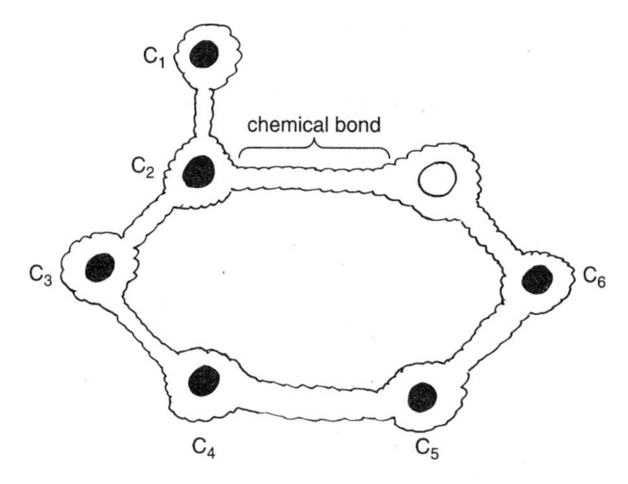

Fig. 6.10 The glucose molecule: some of its atoms and chemical bonds.

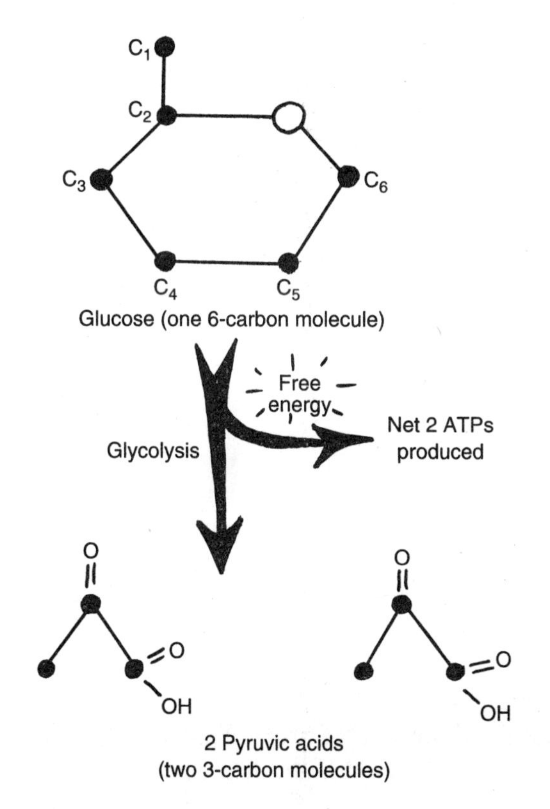

Fig. 6.11 The beginning stages of glycolysis make ATP.

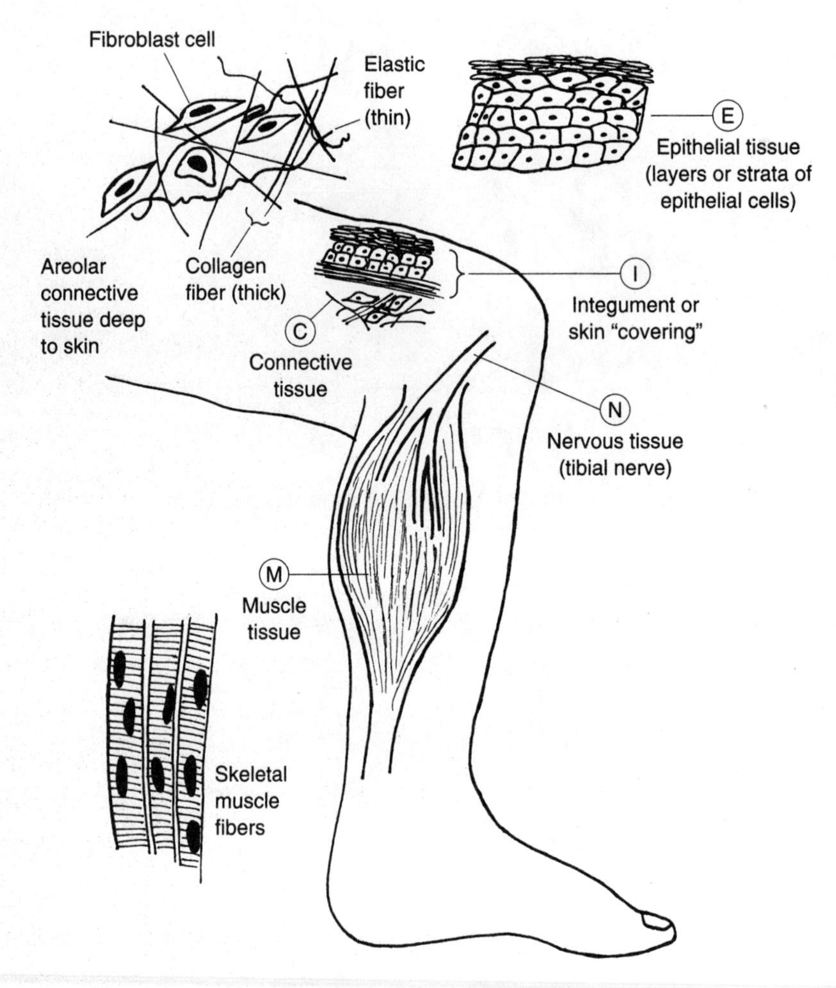

Fig. 6.12 CNEMI: The tissue level of body organization.

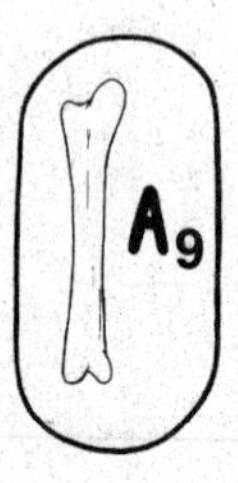

collection of similar cells, plus the *intercellular* (**in**-ter-**SELL**-you-lar) *material* located "between" (*inter-*) them. As is suggested by Figure 6.12, the word *tissue* comes from the Latin for "(something) woven," such as a cloth fabric. Now, you can see a cloth fabric with your naked eyes, right? [**Thinking & memory probe:** Would you classify the tissue level of body organization as microscopic or macroscopic? Why? Check your speculations with the contents of the following sentences.] If you recall, the tissue level (VI) is the level of body organization located immediately above the cell level (V) on the Great Body Pyramid. It is also the first level to be classified as gross or macroscopic.

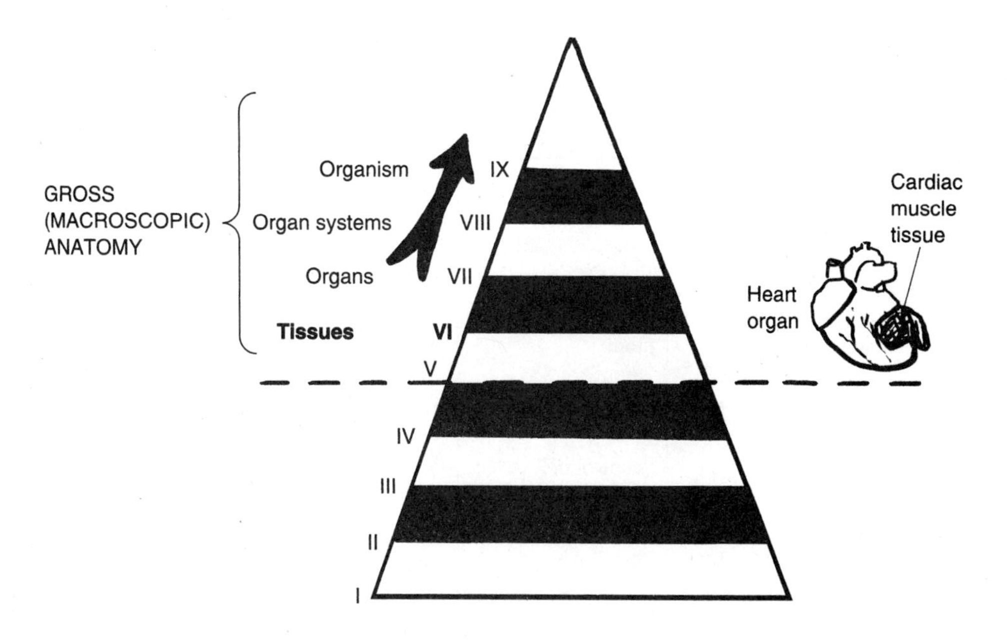

"But don't you usually have to use a microscope to see the individual cells within a tissue?" the inquiring reader may probe. Yes, you must use a microscope to view the *individual* cells *within* a particular body tissue, but you can still see the *whole* tissue with your naked eyes! We will explain more about this vital distinction, shortly.

SUMMARY TABLE 6.1

Consult Summary Table 6.1 for a quick review of some important words and word parts.

C is for connective tissue

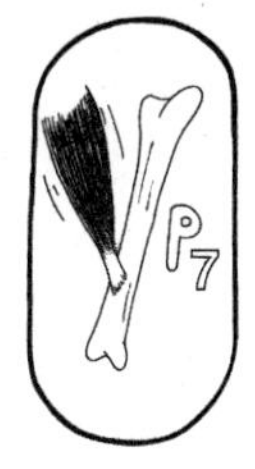

The picture labeled *C* in Figure 6.12 is a specific type of *connective tissue*. In general, connective tissue is a tissue that directly or indirectly *connects* body parts together. The specific example shown is *areolar* (uh-**REE**-uh-ler) *connective tissue*. The word, *areolar*, "refers to" (*-ar*) "little areas" (*areol*). In the case of areolar connective tissue, the "little areas" are those spaces of intercellular material located between the many criss-crossing thick *collagen* and thin *elastic fibers*. The tapered cells shown are called *fibroblasts* (**FEYE**-broh-**blasts**)—that is, "fiber" (*fibr*) "formers" (*blasts*). The fibroblasts form or secrete the numerous collagen and elastic fibers. Doesn't their extensively criss-crossing pattern

Summary Table 6.1 Words and Word Parts

Write in the *exact* meaning (literal English translation) for up to 10 key terms selected from the preceding block of text. After you are done, check your word meanings with the correct answers, which are given at the end of this chapter.

Key Terms	Prefixes	Roots	Suffixes	Exact Meanings
cellular	(none)	cellul "little boxes"	-ar "referring to"	1. ________
subatomic	sub- "below"	atom "atom"	-ic "pertaining to"	2. ________
homeostasis	(none)	homeo "control of"	-stasis "sameness"	3. ________
normothermia	normo- "normal"	therm "heat"	-ia "condition of"	4. ________
organelle	(none)	organ ("organ")	-elle "tiny"	5. ________
chromosome	(none)	chrom "colored"; som "body"	-e "presence of"	6. ________
lysosome	(none)	lys "break down"; som "body"	-e "presence of"	7. ________
mitochondrion	(none)	mit "thread"; chondr "granule"	-ion "presence of"	8. ________
aerobic	(none)	aer "air"; ob "living"	-ic "relating to"	9. ________
glycolysis	(none)	glyc "sweet"; lys "breaking down"	-is "process of"	10. ________

make areolar connective tissue quite closely reflect the "woven fabric" concept behind the word *tissue?* In fact, the whole discipline of examining tissues is called *histology* (**hiss-TAHL**-uh-jee). This term literally means the "study of" (*-ology*) "tissues or webs" (*hist*). When you cut open part of the body (such as the "leg" or *cnemi* [**NEE**-mee] pictured in Figure 6.12), you can see the

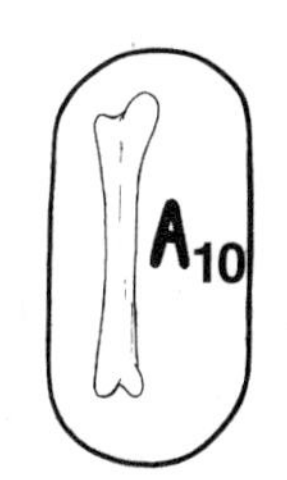

areolar connective tissue forming a clear, shiny, loose web just below the skin and between the various internal organs. [**Study suggestion:** Get a piece of raw chicken. Lift the skin up away from the meat, and you will see a bunch of areolar connective tissue forming a loose, shiny webbing between the meat and skin. You can see this whole tissue with your naked eyes (macroscopically), of course. Now, if you cut a piece of this shiny webbing out of the raw chicken, colored it with a *biological stain*, and examined it *histologically* (**hiss**-toh-**LAHJ**-ik-**lee**) under the microscope, you would see fibroblasts and a criss-crossing network of collagen and elastic fibers.]

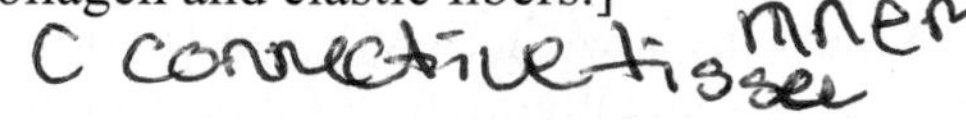

N is for nervous tissue

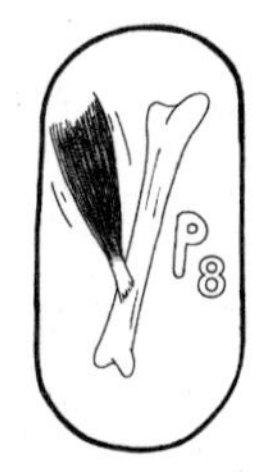

The sketch labeled *N* back in Figure 6.12 is for *nervous tissue*. Such nervous tissue is the body's main communication and control tissue. In particular, the figure displays the *tibial* (**TIB**-ee-al) *nerve*, which runs down the leg just posterior to the *tibia* (**TIB**-ee-ah) or "shin" bone.

E is for epithelial tissue

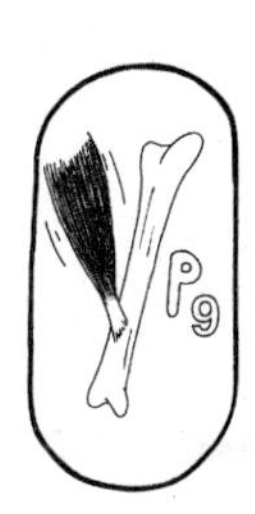

The mini-picture labeled *E* back in Figure 6.12 is for *epithelial* (**eh**-pih-**THEE**-lee-al) *tissue*. The epithelial tissue literally "refers to" (*-al*) tissue that is present "upon" (*epi-*) the "nipples" (*theli*). Broadly speaking, epithelial tissue is the body's major covering and lining tissue. It is arranged in thin sheets called *strata* (**STRAT**-ah). For instance, it makes up the *epidermis* (**ep**-ih-**DER**-mis), the thin layer of epithelial tissue lying "upon" (*epi-*) the surface of the "skin" (*derm*). The epidermis covers the surfaces of not just the nipples, but the entire body.

M is for muscle tissue

The fourth letter in *CNEMI* is *M*, representing *muscle tissue* in Figure 6.12. Muscle tissue occurs in several types. The one depicted in our figure is called *skeletal* (**SKEL**-eh-tal) *muscle tissue* because it is attached to the bones of the "skeleton." Muscle tissue consists of many slender *muscle fibers*, which contract and cause body parts to move.

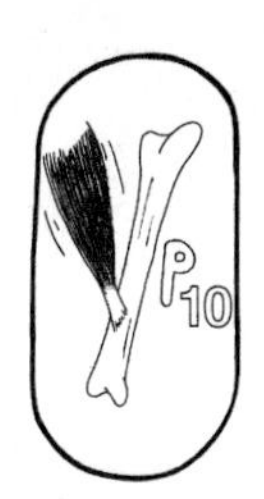

I is for the integument

The fifth and final letter in *CNEMI* is *I*. It symbolizes the *integument* (in-**TEG**-you-**ment**), which is our body's skin or "covering." The integument (skin) is really a major organ that is composed of several types of basic tissue.

BIOLOGICAL DISORDER AND MORBIDITY

We have spent considerable time showing that states of biological order (stable patterns of both normal anatomy and normal physiology) usually underlie states of clinical health. This relationship among order, normality, and health exists from the cell and tissue levels all the way up to the very top of the Great Body Pyramid.

However, the exact opposite relationship exists for conditions of *biological disorder*. Biological disorder is a break or absence of normal patterns in body structure and function. In short, we mean by this that there is a condition of *abnormal anatomy* and/or *abnormal physiology*. Figure 6.13 (in direct contrast to Figure 6.5) pictures some examples of broken patterns of order. [**Thinking probe:** What examples of abnormal *anatomy* are shown in Figure 6.13? What are the examples of abnormal *physiology*?]

Now:

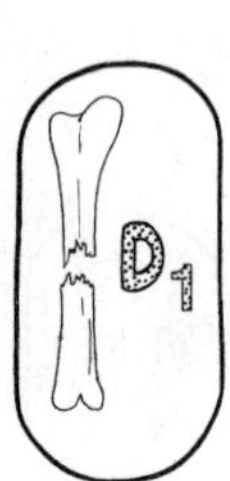

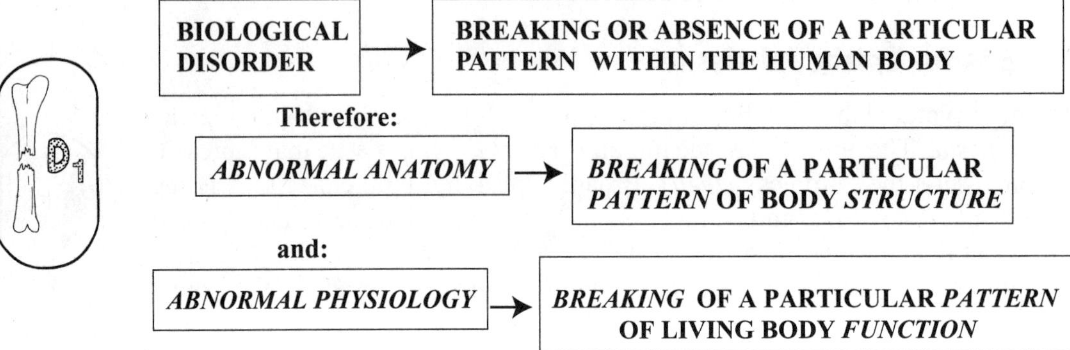

Now the top row in Figure 6.13 shows two dark, wavy lines. You may recall (Figure 6.5) that a wavy line staying within its normal range (between two upper and lower horizontal dashed lines) represents the behavior of a physiological parameter in a state of homeostasis. Such a condition of relative constancy—in the case of oral body temperature—was called *normothermia*, and there was an associated clinical health of body temperature, so that no fever or other morbidity was involved.

In dramatic contrast, the wavy line in the middle of the top row in Figure 6.13 represents a *break* in the normal pattern of an associated physiological parameter. The arrow falls "below" (*hypo-*) the normal range of the body parameter. In the case of oral body temperature, we would have *hypothermia* (**high**-poh-**THERM**-ee-ah). This literally means a "condition of" (*-ia*) "deficient or below normal" (*hypo-*) body "heat or temperature" (*therm*). Hypothermia represents

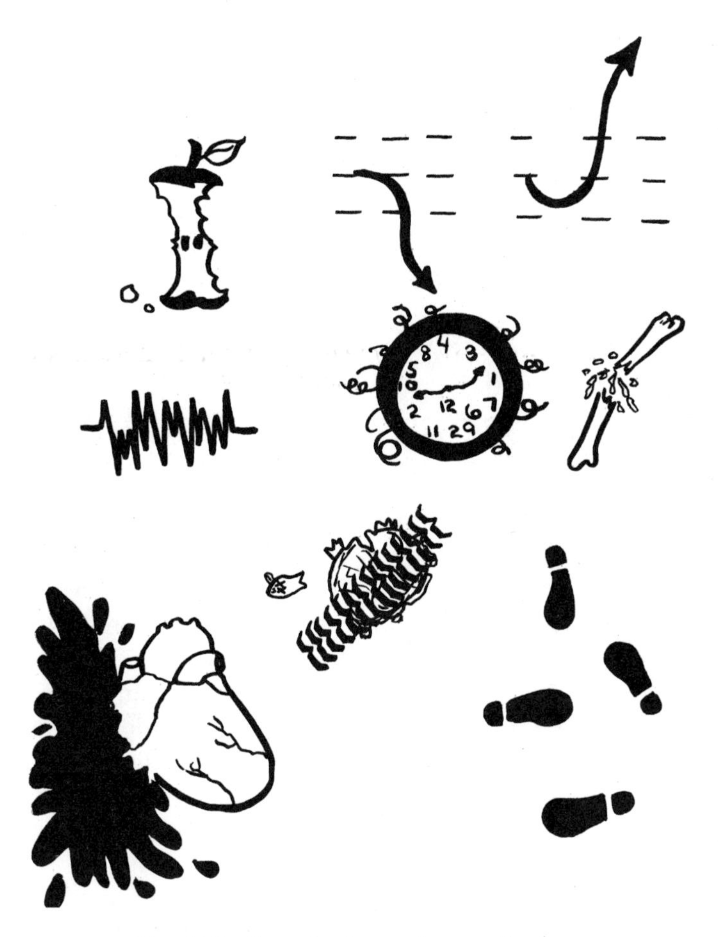

Fig. 6.13 Some broken patterns of order.

any drop in oral body temperature significantly *below* its lower normal limit of about 97.6°F.

In a similar vein, the dark wavy line to the far right of the top row in Figure 6.13 also represents a *break* in the normal pattern of an associated physiological parameter. This time, however, the break or failure lies at the *high* end of the parameter! Specifically, the arrow rises to an "excessive or above normal" (*hyper-*) level. For body temperature, we would use the term *hyperthermia* (**high**-per-**THERM**-ee-ah). This term literally means a "condition of" (*-ia*) "excessive or above normal" (*hyper-*) body "heat or temperature" (*therm*). Hyperthermia represents any rise in oral body temperature significantly *above* its upper normal limit of about 99.6°F.

"So, what's the *big deal* about all this *hyper-* and *hypo-*stuff?" an unsure reader might ask, with some annoyance. "Where is the linkage to *medical* (disease-related) terminology?" The answer is that both the hyper- (above normal or excessive) and hypo- (below normal or deficient) states are pretty tightly linked to the occurrence of morbidity (illness) and mortality (death). Thus, they are closely associated with the medical terminology describing illness and death. To summarize:

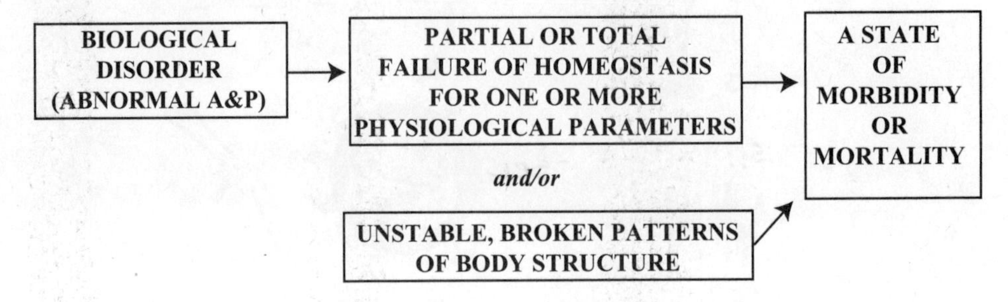

Whenever we are talking about disease, injury, or death in future chapters, therefore, we will essentially be referring back to one or more levels of the *Great Pyramid of Structure-Function **Dis**order*. Figure 6.14 features this Great Pyramid of ***ab**normal anatomy* and ***ab**normal physiology* for each of the nine levels of body organization. Quite appropriately, these levels are given verbal labels of *pathological* (**path**-oh-**LAHJ**-ih-**kal**) *anatomy* for disordered body *structures* and *pathophysiology* (**path**-oh-**fiz**-ee-**AHL**-uh-jee) for disordered *living* body *functions*. Once again, our helpful icon to symbolize such unhealthy body conditions is our poor Professor Joe—but this time he is in a fallen and fractured state!

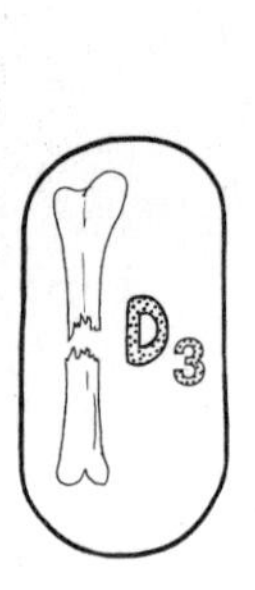

CELLULAR PATHOLOGY AND TISSUE NECROSIS

We have now thoroughly canvassed the entire Pyramid of Body Structure and Function, and we have considered it from two opposite viewpoints: (1) biological order, homeostasis, the *normo-* (normal) state, and clinical health at one end of the spectrum; versus (2) biological disorder, partial or total failures of homeostasis, the *hyper-* (excessive, above normal) and *hypo-* (deficient, below normal) states, and the occurrence of morbidity or mortality at the opposite end.

Zooming in on level V (cells and the Life-line), we are finally ready to discuss medical terminology at the cellular level. In 1855, a German pathologist named *Rudolf Virchow* (**FEER**-koh) stated the *principle of cellular pathology*. This principle says that the individual cell is the fundamental unit of pathology. Dr. Virchow closely examined slides of diseased tissues from hundreds of sick or dead patients. In almost every case of whole-body disease he studied, some abnormality or disorder could be seen in the anatomy of the cells from the

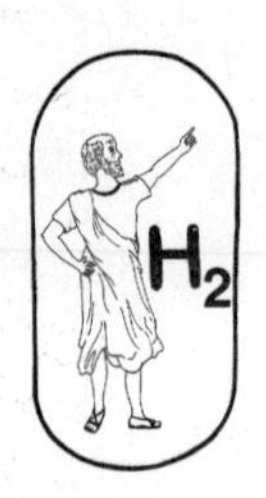

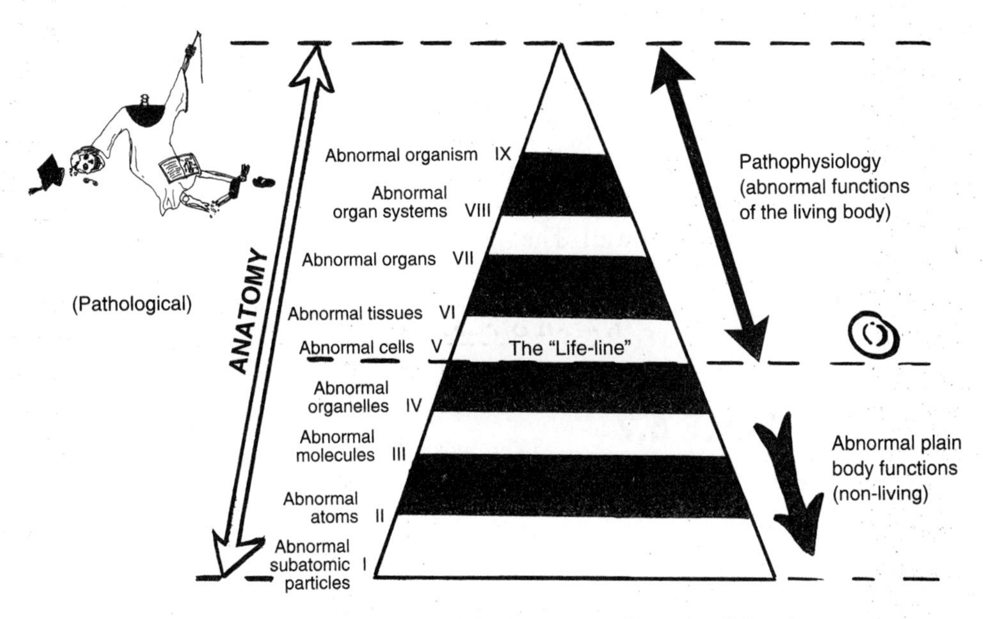

Fig. 6.14 The Great Pyramid of Structure-Function Disorder.

patient! Hence, he concluded that a *systemic* (**sis-TEM**-ik)—or whole body "system"—disease that can kill you, such as *cancer*, usually begins from a single point—one or more diseased *cells*.

The principle of cellular pathology can be considered part of a larger theory. This larger concept is called the *localistic* (**low**-kal-**IS**-tik) *theory of disease causation*. The basic idea is that disease usually begins at a particular "local" level in some relatively small area of the body, such as one or more cells. It then spreads from cells to tissues (families of related cells). Then, from the tissue level (VI) on the Great Body Pyramid, it just keeps spreading biological disorder and morbidity to higher and higher levels.

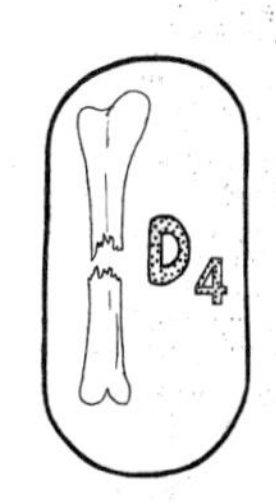

SUMMARY OF LOCALISTIC THEORY OF DISEASE CAUSATION:

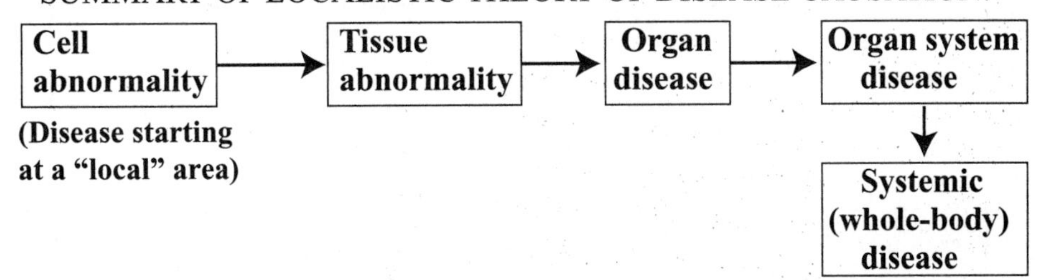

A similar situation exists for *necrosis* (**neh-KROH**-sis). This term indicates an "abnormal condition of" (*-osis*) "death" (*necr*). Let's say, for example, that a few cardiac muscle cells in the heart wall are deprived of oxygen during a so-called “heart attack.” The cardiac muscle cells, because they are starved for O_2 and highly aerobic, can no longer produce ATP energy. Thus, they become *necrotic* (neh-**KRAHT**-ik)—that is, they “die off.” A similar cellular necrosis occurs in neighboring areas of the heart wall. Eventually, the *cellular necrosis* of individual cardiac muscle cells becomes a *tissue necrosis* of the cardiac muscle in the heart wall. The heart pumps less and less blood, until the heart organ itself becomes necrotic. The heart fails to pump enough blood to the rest of the body. The whole circulatory system fails, and the entire body dies.

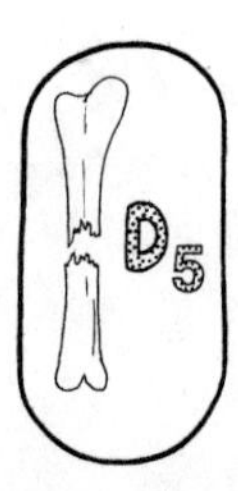

SUMMARY TABLE 6.2

Consult Summary Table 6.2 for a quick review of some important words and word parts.

Summary Table 6.2 Words and Word Parts

Write in the *exact* meaning (literal English translation) for up to 10 key terms selected from the preceding block of text. After you are done, check your word meanings with the correct answers, which are given at the end of this chapter.

Key Terms	Prefixes	Roots	Suffixes	Exact Meanings
fibroblast	(none)	fibr “fiber”	-blast “former”	1. ________
histology	(none)	hist “web or tissue”	-ology “study of”	2. ________
epithelial	epi- “upon”	theli “nipples”	-al “pertaining to”	3. ________
hypothermia	hypo- “deficient; below normal”	therm “heat”	-ia “condition of”	4. ________
hyperthermia	hyper- “excessive; above normal”	therm “heat”	-ia “condition of”	5. ________
necrosis	(none)	necr “death”	-osis “abnormal condition of”	6. ________

Medical Case History: Terminal Lung Cancer in a Chronic Smoker—A Bad Dream of Hyperplasia

Gwendolyn S., age 58, was a chronic smoker. She had smoked 3 1/2 packs per day for more than 20 years! Inhaling deeply, she frequently exclaimed, "Well, ya gotta die of somethin'!" About 6 years ago, Ms. S. was diagnosed with a case of *chronic bronchitis* (**brahn-KEYE**-tis)—an "inflammation of" (*-itis*) the *bronchi* (**BRAHN**-keye). The bronchi are the main air tubes branching off the *trachea* (**TRAY**-kee-ah) or "windpipe." (See Figure 6.15, A) Recently, she has complained of nearly constant and very intense coughing spells that even keep her awake at night! The patient came to see her family doctor after sharp, stabbing, localized chest pains on the left side scared her.

A radiographic exam of the chest cavity was employed to obtain a *bronchogram* (**BRAHN**-koh-**gram**). This is an x-ray "record" (*-gram*) of the "bronchi" (*bronch*). A large oval *neoplasm* (**NEE**-oh-**plazm**) or "new" (*neo-*) "growth" (*plasm*) was visualized in the interior of the *left primary bronchus*. (View Figure 6.15, B.) This new growth was certainly the result of an abnormal *tumorigenesis* (**TOO**-mor-ih-**JEN**-eh-sis)—the "production of" (*-genesis*) a "swelling or enlargement" (*tumor*). It involved an abnormal *hyperplasia* (**high**-per-**PLAY**-zhuh). This term indicates an "excessive" (*hyper-*) amount of tissue "formation" (*plas*).

Neoplasms created by hyperplasia may be either *benign* (bee-**NINE**)—"kind"—or *malignant* (**mah-LIG**-nant)—"wicked." Malignant neoplasms are considered wicked because they often undergo *metastasis* (**muh-TAS**-tuh-sis). This is literally a "process of" (*-is*) "changing over" (*meta-*) to another "place" (*stas*). During metastasis, abnormal cells spread, or *metastasize* (**muh-TAS**-tuh-size), from their original location toward various other parts of the body. Since malignant neoplasms do not function normally, their spreading or metastasis all over the body can often be fatal! In summary:

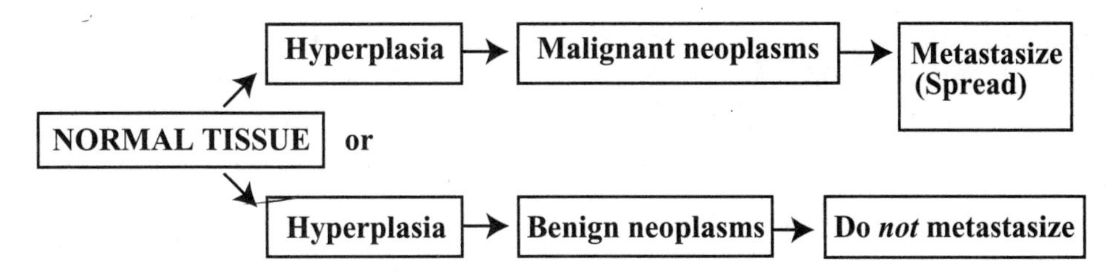

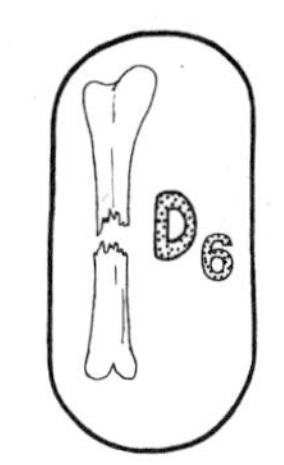

In the case of Gwendolyn S., a small sample of the neoplasm was removed by biopsy. Microscopic examination by a pathologist revealed that the epithelial cells in the neoplasm had strange nuclei that were very *pleomorphic* (**plee**-oh-**MORF**-ik)—occurring in "more than one" (*pleo-*) "shape" (*morph*).

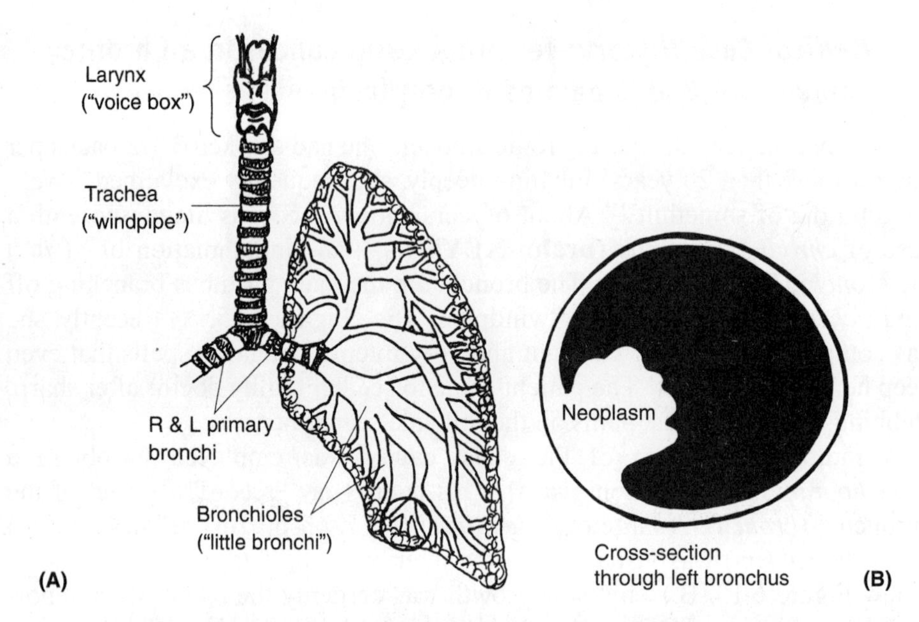

Fig. 6.15 The bronchi in normal and cancerous states. **(A)** Overview showing right and left bronchi branching off from the trachea. **(B)** Interior view of left bronchus via bronchogram, showing neoplasm.

However, most of these cells still had a generally flat and "scaly" or *squamous* (**SKWAH**-mus) form. Such highly abnormal cells confirmed the initial suspicion that the lesion was malignant.

A diagnosis of *squamous cell carcinoma* (**kar**-sin-**OH**-muh) of the lung was made. A carcinoma in general is a "crab" (*carcin*) "tumor" (*-oma*). Carcinoma or cancer is defined as a malignant neoplasm of epithelial tissue. It is symbolized by the crab, which can pinch between its claws and cause lots of body damage! Most unfortunately, metastasis from the primary site—within the left primary bronchus—had already progressed into the ribs and the left lung. The patient was put onto a high dosage of *anticancer* (**an**-tih-**CAN**-sir) *chemotherapy* and tissue-destroying radiation. Only time will tell if she can survive!

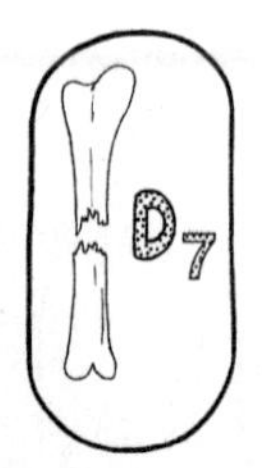

Probe of case history

(**A**) There was a hyperplasia of new, highly abnormal epithelial tissue within the lung tumor. What if there had been a *hypoplasia* instead? Would the mass of tissue become larger, or smaller, than its original size? How would you translate *hypoplasia* into its common English equivalent? (**B**) Assume that the diagnosis had been a *benign squamous neoplasm.* In this situation, what would you *not* have given the patient that she had received for her malignant neoplasm? Why? [Check your short answers with the key near the end of this chapter.]

Quiz

Refer to the text in this chapter if necessary. A good score is at least 8 correct answers out of these 10 questions. The answers are listed in the back of this book.

1. The so-called Life-line occurs at what particular level of body organization?
   (a) Molecule
   (b) Tissue
   (c) Cell
   (d) Atom
2. *Biological order* is best defined as:
   (a) Disruption of normal organ behaviors
   (b) Existence of a recognizable pattern within an organism
   (c) Random changes in the body's external environment
   (d) Morbidity and mortality
3. Involves a parameter that does not rise above its upper normal limit:
   (a) Homeostasis
   (b) Plain body functions
   (c) Blood glucose concentration
   (d) Necrotic tissue
4. "A condition of deficient or below-normal heat":
   (a) Hydronephrosis
   (b) Cephalalgia
   (c) Normothermia
   (d) Hypothermia
5. Dark, wormlike bodies that contain the genes:
   (a) Mitochondria
   (b) Chromosomes
   (c) Lysosomes
   (d) Cytoplasms
6. The so-called Powerhouse of the Cell:
   (a) Electric light plant
   (b) Nucleolus

(c) Ribosome
(d) Mitochondrion

7. The fibroblast occurs in what general type of body tissue?
(a) Connective
(b) Blood plasma
(c) Nervous
(d) Muscle

8. Histology is best described as:
(a) The study of wounds and injuries
(b) Adventures in macroscopic thinking
(c) The study of tissues
(d) A collection of specialized therapeutic techniques

9. Rudolf Virchow is known for this scientific contribution:
(a) First stated the concept of homeostasis
(b) Cured the ill with radiological wizardry
(c) Put forward the principle of cellular pathology
(d) Disease most often begins at the full systemic level

10. Benign neoplasms differ from malignant ones in that they:
(a) Frequently metastasize to outlying body areas
(b) Contain cells with normal nuclei, rather than pleomorphic ones
(c) Always stay very small in size
(d) Never cause the organism any physiological problems

Memory Pillboxes for Chapter 6

Several key facts were tagged with numbered icons in the page margins of this chapter. Write a short summary of each of these key facts into a numbered cell or compartment within the appropriate type of *Memory Pillbox* that appears below.

Background and History **Pillboxes for Chapter 6:**

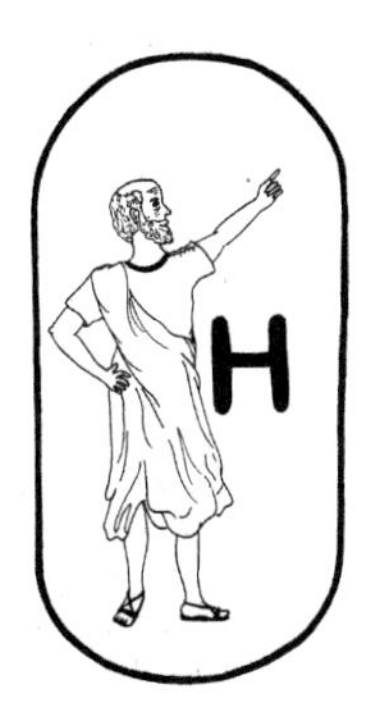

1	2

Anatomy **Pillboxes for Chapter 6:**

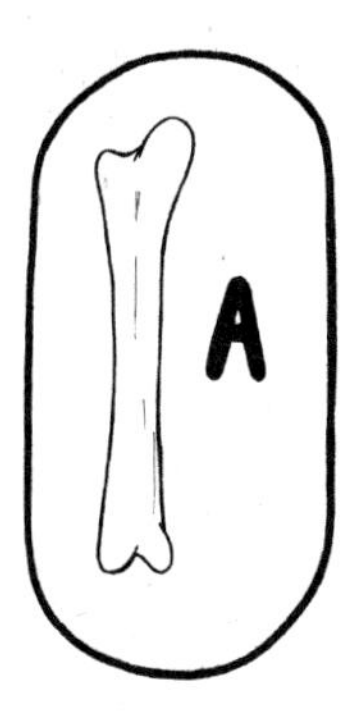

1	2

3	4
5	6
7	8
9	10

***Physiology* Pillboxes for Chapter 6:**

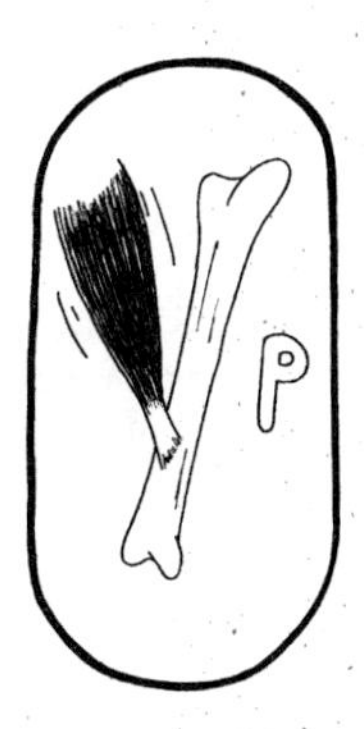

1	2
3	4
5	6

7	8

9	10

Disease/Injury **Pillboxes for Chapter 6:**

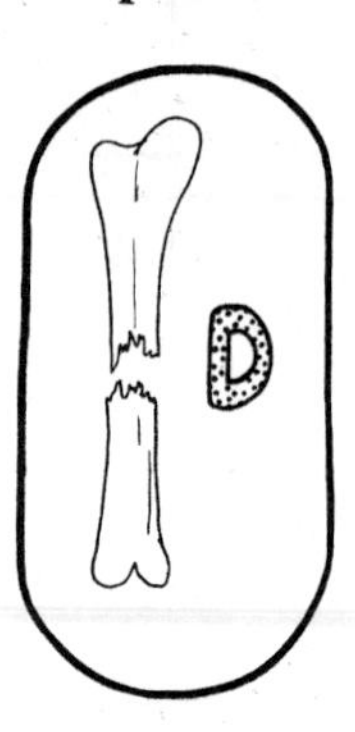

1	2

3	4

5	6

7

Answers for Chapter 6 Summary Tables

FOR SUMMARY TABLE 6.1

1. "referring to little boxes"
2. "pertaining to (something) below the atom"
3. "control of sameness"
4. "condition of normal heat"
5. "tiny organ"
6. "presence of a colored body"
7. "presence of a breakdown body"
8. "presence of a thread-granule"
9. "relating to (something) living air"
10. "process of breaking down (something) sweet"

FOR SUMMARY TABLE 6.2

1. "fiber-former"
2. "study of a web or tissue"
3. "pertaining to (something) upon nipples"
4. "condition of deficient or below normal heat"
5. "condition of excessive or above normal heat"
6. "abnormal condition of death"

Answers to Probe of Case History

(**A**) The tissue would be smaller, since hypoplasia is a "deficient or below normal" (*hypo-*) amount of tissue "formation" (*plas*). (**B**) You would not give her anticancer chemotherapy, since the tumor was a benign (noncancerous) neoplasm of epithelial tissue.

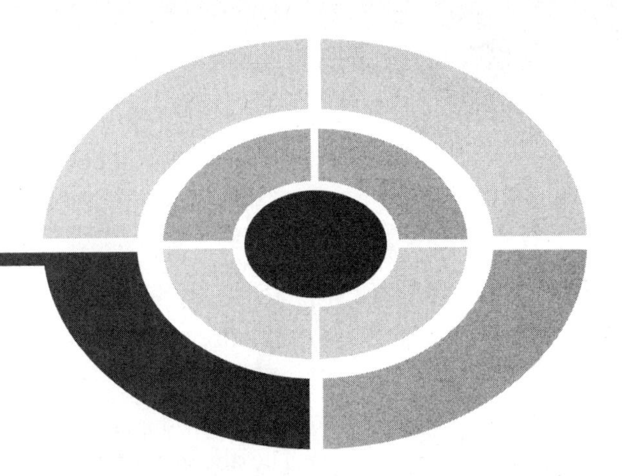

Test: Part 2

DO NOT REFER TO THE TEXT WHEN TAKING THIS TEST. A good score is at least 18 (out of 25 questions) correct. The answers are in the back of the book. It's best to have a friend check your score the first time so you won't memorize the answers if you want to take the test again.

1. Acute is the opposite of:
   - (a) Auscultation
   - (b) Diathermic
   - (c) Chronic
   - (d) Malaise
   - (e) Painful

2. Phagocytosis by macrophages tends to have a prophylactic effect, because:
   - (a) It helps promote pathogenesis
   - (b) Phagocytosis eliminates many pathogenic bacteria
   - (c) This process significantly depresses the actions of many antibodies
   - (d) Affected cells increase their secretion of hormones
   - (e) The common cold is frequently cured by phagocytosis alone

3. A foreign protein or chemical marker that identifies a given cell as either being "self" (part of the body) or "non-self" (not part of the body):
   (a) Antigen
   (b) Enzyme
   (c) Nucleolus
   (d) Glucose
   (e) Lymph
4. *Clinical health* basically represents:
   (a) The absence of any disease requiring medical care
   (b) Abnormal anatomy, but normal physiology
   (c) Only the cell level of body organization
   (d) Severe disruptions of biological order of many body parameters
   (e) Sickening episodes of severe edema
5. "You may soon have a severe fever and the chills" is best categorized as a:
   (a) Diagnosis
   (b) Prodrome
   (c) Sign
   (d) Prognosis
   (e) Zoonosis
6. Clinical __________ are problems that the patient usually notices:
   (a) Symptoms
   (b) Parameters
   (c) Diagnoses
   (d) Signs
   (e) Metastases
7. P&A can be useful in diagnosing chest problems, owing to the fact that:
   (a) Softly touching the chest may reveal underlying lesions
   (b) Ultraviolet rays can penetrate deeply through the skin
   (c) Tapping and listening are simple yet very effective clinical skills
   (d) Regular exercise can reduce the incidence of anginal chest pain
   (e) It removes any doubt about the physician's judgment
8. LYMPHATIC-IMMUNE SYSTEM = THE:
   (a) MACROPHAGES + PHAGOCYTES
   (b) LYMPHATIC VESSELS + ALL THE BLOOD VESSELS
   (c) INVADING ANTIGENS + ANTIGEN-ANTIBODY REACTION
   (d) CARDIAC MUSCLE FIBERS + FIBROBLASTS
   (e) LYMPHATIC SYSTEM + IMMUNE SYSTEM

9. The professional person you should most likely consult in helping you interpret your x-rays:
   (a) Radiologist
   (b) Oncologist
   (c) Pathologist
   (d) Histologist
   (e) Cytologist

10. Organelle mainly responsible for aerobic production of ATP:
   (a) Nucleolus
   (b) Ribosome
   (c) Nucleus
   (d) Mitochondrion
   (e) Plasma membrane

11. ______________ is the process whereby material is pushed out of the blood capillaries (due to the force of the blood pressure) and eventually becomes the lymph.
   (a) Simple diffusion
   (b) Filtration
   (c) Osmosis
   (d) Radiation
   (e) Urination

12. Circulating proteins in blood and lymph that attack and destroy foreign invaders:
   (a) Leukocytes
   (b) Antibodies
   (c) Fibroblasts
   (d) Antigens
   (e) Wandering macrophages

13. Theoretically speaking, a parameter rising above its upper normal limit indicates a state of:
   (a) Biological order
   (b) Clinical health
   (c) Hypertrophy
   (d) Homeostasis
   (e) Biological disorder

14. Literally translates to mean "crab tumor":
   (a) Cancer
   (b) Squamous

(c) Carcinoma
(d) Epithelium
(e) Bronchus

15. The very lowest level of the Great Body Pyramid:
    (a) Organelle
    (b) Cell
    (c) Atom
    (d) Tissue
    (e) Subatomic
16. A cell abnormality leads to a tissue abnormality, which leads to organ disease; this in turn leads to organ system disease, which leads to systemic (whole body) disease:
    (a) The cell theory
    (b) Principle of least resistance
    (c) The theory of homeostasis
    (d) Localistic theory of disease causation
    (e) The Gulf War Syndrome
17. Diagnosis most likely to compel you to write your last will and testament!
    (a) Benign neoplasm of the lung
    (b) Moderate hypoplasis of dividing mast cells
    (c) Optimal normotension of BP
    (d) Acute coryza or rhinitis
    (e) Malignant neoplasm of the skin
18. A pathologist viewing a biopsied piece of tumor would probably become most alarmed if he saw ______________ cells under the microscope.
    (a) Pleomorphic
    (b) Chromosomal
    (c) Aerobic
    (d) Nerve
    (e) Muscle
19. Discovering a network of tiny blood capillaries in your hand would cause you to search for lymphatic capillaries running:
    (a) Far away from them
    (b) Right through their walls
    (c) Parallel and quite close to them
    (d) Way above and beyond them
    (e) Only in the hand on the opposite side of the body
20. "My little boy has hypertrophied adenoids! So, he just can't ________".
    (a) Swim
    (b) Breathe

(c) Swallow
(d) Walk
(e) Think

21. A nurse reading a patient history that included an entry of *FUO* (*fever of unknown origin*) should interpret this finding to mean that the fever:
    (a) Just wouldn't respond to antibiotic chemotherapy
    (b) Never resulted in serious morbidity
    (c) Had an idiopathic or essential origin
    (d) Was correctly diagnosed as marginal hypothermia
    (e) Frequently interrupted the homeostatic balance of many other organic functions

22. The first gross or macroscopic level of body organization on the Great Pyramid:
    (a) Tissue
    (b) Cell
    (c) Molecule
    (d) Organelle
    (e) Organ

23. Both the nucleolus and ribosomes within a cell are composed mainly of:
    (a) Glucose
    (b) RNA
    (c) Chromosomes
    (d) Genes
    (e) DNA

24. A flock of geese is flying in a V formation across the sky. A hunter shoots down three of them that are flying on the same side of the V. Hence, a condition of __________ has been created.
    (a) Homeostasis
    (b) Morbidity
    (c) Biological order
    (d) Hypothermia
    (e) Biological disorder and mortality

25. Every time you see this prefix, you know that the rest of the medical term involves something that is "below normal or deficient":
    (a) Neo-
    (b) Pre-
    (c) Hypo-
    (d) Uni-
    (e) Hyper-

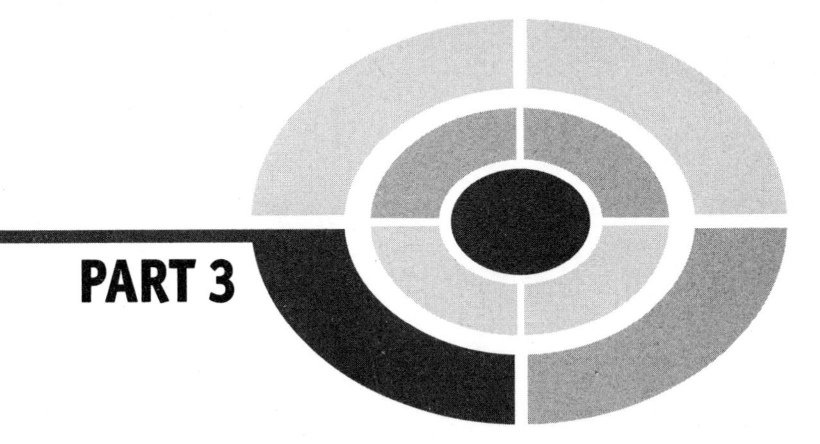

PART 3

Bones and Muscles

CHAPTER 7

Terms of Skeletal and Muscular Disorders, or "There's Too Much Trouble in This *Joint*!"

In Part 2, we spent time establishing a sound basis for understanding biological order as patterns involving living organisms, and biological disorder as the breaking or absence of such patterns. This gave us a solid skeleton upon which to hang our growing knowledge of both normal anatomy and physiology (A&P) (suggesting clinical health and homeostasis) as well as abnormal A&P (suggesting morbidity and mortality). And we were guided to become conscious of the Great Body Pyramid, with its nine major levels of body organization:

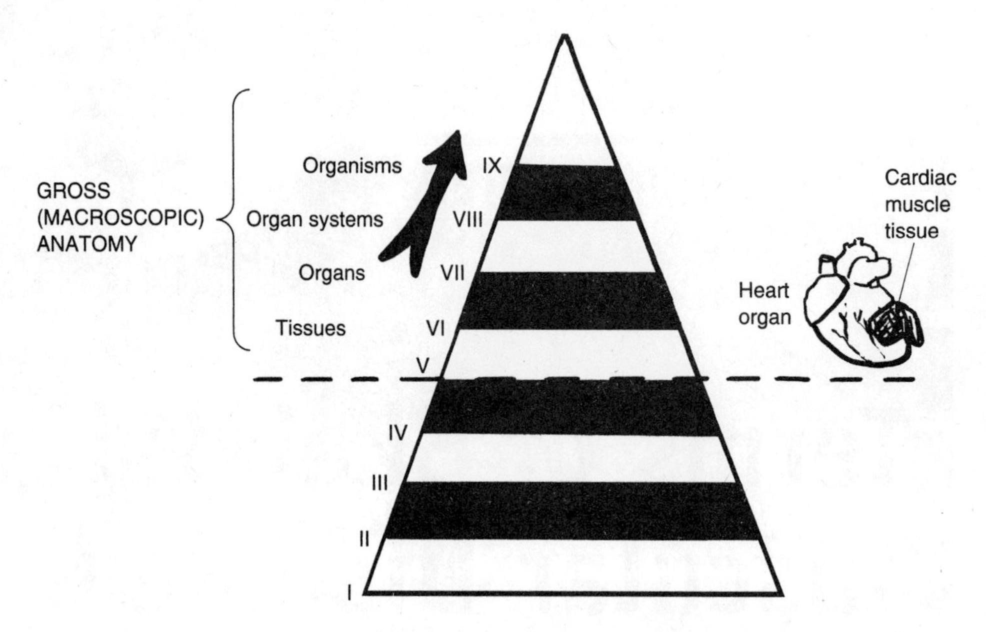

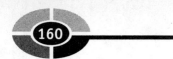

In Part 3, we will now proceed from the tissues (level VI) upward to the organs and organ systems (levels VII and VIII). Here in Chapter 7, our first encounter will be with the organs of the *skeletal* and *muscular systems*. It is with these two closely related organ systems that our study of both normal and medical terminology will continue.

Background and History

Here in Chapter 7, we are basically considering both the normal A&P and the abnormal A&P of two separate but closely related *organ systems*. These are the *skeletal system* and the *muscular system*. These two organ systems, in turn, consist of several different types of *organs*. As we define these concepts, let us orient ourselves by reviewing two schemes: the Great Pyramid of Structure-Function *Order* (Figure 7.1, A) and the Great Pyramid of Structure-Function *Disorder* (Figure 7.1, B).

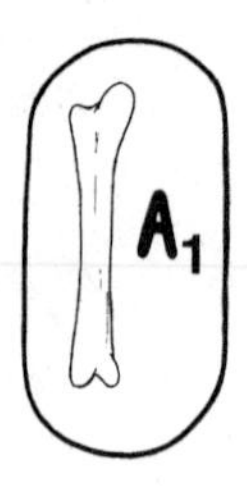

Observe from Figure 7.1 that both *organs* and *abnormal organs* are tagged as level VII on the two Great Pyramids. An organ represents two or more of the basic body tissues that together perform a very specialized body function. (NOTE: You may recall that *CNEMI* identified the first four of these as *connective, nervous, epithelial,* and *muscle* tissue.) At a higher level (VIII), an organ system represents a collection of related organs that together perform some complex body function.

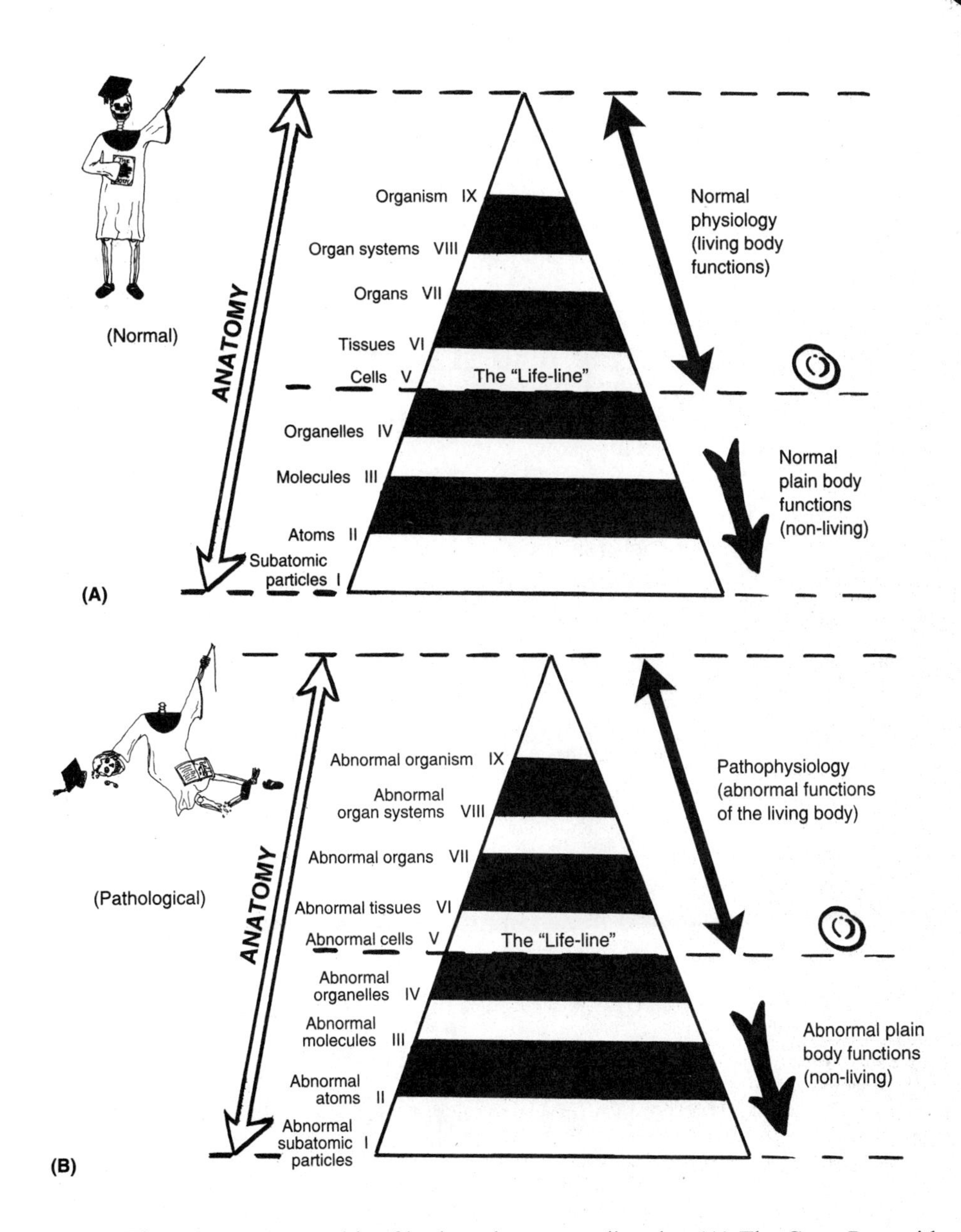

Fig. 7.1 The two great pyramids of body order versus disorder. **(A)** The Great Pyramid of Structure-Function *Order*. **(B)** The Great Pyramid of Structure-Function *Disorder*.

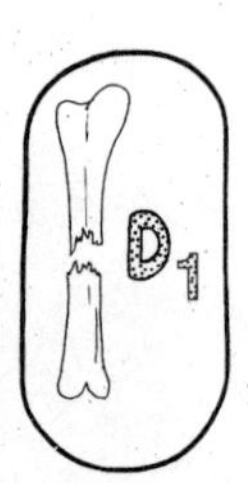

In this chapter, we shall be considering the background of the skeletal and muscular systems (and their major organs) separately from one another. Each time we discuss these systems, you can picture our focus as being mainly upon either the organ level (VII) or organ system level (VIII). For normal organs and organ systems, we will be referring to the Great Pyramid of Structure-Function Order. Conversely, for abnormal, injured, or diseased organs and organ systems, we shall be looking at the Great Pyramid of Structure-Function Disorder.

THE SKELETAL SYSTEM AND ITS ORGANS

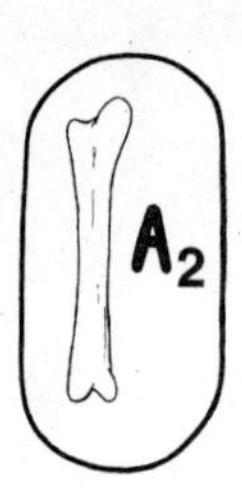

The human skeletal system is correctly classified as a type of *endoskeleton* (**en**-doh-**SKEL**-eh-ton). This exactly translates to mean "a hard dried body" (*skeleton*) lying "within" (*endo-*). Figure 7.2 makes an imaginative comparison between the human endoskeleton and the pit of a peach. What is the connection? Well, for both of these structures, the hard dried "body" (skeleton or pit) is buried within a soft padding of fleshy material! [**Word practice suggestion:** The prefix, *exo-*, means "outside of" (something). See if you can use this fact to help you write a new term, ______________, which exactly means "presence of a hard dried body outside."]

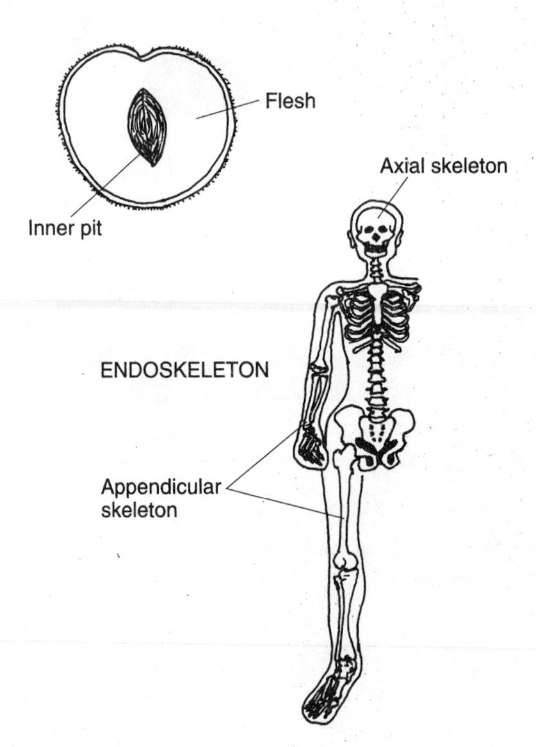

Fig. 7.2 The human endoskeleton: What a peach!

Observe from Figure 7.2 that the total endoskeleton in an adult is artificially subdivided into two smaller skeletons for study. These are the *axial* (**AX**-ee-ul) *skeleton* plus the *appendicular* (**ah**-pen-**DIK**-you-ler) *skeleton*. The axial skeleton "pertains to an axis" or central turning rod. Like the two axles on the wheels of your car or the central axis of a globe, the axial skeleton is the central turning rod or line around which your body pivots. The appendicular skeleton is the one that includes your body *appendages* (ah-**PEN**-dah-jes); that is, it includes your limbs or "attachments" to the axial skeleton.

Both of these major subdivisions of the skeleton are composed of two types of organs: 206 *bones* and the *joints* made between them. Profiling this relationship yields:

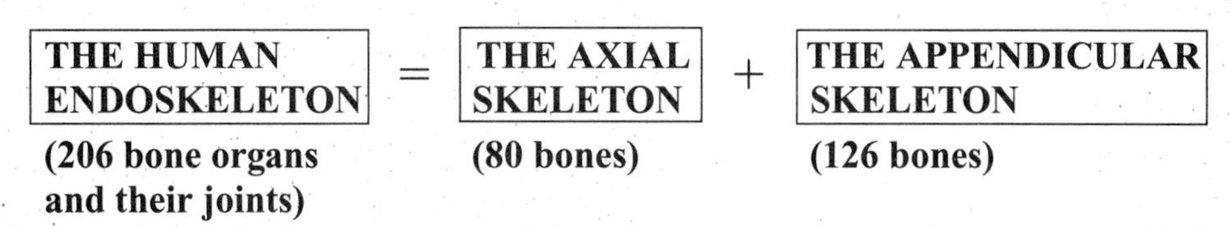

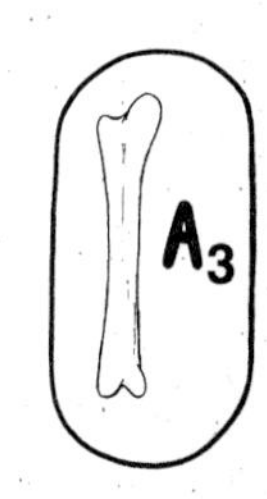

and

ORGANS OF THE SKELETAL SYSTEM (HUMAN ENDOSKELETON) = BONES + JOINTS (between bones)

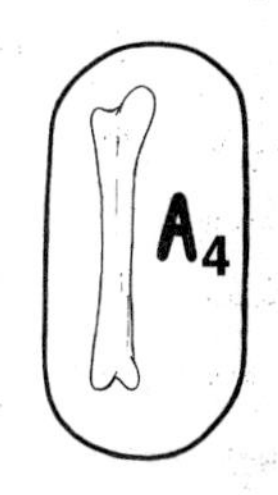

A brief overview of these two organ types is provided by a look at Figure 7.3. The three bones pictured are called *phalanges* (fuh-**LAN**-jees). Each individual bone is called a *phalanx* (**FAY**-lanks). The phalanges are the bones located within our fingers and toes. They are classified as *long bones*, since they are much longer than they are wide. The phalanges resemble hard, white, slender sticks—a result of their calcium-rich bone *matrix* (**MAY**-tricks).

The phalanges, because they are hard like rocks, would rub and scrape against one another during movement of the fingers or toes if it were not for the presence of the *interphalangeal* (**in**-ter-fah-lan-**JEEL**) *joints*. A joint in general is a "joining place" between two bones. The interphalangeal joints are the joining places located "between" (*inter-*) the "phalanges" (*phalange*). These joints are where the phalanges do one of their essential functions: helping to carry out movements of the fingers and toes.

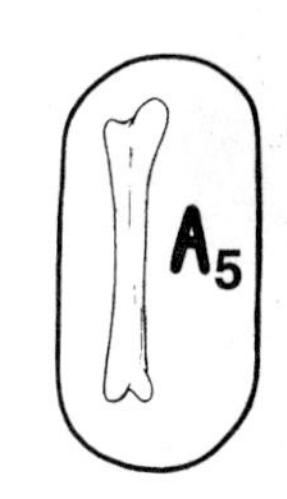

Figure 7.3 also uses the interphalangeal joint as a typical example of a *synovial* (**sih-NOHV**-ee-al) *joint*. The synovial joints are the broad category of freely movable joints in the body. They include (in addition to the interphalangeal joints) many very familiar joints, such as the knee, hip, and shoulder. The joint name reflects their internal anatomy. Consider, for instance, the *fibrous* (**FEYE**-brus) *joint capsule* that surrounds and encloses the meeting

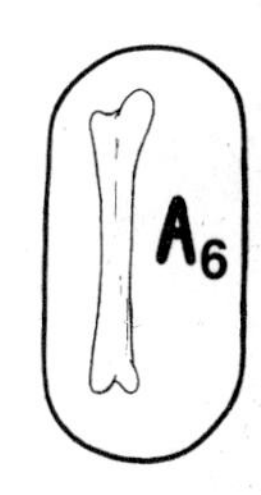

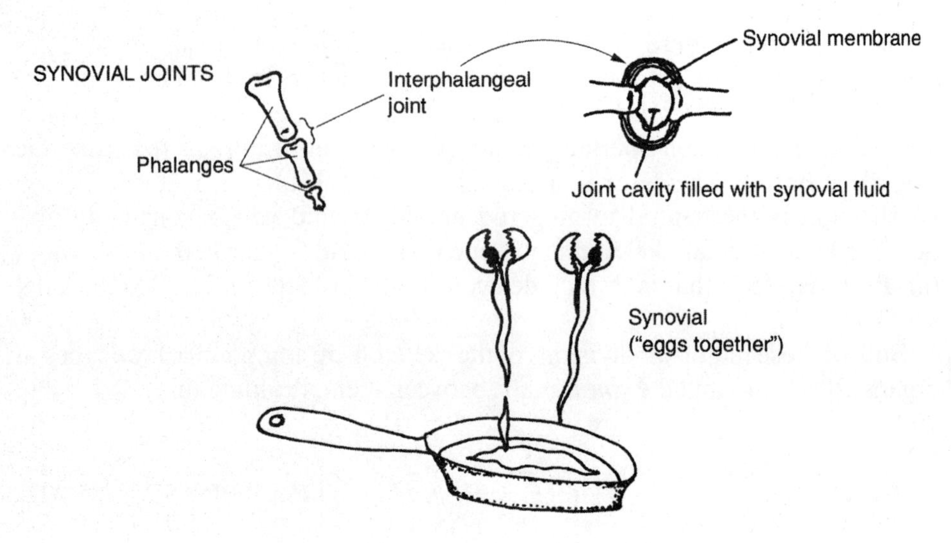

Fig. 7.3 The phalanges and their joints.

ends of two adjacent phalanges. The hollow *joint cavity* within this capsule is lined by a *synovial membrane*. Special cells in the membrane secrete *synovial fluid*. It literally resembles the raw whites of many "eggs" (*ovi*) that have been poured "together" (*syn-*). This thick, slimy, egg white–like fluid serves to lubricate the ends of bones, thereby greatly reducing their friction and wear during free body movements. [**Visualization suggestion:** Imagine a baseball pitcher winding up his arm to throw a ball. Again and again, throughout the entire afternoon, the pitcher keeps using the shoulder joint. Why don't the bones in his shoulder just chip away from all this friction?]

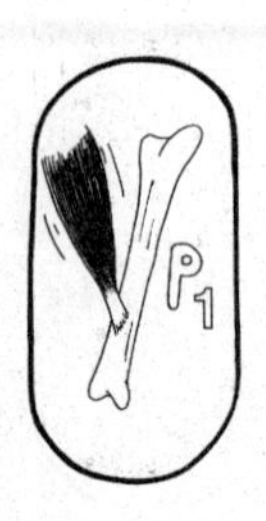

Take a moment and look at one of your fingers. Now bend it. This movement is called *flexion*—a "process of" (*-ion*) "bending" (*flex*). After *flexing* (**FLEKS**-ing) your finger, straighten it back out. This movement is called *extension*—a "process of" (*-ion*) "straightening" (*extens*). Observe that the two major motions of the fingers and their jointed phalanges are flexion and extension. Overall, the interphalangeal joints are synovial ones, but they are further classified as *hinge joints*. The reason, of course, is that they move back and forth in one direction or plane only, just like a door hinge.

Some bones of the upper limb

Figure 7.4 shows the phalanges in the fingers, plus a number of other interesting bones in the upper limb of the body. This figure reveals that the name for the phalanges comes from the Latin word for a "battle line of soldiers" or a "closely

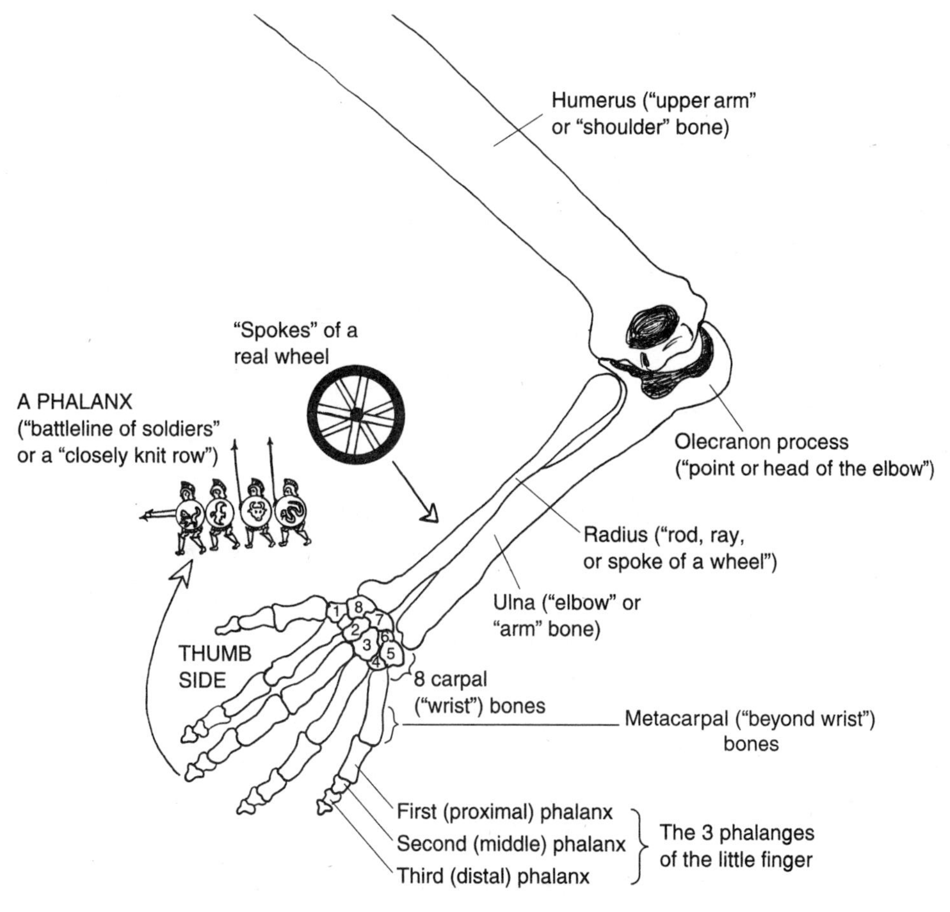

Fig. 7.4 Some bones in the upper limb.

knit row." From the positions of these phalanges within the hand, the etymology (original meaning) of their name becomes quite evident.

The wrist is called the *carpus* (**KAR**-pus); hence, the *carpals* (**KAR**-puls) are a group of eight bones in the wrist. Lying just "beyond" (*meta-*) these "carpals" (wrist bones) are the five *metacarpal* (**met**-ah-**KAR**-pal) *bones*. [**Self-discovery probe:** Look at your own hand. Now, the phalanges are in your fingers, and the carpals are in your wrists. The metacarpals are therefore located within what specific part of your hand?]

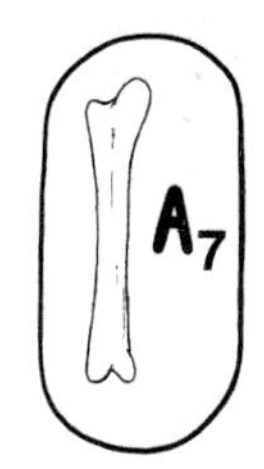

The forearm consists of two long bones: the *radius* (**RAY**-dee-us) and the *ulna* (**UL**-nuh). Look at Figure 7.4 and discover for yourself the original Latin meaning or etymology for these forearm bones. You can see why ulna means "elbow," since the *olecranon* (oh-**LEK**-ruh-nahn) *process* forms the bony point of your elbow. (The word, *olecranon*, means "elbow.") Finally, situated immediately superior to the radius and ulna is the *humerus* (**HYOO**-mer-us). You can see why its exact meaning is "upper arm."

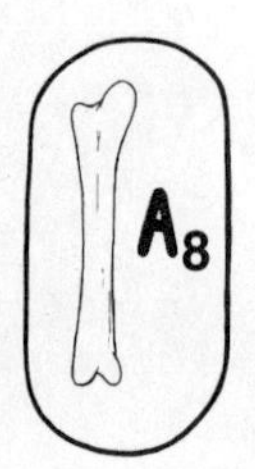

A few other bones in the body

Figure 7.5 provides an overview of the entire skeleton. Observe that the axial skeleton is centrally located. It includes the skull and facial bones, the *sternum* (**STERN**-um, meaning "chest" or breastplate), the ribs, and the *vertebral column* or backbones. The *cranial bones* are very thin, flat bones that form

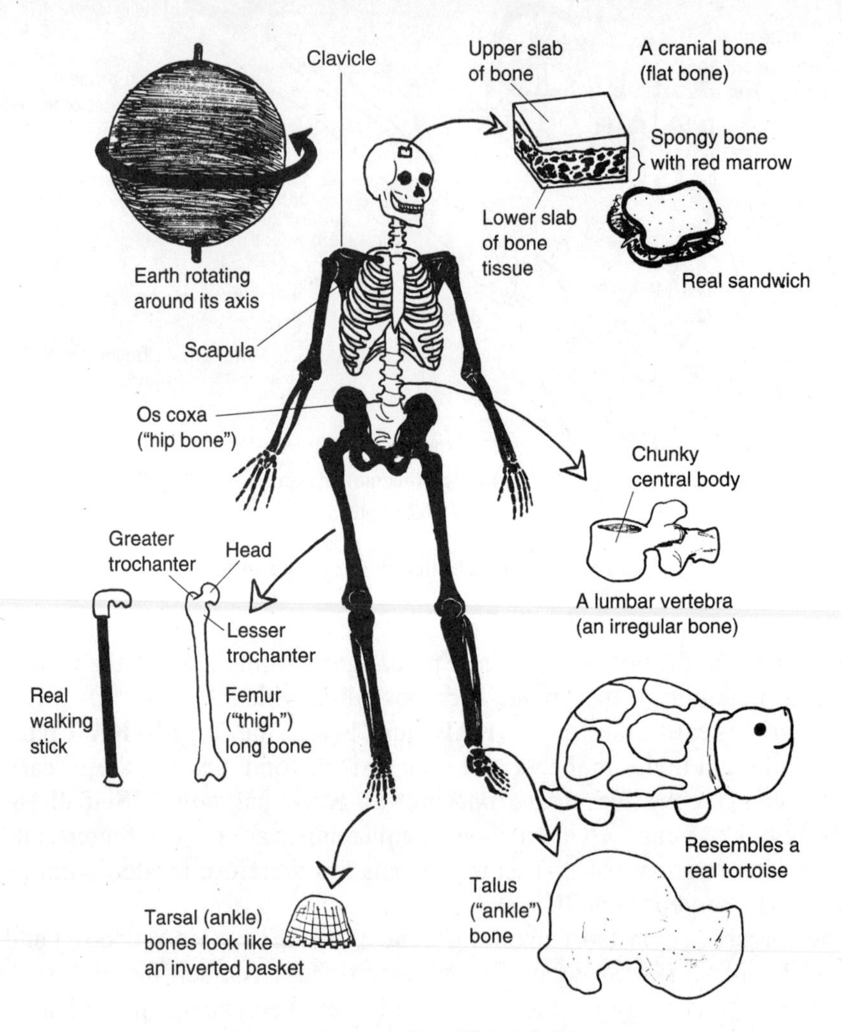

Fig. 7.5 An overview of the skeleton.

a dome over the top of the brain. Figure 7.5 shows a small section cut from one of these cranial bones. In the middle of this bony sandwich is the *spongy bone*. Its lattice or matrix of bony projections contains *red marrow* within its holes.

The *scapula* (**SKAP**-you-lah), or "shoulder blade," along with the *clavicle* (**KLAV**-ih-kl)—the "little key" or "collarbone"—help make up the *shoulder girdle*. The shoulder girdle is a curved arch that forms a joint with the top of the humerus. The *os coxa* (**AHKS KAHKS**-ah) or "bone of the hip," in contrast, creates a curved and indented *hip girdle* that receives the rounded *head* of the *femur*.

Femor (**FEH**-mor) is a word root that means "thigh." Hence, the word, *femoral* (**FEM**-er-al), "pertains to the thigh or the femur." The *femoral shaft* is the long stick-like portion of the femur. Along with its rounded head, which slants toward the middle, doesn't the femur somewhat resemble a walking stick?

Just above the foot lies the *tarsus* (**TAR**-sus) or ankle. Taken altogether, the *tarsal* (**TAR**-sal) bones in the ankle look like an inverted (upside-down) wicker basket! The *talus* (**TAY**-lus) bone, which supports much of the body's weight in the tarsal group, quite closely resembles a squat little tortoise! (Review Figure 7.5.)

Summary of bone and joint comments

In this book, we can only provide a brief overview of some of the main bones and joints. Please consult our close cousins, *ANATOMY DEMYSTIFIED* and *PHYSIOLOGY DEMYSTIFED*, for many more fun and interesting details!

DISORDERS OF BONES AND JOINTS

Now that we have looked at the biological order (normal A&P) of bones and joints, it is time we became more clinical. Specifically, we need to address some of the common biological disorders that can occur in these organs.

Bone fractures

What is the first thing that comes to mind when we speak of bone disorders? Probably *bone fractures*, right? A fracture is a "break" in a bone. What causes this break or fracture? The answer is: excessive *bone stress* or *bone strain*.

Bone stress is the amount of physical force being applied to a bone. It can be measured in units of pounds of pressure per square inch of bone surface. Every time you get up out of your chair, for example, and rise into a standing position, the amount of *femoral stress* greatly increases. This increased stress

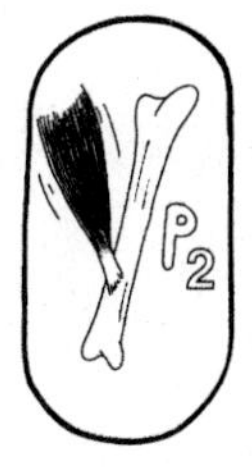

exerted upon the femur is a result of such things as the force of gravity acting upon your body weight. Nevertheless, *normostress* (**NOR**-moh-stress)—bone stress that remains within a "normal" range—is a quite appropriate and even healthy situation (Figure 7.6, A). [**Visualization suggestion:** Imagine a long wooden stick or tree limb. Now bend both ends of the stick with your hands. This creates a condition of stick stress.]

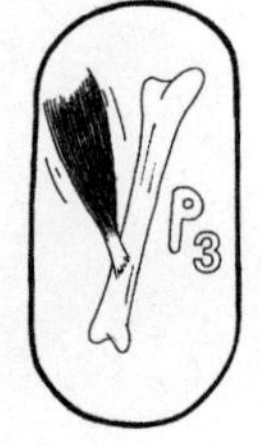

Bone strain is the amount of deformation or change in shape that occurs as a result of bone stress. If you could observe your femurs closely enough when you first stand up, for instance, you would see them undergo a small

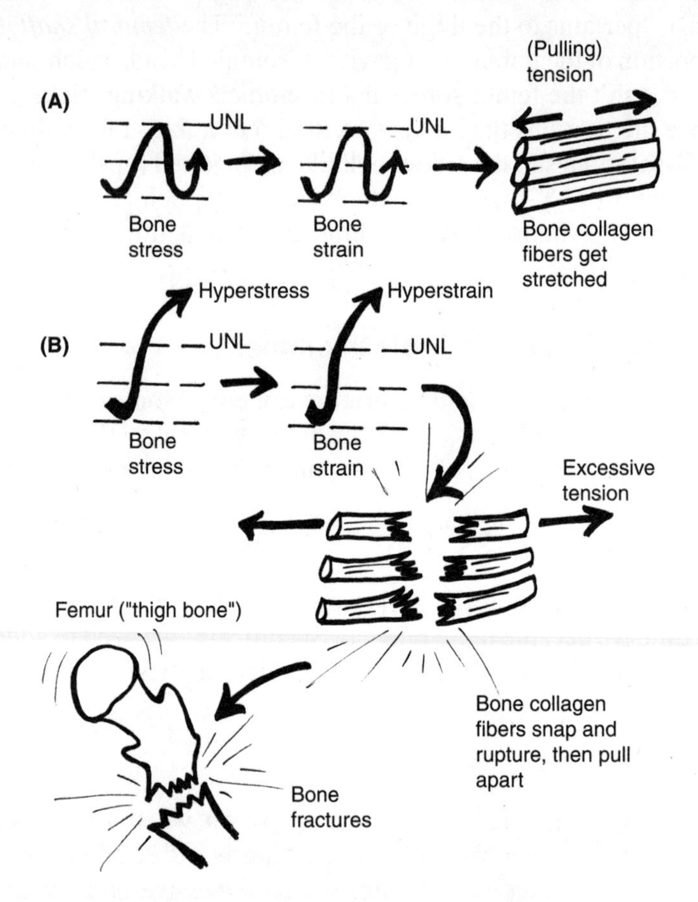

Fig. 7.6 Bone stress, bone strain, and bone fracture. **(A)** Bone *normo*stress results in bone *normo*strain. Tension is placed upon bone collagen fibers, but only up to the upper normal limit (UNL), not enough to make them snap. **(B)** Bone *hyper*stress results in bone *hyper*strain (*beyond* the UNL). Excessive tension upon bone collagen fibers makes them snap, rupture, and pull apart. Bone fracture results.

amount of bone strain, bending and bowing out a bit. But like normostress, bone *normostrain* (**NOR**-moh-strain) is quite ordinary and appropriate in everyday life. [**Visualization suggestion:** Take that imaginary stick of yours and again apply force to both ends of it. When you see the stick bend, it represents the occurrence of stick strain.]

The potential problems arise when bone stress rises far above its *upper normal limit* (Figure 7.6, B). This situation might occur, say, if you fell off a high roof and landed on both feet! The resulting impact with the ground would result in *hyperstress* (**HIGH**-per-stress)—an "excessive or above normal" (*hyper-*) amount of bone stress. Such large impact forces upon the femur would likely result in bone *hyperstrain*. This word means, of course, an "excessive or above normal" amount of bone strain.

Such an excessive amount of bone strain would probably overstretch and tear the many collagen fibers located within the bone matrix. (Visualize collagen fibers as thick ropes that snap when overstretched.) When the overstretched collagen fibers rupture and separate, the resulting crack shows up on the surface as a bone fracture.

DIFFERENT TYPES OF BONE FRACTURES

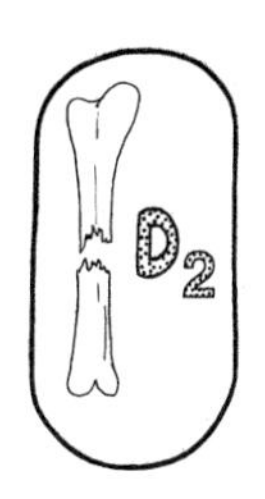

As you might suspect, bones can fracture in several different ways. Figure 7.7 provides an orienting framework. One way of classifying fractures is by the degree of bone breakage. A *complete fracture* is a break all the way through a bone, such that two or more separate pieces result. Conversely, an *incomplete* or *greenstick fracture* is a break that extends only partway through a bone, such that the bone still remains in one piece. The colorful term, *greenstick*, suggests a comparison to a young, green stick growing on a tree. When you apply hyperstress and hyperstrain to the green stick with both your hands, it usually doesn't fracture cleanly. More likely, it will just partially tear and shred. [**Thinking suggestion:** Who would be more likely to suffer a greenstick fracture of the femur: an adult, or a young child? Explain your reasoning.]

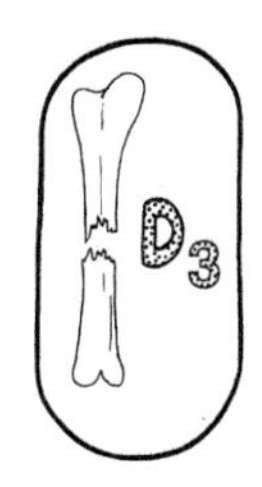

Another way of classifying fractures is according to the amount of damage to the overlying skin. A *simple fracture* is one that involves only a break in a bone, with no damage to the overlying skin. A *compound fracture*, in comparison, is a fracture where a break in the bone is "compounded" or made worse by a break in the overlying skin. [**Thinking probe:** *Toxemia* (**tahk-SEE**-mee-uh) is a "condition of blood" (*-emia*) "poisoning" (*tox*). *Bacterial* toxemia, for instance, occurs when the poisons of infecting bacteria get into the bloodstream. Now, which type of fracture is most likely to lead to a case of bacterial toxemia: simple fractures, or compound fractures? Why?]

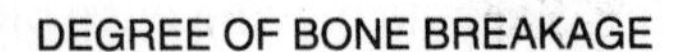

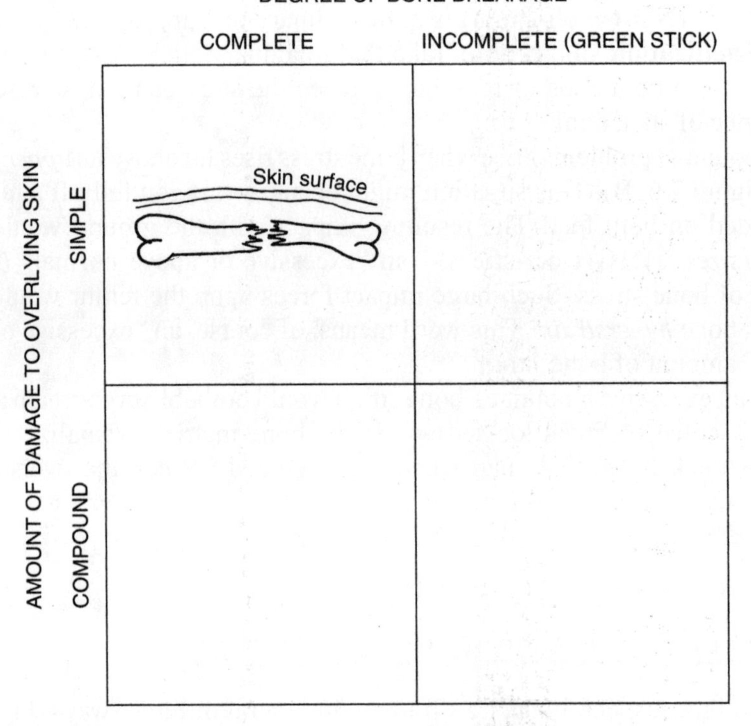

Fig. 7.7 The four general types of bone fractures. (**Note**: Only the first box or cell contains an illustration. The reader is asked to fill in the other 3 boxes in the figure.)

In real life, we usually deal with some particular combination of fracture types. In the first square cell shown in Figure 7.7, specifically, we see drawn a *simple complete fracture*. This type involves a break entirely through the bone, but with no damage to the skin overlying the bone. [**Study suggestion:** Now, *you* go ahead and name the other three broad combinations of fracture types. Make a quick sketch of each in the cells of Figure 7.7, then check your answers with a friend.]

Osteoporosis

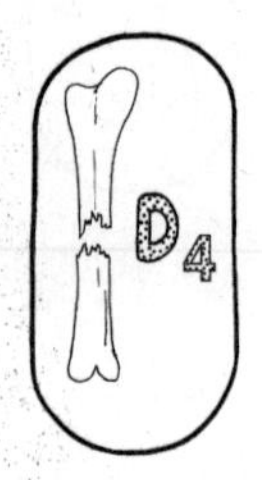

As you read the preceding material about bone fractures, you may have asked yourself this question: "Why do some elderly people get fractures so much easier than younger people?" Part of the answer comes from a single medical term: *osteoporosis* (**ahs**-tee-oh-por-**OH**-sis). This word literally translates to mean an "abnormal condition of" (*-osis*) "pores" or holes (*por*) in "bones" (*oste*).

Figure 7.8 (A) reveals the normal *microanatomy* of bone connective tissue. Three *Haversian* (hah-**VER**-shun) *systems* or *osteons* (**AHS**-tee-**ahns**) are

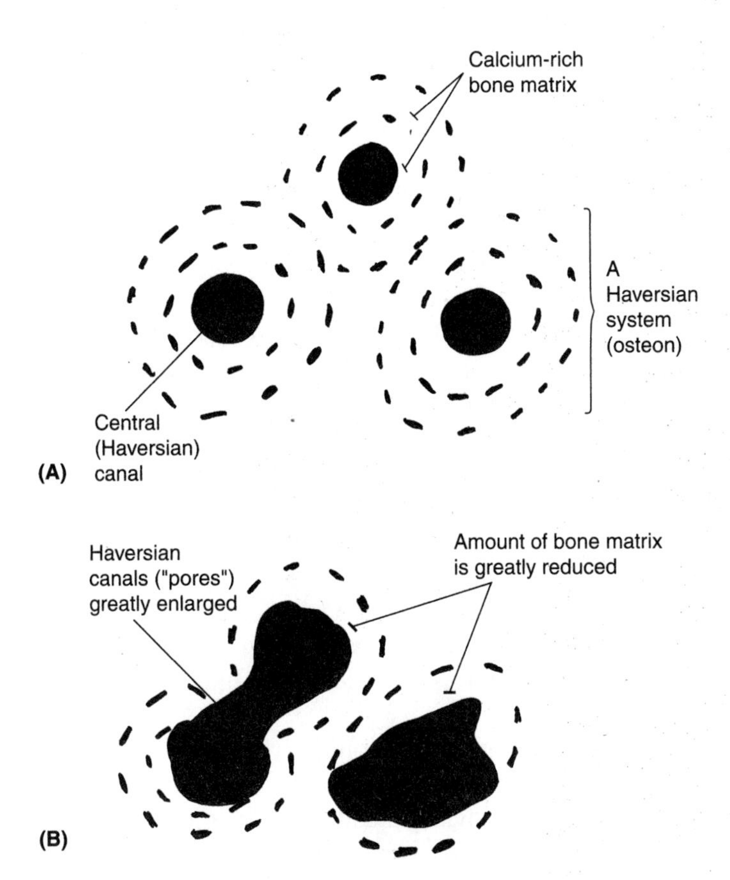

Fig. 7.8 Holes in normal bone tissue versus osteoporotic bone tissue. **(A)** Normal bone matrix showing three Haversian systems (osteons). **(B)** Abnormal bone matrix showing dramatic effects upon the same three Haversian systems in osteoporosis: Greatly enlarged "pores" (Haversian canals), with some merging together.

pictured. These Haversian systems (osteons) are the repeating structural units that make up *dense bone tissue*. Observe that a large black hole, called a *central* or *Haversian canal*, is found in the middle of each Haversian system. These Haversian or central canals are completely normal. In fact, they serve as the vital channels through which *nutrient* or "feeder" *blood vessels* pass.

Figure 7.8 (B) demonstrates the dramatic difference in a bad case of osteoporosis. The Haversian canals have greatly enlarged—in some cases to the extent of even merging with one another! The result is a very hole-ridden bone tissue. Very little hard, white, calcium-rich bone matrix still remains. Thus, *osteoporotic* (**ahs**-tee-oh-por-**AH**-tik) bones are very weak, brittle, and easily fractured. One potentially valuable prophylactic behavior to protect

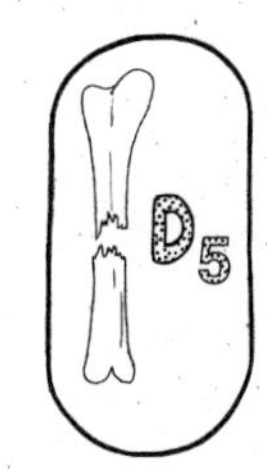

yourself from osteoporosis is to take a large oral dose of calcium (about 1,000 milligrams per day). This simple daily ritual helps retard the breakdown and dissolving of the calcium-rich bone matrix.

Bursitis versus arthritis

There are several different types of *-itis* or "inflammations of" tissues that lie in or around the joints. Let us consider two types: *bursitis* (**bur-SIGH**-tis) versus *arthritis* (**arth-RYE**-tis) of the shoulder joint. A *bursa* (**BUR**-sah) is a fluid-filled sac or "purse" (*burs*) "present" (*-a*) between skeletal muscles and their *tendons* and the underlying bones.

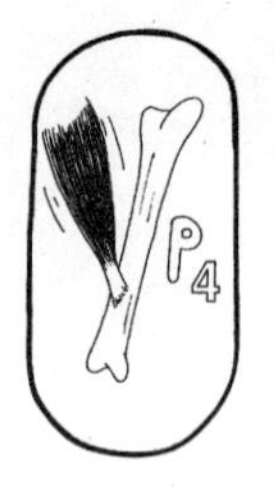

The *bursas* themselves are not part of the freely movable joint. Rather, they often lie around one. The bursas serve to reduce friction between muscles and bones, especially in body areas that perform a lot of movement, such as the shoulder.

The shoulder joint, for instance, has a group of four small bursas around it (Figure 7.9, A). One of the most prominent of these is the *subdeltoid* (**sub-DEL**-toyd) *bursa*. It lies just "below" (*sub-*) the *deltoid* muscle, which forms the fleshy pad of the shoulder. It is the outer purse-like sac on the lateral surface of the head of the humerus.

A frontal section cut through the shoulder (Figure 7.9, B) displays the associated internal anatomy. Note that, in addition to being lined by a synovial membrane and containing synovial fluid, the shoulder joint contains a good deal of *articular* (ar-**TIK**-you-lar) *cartilage*. This is literally soft, rubbery "gristle" (*cartilag*) that is "present" (*-e*) to help make a "little joint" (*articul*). The articular cartilage softens the otherwise rock hard, bony contact surfaces between the head of the humerus and the shoulder socket of the scapula.

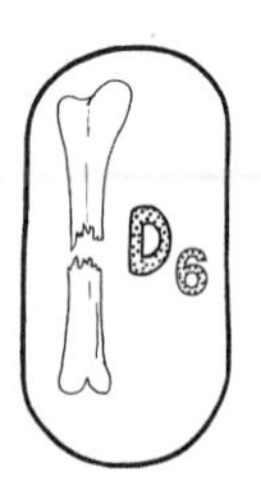

Figure 7.9 (C) shows the very unpleasant effects associated with a *chronic overuse syndrome* of the shoulder joint. After long hours of pitching, a professional baseball player may suffer this type of disorder. The bursas around the joint become severely swollen, reddened, and inflamed. This is *bursitis*. The *bursal* (**BUR**-sal) wall also secretes a "watery" *serous* (**SEER**-us) *fluid* into the surrounding tissues. There is severe pain, tenderness, and limitation of motion of the shoulder. Abnormal calcium deposits may be present beneath the subdeltoid bursa.

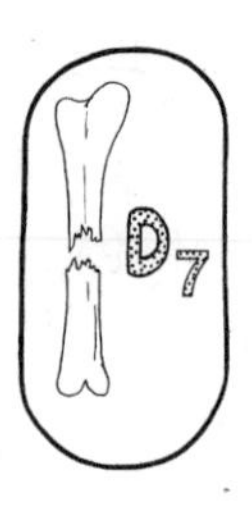

The most frequent type of arthritis—an "inflammation of the joints" themselves—is called *osteoarthritis* (**ahs**-tee-oh-arth-**REYE**-tis) or *OA*. This is common "wear-and-tear" arthritis, often resulting from chronic overuse, or improper use, of particular joints. When joints such as the shoulder are used excessively over a long time, the articular cartilage wears down and the underlying bony tissue becomes eroded and inflamed. (That's why it's called *osteo*arthritis, rather than just plain arthritis.) It is also called *degenerative joint*

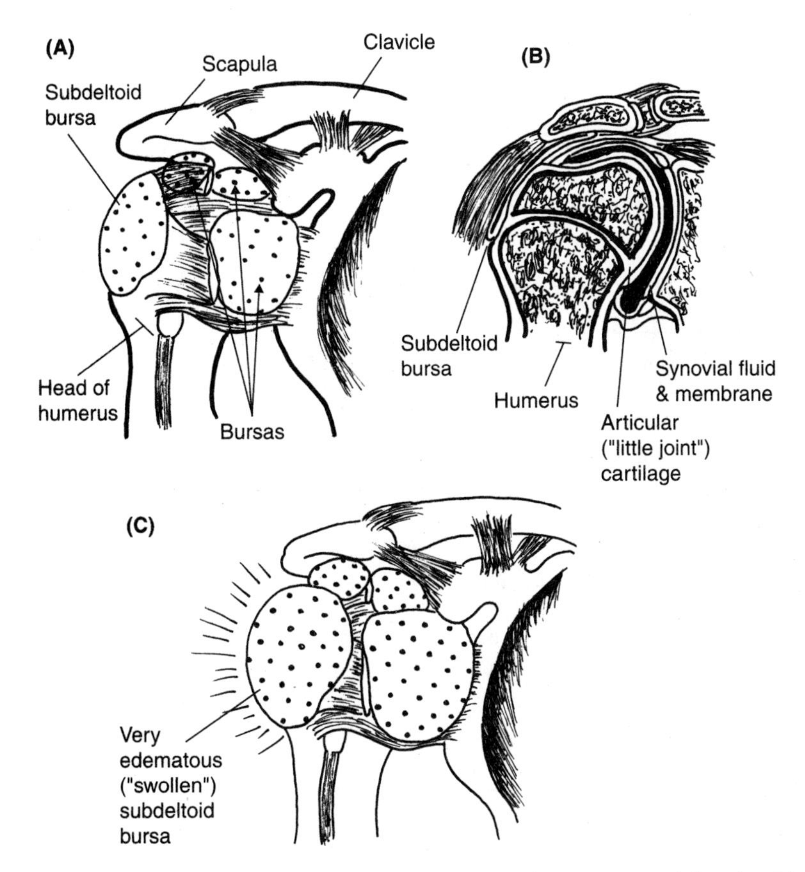

Fig. 7.9 Bursas and the shoulder joint. **(A)** Four small bursas around the shoulder joint. **(B)** Internal anatomy of the shoulder joint. **(C)** Bursitis associated with a *chronic overuse syndrome* of the shoulder joint.

disease, because the entire joint can eventually degenerate or break down. Pain, especially after exercise, is usually the earliest symptom. Severe limitation of joint motion may also occur.

SUMMARY TABLE 7.1

Consult Summary Table 7.1 for a quick review of some important words and word parts.

THE MUSCULAR SYSTEM AND ITS ORGANS

Now that we have introduced the skeletal system, its bones and joints, and some of the disorders of the skeletal system, it is now fitting to look at the muscular system. In humans, the muscular system "refers to" (*-ar*) more than 600 "little

Summary Table 7.1 Words and Word Parts

Write in the *exact* meaning (literal English translation) for up to 10 key terms selected from the preceding block of text. After you are done, check your word meanings with the correct answers, which are given at the end of this chapter.

Key Terms	**Prefixes**	**Roots**	**Suffixes**	**Exact Meanings**
endoskeleton	endo- "within"	skelet "hard dried body"	-on "presence of"	1. ________
axial	(none)	axi "axle"	-al "pertaining to"	2. ________
appendicular	(none)	appendicul "little attachment"	-ar "relating to"	3. ________
interphalangeal	inter- "between"	phalange "phalanges (battle lines of soldiers)"	-al "referring to"	4. ________
synovial	syn- "together"	ovi "eggs"	-al "pertaining to"	5. ________
flexion	(none)	flex "bending"	-ion "process of"	6. ________
extension	(none)	extens "straightening"	-ion "process of"	7. ________
carpals	(none)	carp "wrist"	-als "pertaining to"	8. ________
metacarpals	meta- "beyond"	carp "wrist"	-als "pertaining to"	9. ________
humerus	(none)	humer "upper arm"	-us "presence of"	10. ________

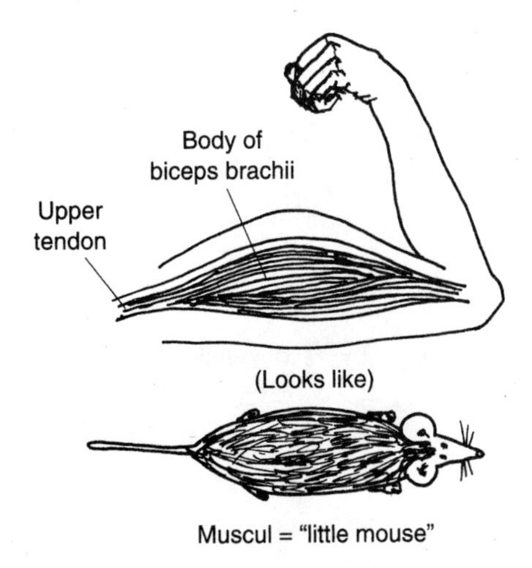

Fig. 7.10 The biceps brachii "mouse" and its "tail".

mice" (*muscul*) attached to the bones of the skeleton! These "little mice" are, in reality, the individual skeletal muscle organs.

Figure 7.10 reveals the highly imaginative thinking behind this strange metaphor. The *biceps* (***BUY***-seps) *brachii* (***BRAY***-kee-*eye*) muscle is pictured as being a mouse-like bulge in the forearm, hidden under the skin. [**Study suggestion:** Go ahead and flex, then extend, your forearm. Doesn't this rather look like a "little mouse" (*muscul*) running back-and-forth beneath your skin?] Note that there is a *tendon* or "stretcher" attached at each end of the muscle (like the tail of a mouse). A tendon is a thin strap of dense *fibrous* (**FEYE**-brus, "fiber"-containing) *connective tissue* that attaches a skeletal muscle to a bone. When the skeletal muscle contracts and shortens, the tendon is stretched longer. But when the muscle relaxes and lengthens, the tendon is unstretched.

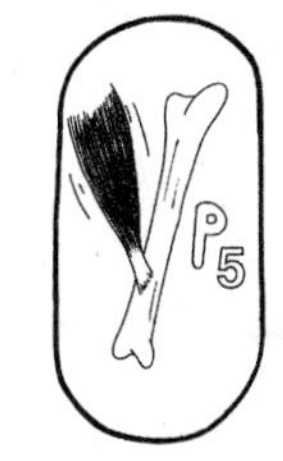

Summarizing, we have:

MUSCULAR SYSTEM = **MORE THAN 600 SKELETAL MUSCLE ORGANS** + **TENDONS (attach muscles to bones)**

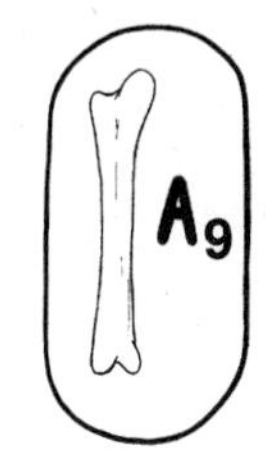

Some muscles of the face and shoulder

Figure 7.11 reveals some representative muscles of the neck and face. There are three *orbicularis* (or-**bik**-you-**LAIR**-is) muscles forming "little orbits" around both the "eyes" (*oculi*) and the "mouth" (*oris*). Helping you eat your

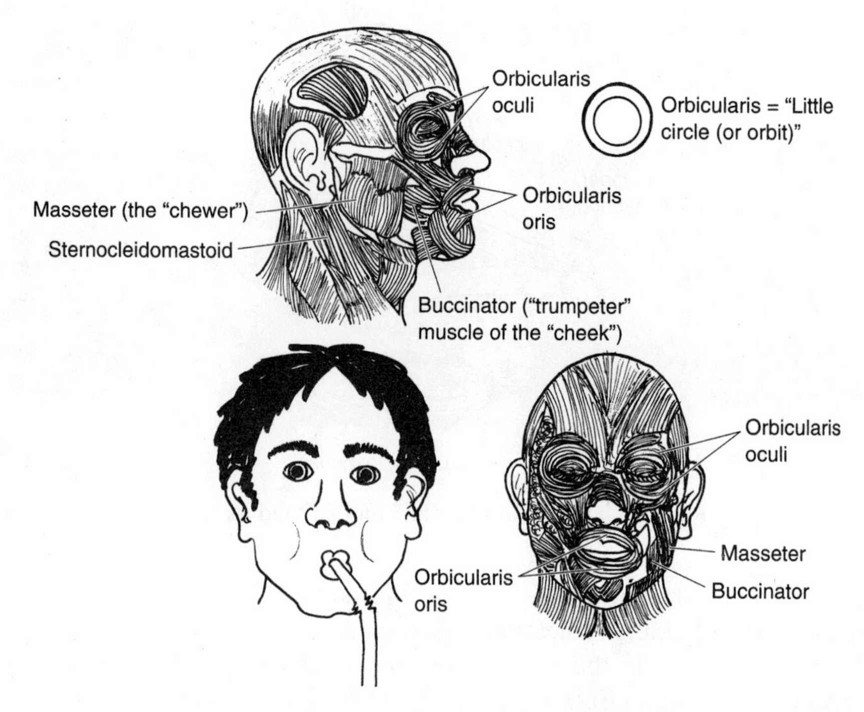

Fig. 7.11 Some muscles of the face and neck.

food is the *masseter* (mah-**SEE**-ter), Latin for "chewer." Assisting you in blowing bubbles is the *buccinator* (**BUK**-sih-**nay**-ter), known as the "trumpeter" muscle in the side of the "cheek." Helping you to nod your head up and down is the *sternocleidomastoid* (**ster**-noh-**kleye**-doh-**MASS**-toyd) muscle.

The tongue-twisting name, *sternocleidomastoid*, is derived from its points of attachment to the skeleton (Figure 7.12). These are the "sternum" (*sterno*), the "clavicle" (*cleido*), and the *mastoid* (**MASS**-toyd) *process*. Mastoid translates to mean "breast" (*mast*) "resembling" (*-oid*). [**Study suggestion:** With your fingertips, palpate for the rounded bottom tip of the mastoid process. It is the bony, breast-like bump you can feel just posterior to your ear.]

Some muscles of the arm and leg

We have already mentioned two muscles of the arm: the biceps brachii and the deltoid. Figure 7.13 shows these and more. As you can see, the deltoid "resembles" (*-oid*) a "triangle" (*delt*) in shape. The biceps brachii has "two" (*bi-*) "heads" (*ceps*) or major divisions with attached tendons. The *brachii*

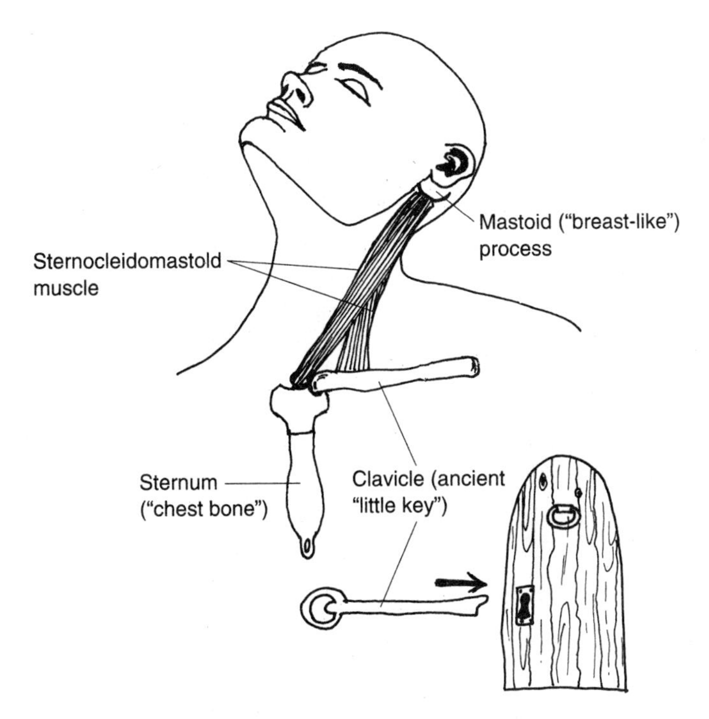

Fig. 7.12 The sternocleidomastoid muscle, named for its attachments.

part of its name indicates its location in the upper "arm" (*brachi*). The biceps brachii is a major *flexor* or "bender" of the forearm. The *brachialis* (**bray**-kee-**AL**-is) muscle, also in the "arm," helps the biceps brachii do its flexing action.

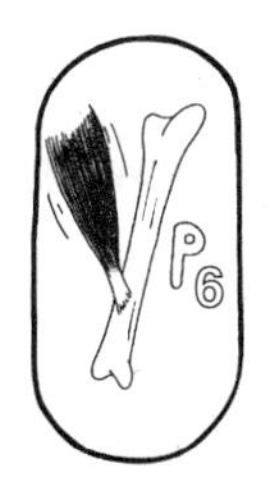

Conversely, note the presence of the *triceps* (**TRY**-seps) *brachii* (**BRAY**-kee-eyez)—a "three" (*tri-*) "headed" (*ceps*) muscle on the back of the upper "arm" (*brachi*). The triceps brachii *extends* or "straightens" out the forearm when it contracts. [**Study suggestion:** Try this action on yourself! Feel the back of your upper arm tighten when you fully extend your forearm.]

Several skeletal muscles of the upper leg are displayed in Figures 7.13 (D) and (E). If we can get off our "big" (*maxim*) "rumps" (*glute*), then we shall be privileged to examine the *gluteus* (**GLOO**-tee-us) *maximus* (**MAX**-ih-**mus**), which is "present" (*-us*)! Inferior to it, on the posterior aspect of the thigh, discover the *biceps femoris* (**FEM**-or-is). This is a "two-headed" (*biceps*) muscle behind the "femur" located on the back of the "thigh" (*femor*). The biceps femoris of the thigh (like the biceps brachii of the upper arm) is a flexor muscle. [**Reading & understanding probe:** So, what specific body action, exactly, does the biceps femoris carry out?]

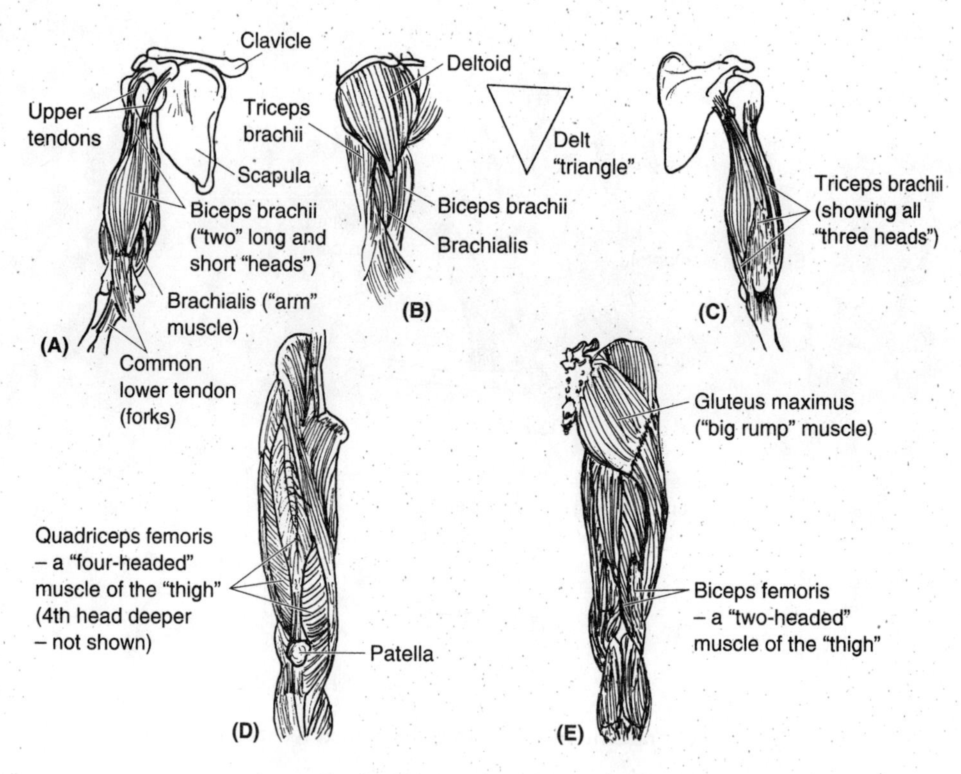

Fig. 7.13 Some muscles of the arm and leg.

On the anterior surface of the thigh, note the large *quadriceps* (**KWAHD**-rih-seps) *femoris* (**FEM**-or-is) group. This "four-headed" (*quadriceps*) group runs down the front of the thigh and acts as a powerful extensor of the lower leg. [**Advice for additional study:** A much more thorough discussion of the normal structure and function of the skeletal muscles is provided in our friendly tablemates, *ANATOMY DEMYSTIFIED* and *PHYSIOLOGY DEMYSTIFIED*. So why don't you go get them, and dig in?]

DISORDERS OF SKELETAL MUSCLES

Skeletal muscles and their tendons, like their partnering bones and joints, have particular weaknesses that make them susceptible to disease or injury.

Muscles strain, but ligaments sprain

Probably the most common *musculoskeletal* (**musk**-you-loh-**SKEL**-eh-tal)—"muscle" (*muscul*) and bony "skeleton" (*skelet*)—problems we experience are various *strains* and *sprains*. The terminology is similar and therefore confusing. A *muscle strain*, also called a *muscle pull*, is literally a "drawing [out] tight" or overstretching of a skeletal muscle. The muscle is abnormally pulled beyond the normal range of its usual length (Figure 7.14, A). In technical terms, there is a muscular *hyperextension* (**high**-per-eks-**TEN**-shun) or "process of" (*-ion*) "excessive or above normal" (*hyper-*) "stretching out" (*extens*). Because the muscle is pulled beyond its normal range, some of its individual *muscle fibers*

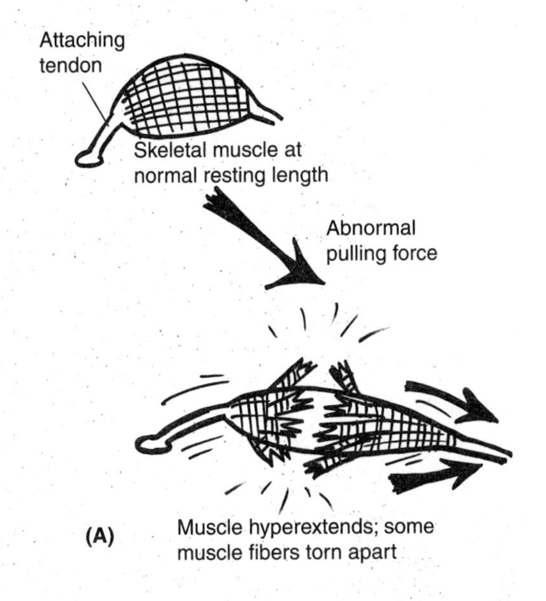

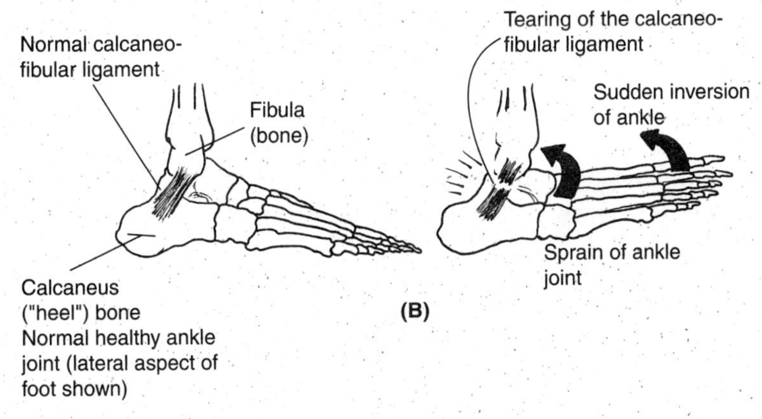

Fig. 7.14 Muscle strain versus ligament sprain. **(A)** Muscle *strain*: A skeletal muscle gets overstretched and hyperextended, resulting in tearing of the muscle fibers **(B)** Ligament *sprain* in the ankle joint: Tearing of the *calcaneo-fibular ligament*.

(thin, fiber-shaped cells) get torn. This results in muscular pain and, depending upon the severity of the muscle tear, some degree of *internal bleeding*.

A *back strain*, for instance, could involve a sudden overstretching (hyperextension) and tearing of fibers in the low muscles of the back, as when slipping and falling on the ice.

Summarizing the basic course of events, we have:

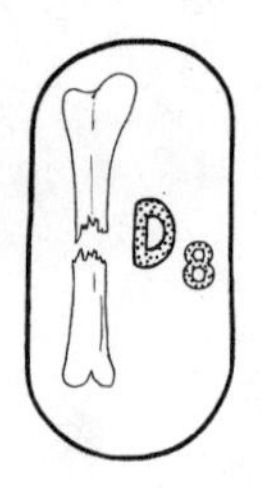

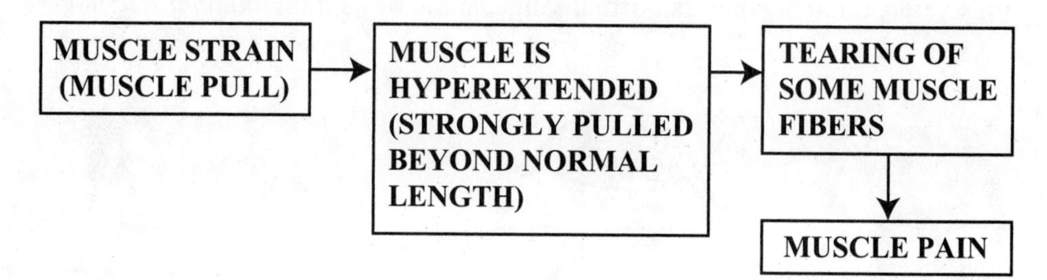

Now we know that strains happen to skeletal muscles. A *ligament* (**LIG**-ah-**ment**), in contrast, is a narrow "band" of tough collagen and stretchy elastic fibers that connects bones to each other. Especially common problems involve the *ligamentous* (**lig**-ah-**MEN**-tus) tissue of the tarsals (ankle bones). These are illustrated in Figure 7.14 (B).

In particular, there is the very common problem of *tendon* or *ligament sprain*. The actual word, *sprain*, means to "force out." A sprain is thus a sudden "forcing out of place" of a tendon or ligament near a joint. Specifically, the tendon/ligament is hyperextended far beyond its normal length. Some of the connective tissue fibers within these "forced out," abnormally hyperextended ligaments or tendons may rupture or tear. However, there is no bone fracture or actual dislocation of the nearby joint. Sprains are graded into *first-degree*, *second-degree*, and *third-degree* sprains, with the higher degrees indicating more severe ligament damage.

Figure 7.14 (B) shows the dynamics of an *ankle sprain*. The more *lateral* ligaments strapping the ankle bones together on the *outside* of the foot are the ones most frequently sprained. Consider the *calcaneo-fibular* (**kal-KAY**-nee-oh-**FIB**-you-lar) *ligament*, for example. It is the ligament that attaches the outer surface of the *calcaneus* (**kal-KAY**-nee-us) or "heel bone" to the *fibula* (**FIB**-you-lah) bone in the lower leg. The most frequent cause of ankle sprain (especially of the calcaneo-fibular ligament) is a sudden *inversion* (**in-VER**-zhun) or "turning" (*vers*) "inward" (*in-*) of the ankle. The connective tissue fibers in the calcaneo-fibular ligament are overstretched and may rupture or tear. This results in pain, swelling, and limitation of ankle motion. Such ankle inversion (sudden turning inward) can occur during various running sports. At other times, however, it may involve an accident as simple as twisting your ankle inward when you step off a curb into the street!

Summarizing sprains, we have:

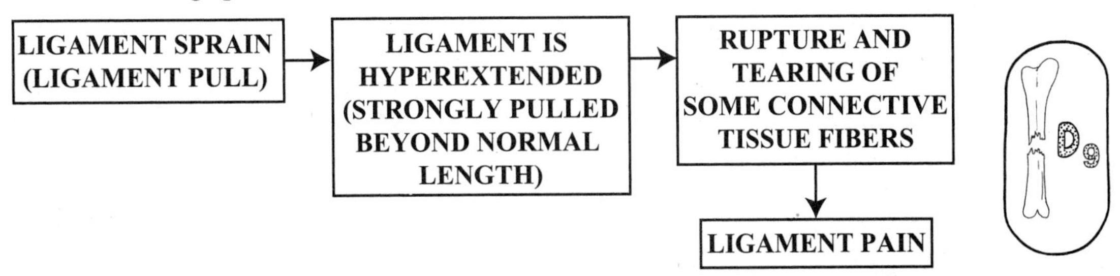

It is good to remember this helpful *"Strain and Sprain Rule": **Skeletal muscles** are **strained,** while **ligaments** are **sprained,** but both of these can give you a lot of pain!"*

SUMMARY TABLE 7.2

Consult Summary Table 7.2 for a quick review of some important words and word parts.

Summary Table 7.2 Words and Word Parts

Write in the *exact* meaning (literal English translation) for up to 10 key terms selected from the preceding block of text. After you are done, check your word meanings with the correct answers, which are given at the end of this chapter.

Key Terms	Prefixes	Roots	Suffixes	Exact Meanings
muscular	(none)	muscul "little mouse"	-ar "referring to"	1. ________
deltoid	(none)	delt "triangle"	-oid "resembling"	2. ________
biceps brachii	bi- "two"	ceps "heads"; brachi "arm"	-i (plural)	3. ________
triceps brachii	tri- "three"	ceps "head"; brachi "arm"	-i (plural)	4. ________
hyperextension	hyper- "excessive"	extens "straightening"	-ion "process of"	5. ________

Medical Case History: Arthroscopy of the Knee Joint in an Injured Runner

Bob F., a very committed long-distance runner, recently suffered a severe incident of *arthralgia* (**arth-RAL**-juh)—an "abnormal condition of pain" (*-algia*) in the "joint" (*arthr*) of his right knee. During clinical examination, the pain was quite severe on both extension and flexion of the knee. Bob explained that his right foot had fallen off the edge of some steep pavement during his last marathon, wrenching his right knee outward and dramatically *everting* (e-**VERT**-ting) his right foot in the process. In addition, Bob heard a loud "popping" noise as he fell. About two hours after the accident, the knee region became severely *edematous* (eh-**DEM**-ah-**tus**) or "swollen."

Background on the knee joint

To provide an overview, we can say that the knee joint is the largest and one of the most complex joints within the entire body. And because of its heavy weight-bearing responsibility, it is also one of the most frequently injured joints.

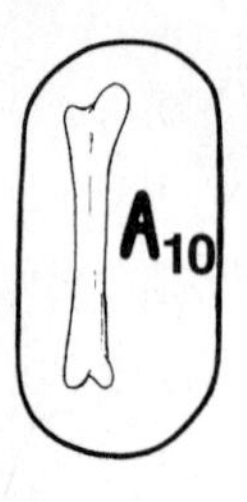

The knee is technically called the *tibiofemoral* (**TIB**-e-oh-**FEM**-or-al) *joint*. This is because the joint connects the "femur" (*femor*) above and the *tibia* (**TIB**-ee-ah) or "shin" bone below (Figure 7.15). The joint cavity of the knee contains two plates of cartilage: the *lateral meniscus* (men-**IS**-kus) more to the "side" (*later*), plus a *medial meniscus* located more toward the "middle" (*medi*) of the body. Each meniscus is named for its shallow, curved "crescent" (*menisc*)

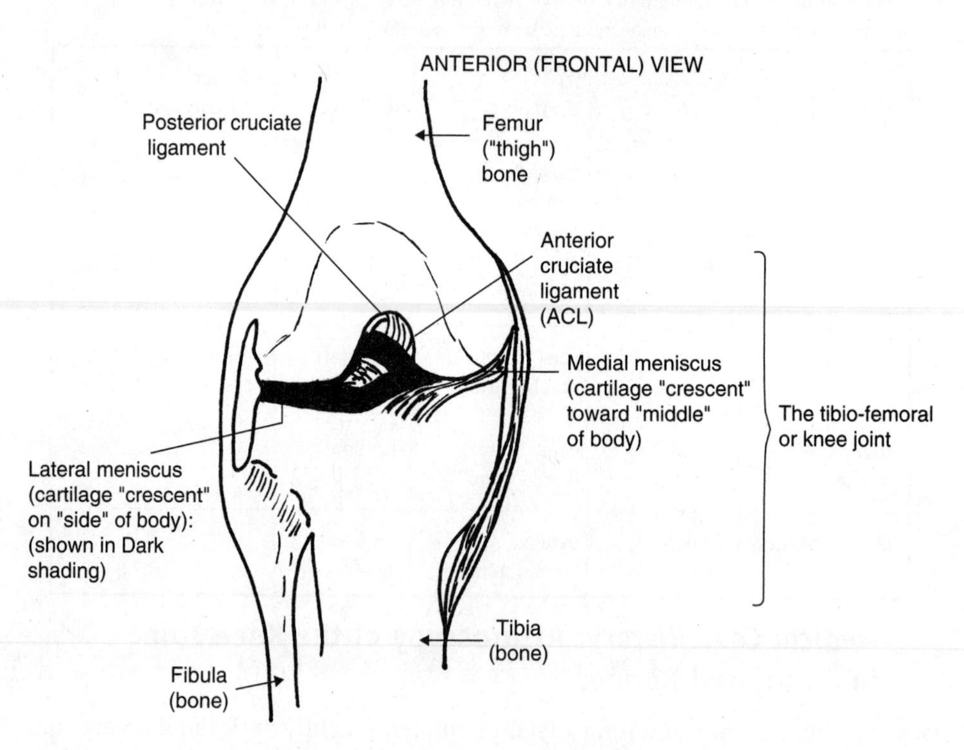

Fig. 7.15 Some of the cartilage and ligaments in the normal knee (*tibiofemoral*) joint.

shape. These two *menisci* (**MEN**-ih-**see**), or cartilage "crescents," function as shallow sockets that hold the bottom of the femur. They also serve as effective shock absorbers within the knee joint. Finally, they keep the femur from rocking from side to side upon the tibia.

Several ligaments strap the bones and cartilages together within the knee joint. From an anterior (frontal) view (Figure 7.15), we can see two of the most important. These are the *anterior cruciate* (**KROO**-she-**it**) *ligament,* which is more in "front" (*anteri*), and the *posterior cruciate* (**KROO**-she-**it**) *ligament,* located farther "behind" (*posteri*). Figure 7.15 shows that these two ligaments are called cruciate because they "cross" (*cruci*) over one another as they run from the tibia up to the femur. The cruciate ligaments help prevent the jointed bone surfaces from sliding out of their normal positions.

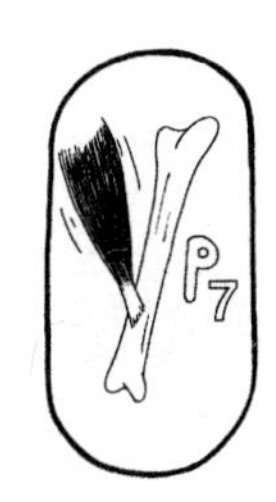

Clinical activities involving the patient

In the case of Bob F., the injured marathon runner, his *general practitioner* (*GP*) applied an ice pack to the damaged right knee. He also prescribed some oral analgesics, and referred him to a local *orthopedist* (**or**-thoh-**PEA**-dist). This is literally "one who specializes in" (*-ist*) "correcting or straightening" (*ortho-*) injuries or deformities in the muscles, bones, and joints. The *ped* part of *orthopedics* (**or**-thoh-**PEA**-diks) reflects the fact that this discipline began as a specialty for treating deformities in "children."

A series of knee *arthrograms* (**ARTH**-roh-**grams**)—x-ray "records" (*-gram*) of the knee "joint" (*arthr*)—suggested severe tearing of the lateral meniscus. "Bob, we're going to scope you," the orthopedist explained. Bob was given a local anesthetic in the knee area, as part of a preoperative procedure for *arthroscopy* (**arth-RAH**-skoh-pea). Arthroscopy is literally—a "process of examining" (*-scopy*) the knee "joint" (*arthr*). (A crude overview of this procedure is provided in Figure 7.16.)

A narrow, tube-like *arthroscope* (**ARTH**-roh-**skohp**), or "instrument used for examining a joint," was inserted through a small incision in the knee. Above it, another needle was inserted, which injected a quantity of *saline* (**SAY**-leen)—"salt" water. The saline expanded the knee joint and provided a clear view of its internal anatomy. In addition to a torn lateral meniscus, a rupture in the *ACL* (*anterior cruciate ligament*) was also observed *arthroscopically* (**arth**-roh-**SKAHP**-ik-lee). The orthopedist concluded that *arthroplasty* (**ARTH**-roh-**plas**-tee) or "surgical repair" (*-plasty*) of the knee "joint" (*arthr*), was required. Several small new incisions were made in the knee, and a variety of *arthroscopic* (**arth**-roh-**SKAHP**-ik) surgical instruments were inserted into the knee joint cavity.

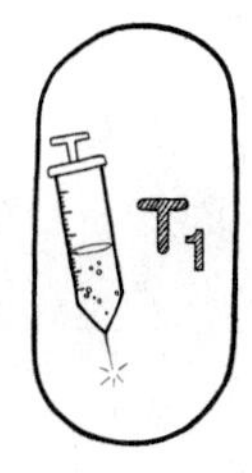

The *orthopedic* (**or**-thoh-**PEA**-dik) *surgeon* sutured the torn lateral meniscus, but he decided to replace the damaged ACL with a *graft* (another name for

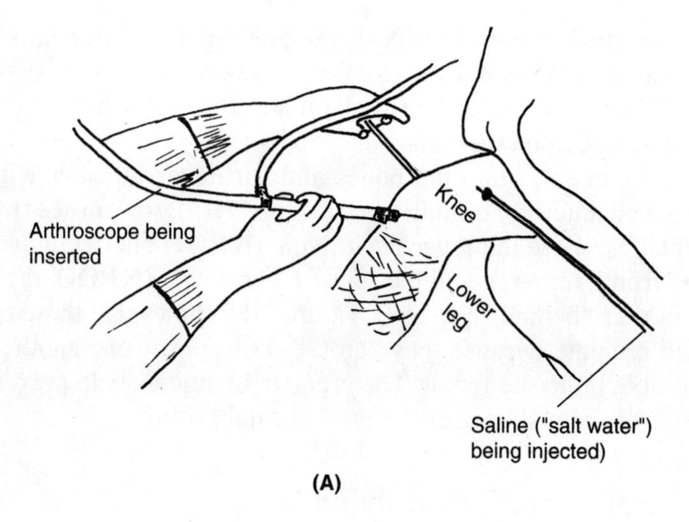

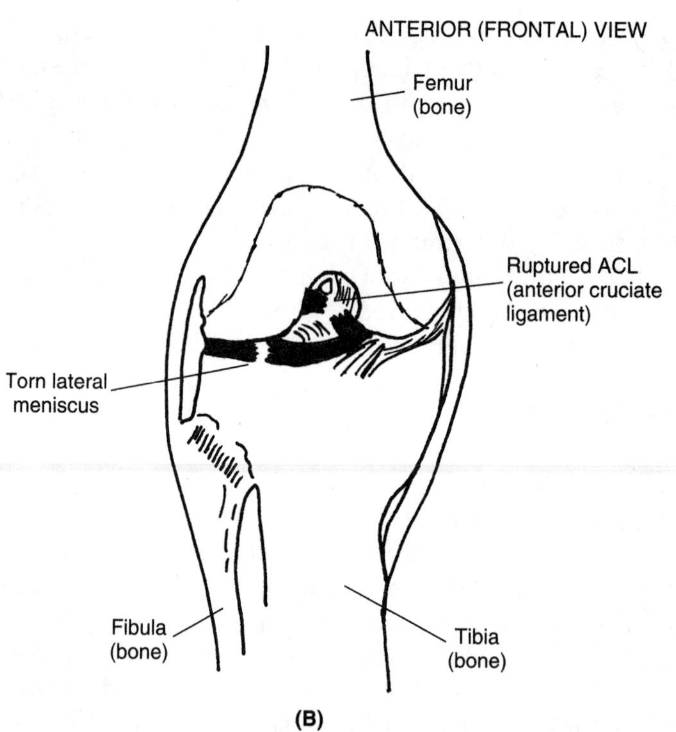

Fig. 7.16 Getting a feeling for arthroscopy. **(A)** Arthroscopy for the knee joint. **(B)** Arthroscopic view of torn *lateral meniscus* and ruptured *anterior cruciate ligament* (*ACL*) within the knee joint.

a *tissue transplant*). He took the graft (transplant) from the nearby *patellar* (pah-**TEL**-ar) *ligament*. This ligament hooks onto the *patella*—the "kneecap or kneepan" bone. The transplanted piece of patellar ligament eventually became ingrown with blood vessels and was thickened and strengthened naturally with additional collagen fibers.

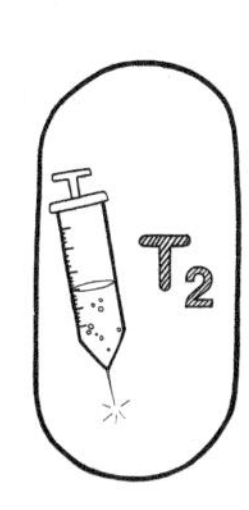

Probe of case history

(**A**) Suppose that the patient was suffering from *tendinalgia* (**TEN**-din-**AL**-juh), as well as arthralgia. What would this exactly mean, in common English? (**B**) Build a single term for "surgical repair of a muscle." [Check your short answers with the key near the end of this chapter.]

Quiz

Refer to the text in this chapter if necessary. A good score is at least 8 correct answers out of these 10 questions. The answers are listed in the back of this book.

1. The human skeletal system is most correctly classified as:
   (a) An exoskeleton
   (b) A collection of uncoordinated bones and cartilages
   (c) Just a bunch of bones
   (d) An endoskeleton
2. The portion of the skeletal system located within the body limbs:
   (a) Cranial bones
   (b) Appendicular
   (c) Mandibular
   (d) Axial
3. By definition, the interphalangeal joints would be found:
   (a) "Between the battle lines of soldiers"
   (b) "Within the little cartilages of the ankle"
   (c) "Around a three-headed muscle"
   (d) "Below the bones of the fingers and toes"
4. Osteoporotic bones are more likely to fracture than normal ones, because they:
   (a) Contain Haversian canals
   (b) Are now more weight-bearing than before
   (c) Only occur in young children, whose bones are softer
   (d) Hold central or Haversian canals that have greatly enlarged

5. These bones lie "beyond" those in the ankle:
   (a) Cranial
   (b) Tarsals
   (c) Metatarsals
   (d) Metacarpals
6. The main extensor muscle in the upper arm:
   (a) Biceps femoris
   (b) Buccinator
   (c) Triceps brachii
   (d) Sternocleidomastoid
7. "Pertains to the thigh":
   (a) Femoral
   (b) Mastoid
   (c) Talar
   (d) Carpal
8. Hyperstress causes bone fracture because it also causes bone:
   (a) Physiology
   (b) Tumors
   (c) Hyperstrain
   (d) Normostress
9. If you were a nurse trying to reassure a patient, you would most likely say, "Don't worry! Your fracture is just a ______ one!"
   (a) Simple greenstick
   (b) Compound complete
   (c) Simple but extensively fragmented
   (d) Compound incomplete
10. A *musculitis* (**mus**-kyoo-**LIE**-tis) is a technical term for:
    (a) An x-ray record of some skeletal muscle
    (b) Removal of a bone
    (c) Inflammation of a muscle
    (d) Hyperextension of a tendon

Memory Pillboxes for Chapter 7

Several key facts were tagged with numbered icons in the page margins of this chapter. Write a short summary of each of these key facts into a numbered cell or compartment within the appropriate type of *Memory Pillbox* that appears below.

Anatomy Pillboxes for Chapter 7:

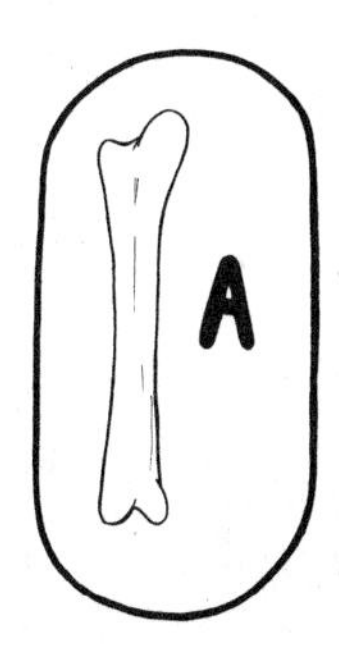

1	2
3	4
5	6
7	8

9	10

Physiology Pillboxes for Chapter 7:

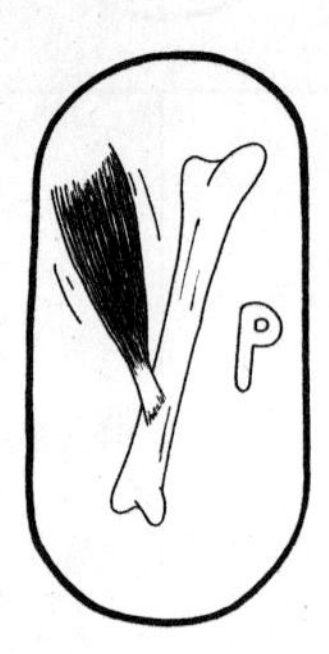

1	2

3	4

5	6

7

Disease/Injury **Pillboxes for Chapter 7:**

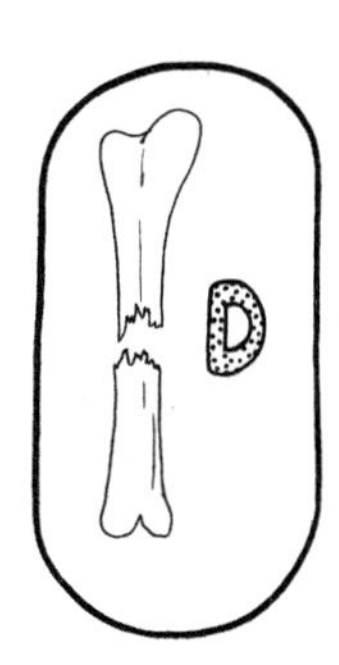

1

2	3
4	5
6	7
8	9

***Treatment/Therapy* Pillboxes for Chapter 7:**

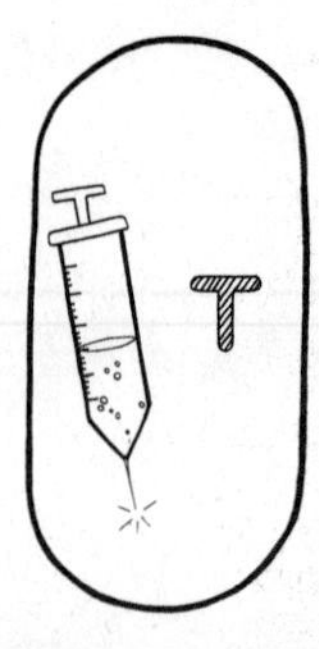

1	2

Answers for Chapter 7 Summary Tables

FOR SUMMARY TABLE 7.1

1. "presence of a hard dried body within"
2. "pertaining to an axle"
3. "relating to a little attachment"
4. "referring to (something) between phalanges"
5. "pertaining to eggs together"
6. "process of bending"
7. "process of straightening"
8. "pertaining to the wrist"
9. "pertaining to (something) beyond the wrist"
10. "presence of the upper arm"

FOR SUMMARY TABLE 7.2

1. "referring to a little mouse"
2. "resembling a triangle"
3. "two-headed" (muscle) in "arm"
4. "three-headed (muscle) in "arm"
5. "process of excessive straightening"

Answers to Probe of Case History

(**A**) "A condition of pain in a tendon." (**B**) Musculoplasty.

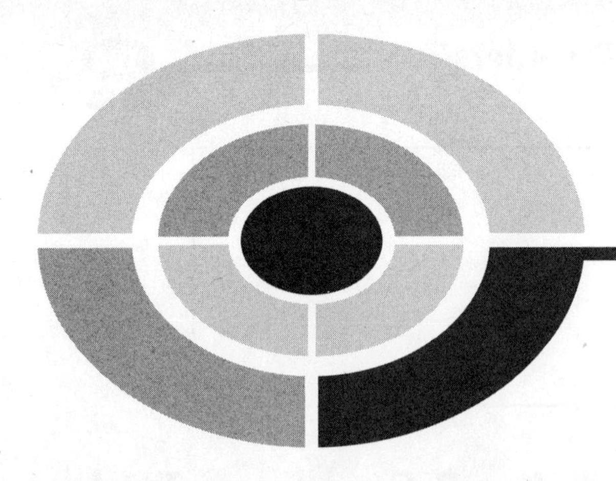

Test: Part 3

DO NOT REFER TO THE TEXT WHEN TAKING THIS TEST. A good score is at least 18 (out of 25 questions) correct. The answers are in the back of the book. It's best to have a friend check your score the first time so you won't memorize the answers if you want to take the test again.

1. The central turning line around which the body pivots:
   (a) Appendix
   (b) Transverse plane
   (c) Appendicular skeleton
   (d) Articular cartilage
   (e) Axial skeleton

2. Freely movable joints are also classified as:
   (a) Fibrous
   (b) Synovial
   (c) Bursas
   (d) Sutures
   (e) Biceps

3. Cutting a _______ would cause one end of a skeletal muscle to droop.
   (a) Joint
   (b) Stone
   (c) Tendon
   (d) Ligament
   (e) Valve

4. A root for "bend":
   (a) Flex
   (b) Oste
   (c) Extens
   (d) Contract
   (e) Ligat

5. There are fewer than _______ skeletal muscles in the adult body.
   (a) 100
   (b) 200
   (c) 400
   (d) 500
   (e) 7,000

6. An individual long bone, such as the femur, is properly assigned to the _______ level of the Great Body Pyramid.
   (a) Tissue
   (b) Organ
   (c) Molecule
   (d) Organ system
   (e) Entire organism

7. *Intercarpal* joints would be found where?
   (a) Between the bones of the wrist
   (b) Around the knee joint
   (c) Flanking either side of the gonads
   (d) Creating a "little circle" around the lips
   (e) Serving as a rod in the back

8. The word, muscular, is properly subdivided into its word parts as:
   (a) Mus/cu/lar
   (b) M/uscula/r
   (c) Muscul/ar
   (d) Mu/scu/lar
   (e) Muscula/r

9. Joint type that permits back-and-forth movement in one plane or direction only:
   (a) Shoulder
   (b) Hip
   (c) Suture
   (d) Hinge
   (e) Appendicular

10. The prefix, quadri-, indicates the fact that:
   (a) There is only one thing present
   (b) A muscle has split in half
   (c) Four things are present
   (d) You are simply rhyming with "fwah-drih"
   (e) Two or three muscle heads are involved

11. A joint is:
   (a) An example of a tissue
   (b) The place where a bone breaks down when it fractures
   (c) The usual location of red marrow
   (d) An organ of the musculoskeletal system
   (e) A type of phalanx

12. The normal range of bone stress:
   (a) Generally reflects homeostasis of the impact forces upon a bone
   (b) Frequently results in bone fracture
   (c) Inhibits the release of synovial fluid
   (d) Results in hyperstrain
   (e) Is almost constantly exceeded during normal ROM (range of motion)

13. In the phrase, *biceps brachii*, the word, *brachii*:
   (a) Translates as "arm"
   (b) Indicates muscle location in the leg
   (c) Suggests that rotation is the muscle's major movement
   (d) Reveals the number of muscle heads
   (e) Means the exact opposite of the word *trachei*

14. Which of the following bones is *not* in the axial skeleton?
   (a) Vertebra
   (b) Cranial
   (c) Mastoid process
   (d) Ulna
   (e) Wisdom tooth

15. A sprain is:
    (a) A tearing effect upon some ligaments
    (b) Disturbance of the position of the vertebral column
    (c) Too much calcium in the bloodstream
    (d) The same as a fracture
    (e) Essentially identical to a muscle strain

16. A new term created by taking the suffix of *squamous* (Chapter 6) and combining it with the root in extensor:
    (a) Extensous
    (b) Exus
    (c) Exteous
    (d) Ecstasy
    (e) Extenous

17. The formal anatomic name for "heel bone":
    (a) Talus
    (b) Deltoid
    (c) Calcaneous
    (d) Heelious
    (e) Gastrocnemius

18. If a person's ankle inverts, then it is going in what specific direction?
    (a) Revolves completely around its axis
    (b) Leaves the ground at a 90-degree angle
    (c) Turns outward
    (d) Plants the foot to the earth
    (e) Turns inward

19. A new term built by taking the prefix from *analgesia* (Chapter 2), the root from *anesthesia* (Chapter 2), and the suffix from *calcaneo-fibular*:
    (a) Anesular
    (b) Analgesular
    (c) Anesthesiar
    (d) Agesiar
    (e) Analthesiar

20. The long term, *sternocleidomastoid*, is correctly subdivided with slash marks as:
    (a) Stern/o/cleidom/as/toid
    (b) Stern/o/cleid/o/mastoid
    (c) Ste/rnocl/eidomastoid

(d) Sternocleido/mast/oid
(e) Ster/no/cleid/o/mastoid

21. The correct number of roots found in the word, *sternocleidomastoid*:
(a) One
(b) Two
(c) Three
(d) Four
(e) Five

22. "One who specializes in correcting or straightening children":
(a) ENT woman
(b) Orthodontist
(c) Pharmacologician
(d) GP
(e) Orthopedist

23. Extracting the suffix in *arthroplasty* and combining it with the root in *cruciate* (along with a combining vowel) yields:
(a) Arthrocruciate
(b) Crucioplasty
(c) Arthrocruciatology
(d) Arthriatc
(e) Crucioarthritis

24. The two menisci within the knee joint are named for their _____ shape.
(a) Crescent
(b) Bowl
(c) Triangular
(d) "Three-sided"
(e) Square

25. An acceptable alternate name for common "wear-and-tear" inflammation of joints:
(a) Epicondylitis
(b) Osteosarcoma
(c) Arthroscopy
(d) Osteoarticulitis
(e) Musculoligamentosis

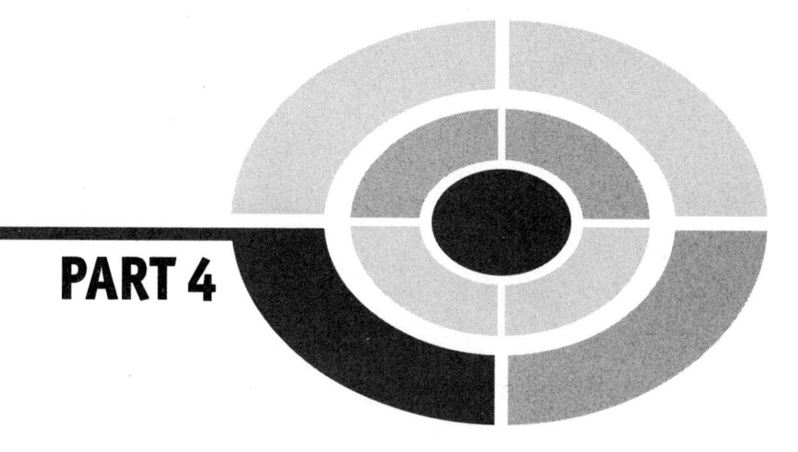

PART 4

Moving Our Blood and Air

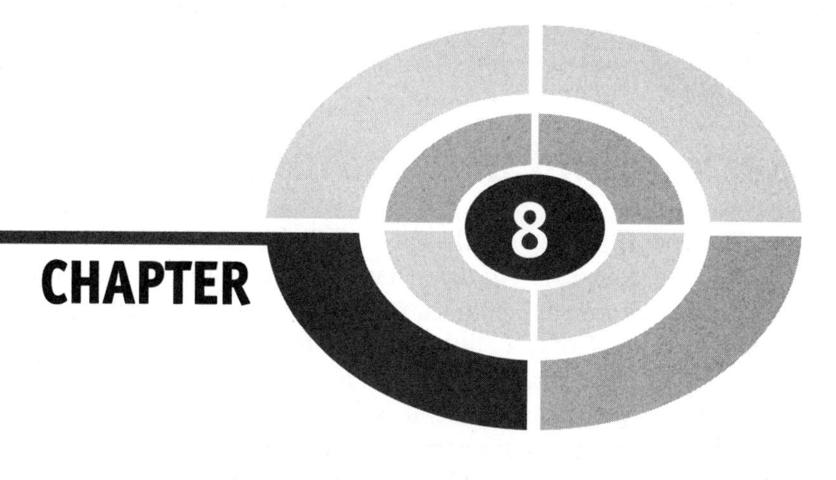

Terms Related to Disorders of the Heart and Blood Vessels

In Part 3, the normal and abnormal aspects of bones and skeletal muscles were discussed. When skeletal muscles contract and shorten, they pull upon their tendons. These tendons, in turn, pull upon certain bones. And as a final result, body movement occurs at the joints.

But skeletal muscles are definitely *not* the only kind of muscles in the body! We have *cardiac muscle* in the walls of the "heart" (*cardi*), as well as *smooth muscle* in the walls of various other viscera (internal organs), such as the *blood vessels*. In Chapter 8, we will dissect the normal and abnormal anatomy and physiology (A&P) of cardiac and smooth muscle tissue, along with the organs that contain them.

Background and History

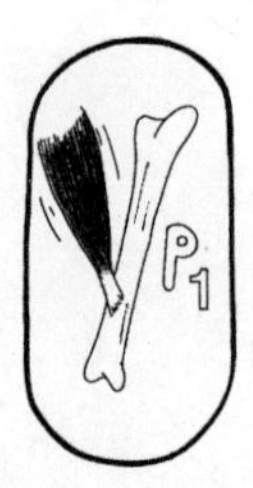

This chapter tells the story of a moving fluid tissue: the blood. The blood, of course, *circulates*. That is, it moves around the body in a "little circle" (*circul*). Figure 8.1 demonstrates this *circulatory* (**SIR**-kyuh-luh-**tor**-ee)—"pertaining to" (-ory) a "little circle"—movement. The main reason that the blood moves at all, certainly, is that it is being pumped out of one side of the "heart" (*cardi*). At the same time, it is flowing back into the opposite side of the heart. What structures are carrying the blood out of, and back toward, the heart? There is a *vascular* (**VAS**-kyoo-lar) *network*—a collection of "little vessels" (*vascul*) with open *lumens* (*Loo*-mens) or "light spaces"—that performs this absolutely critical body function.

Therefore, the organ system we are talking about is formally named the *circulatory* or *cardiovascular* (**kar**-dee-oh-**VAS**-kyuh-lar) *system*. Cardiovascular literally "pertains to" (*-ar*) the "heart" (*cardi*) and "little vessels" (*vascul*) carrying the blood. [**Thinking probe:** So, which of these two organ system names is an anatomic (body structural) name? Which is a physiological (living body function) name?]

Both the heart and the blood vessels represent the organ level of the Great Body Pyramid. The blood itself, in distinction, is a very specialized type of

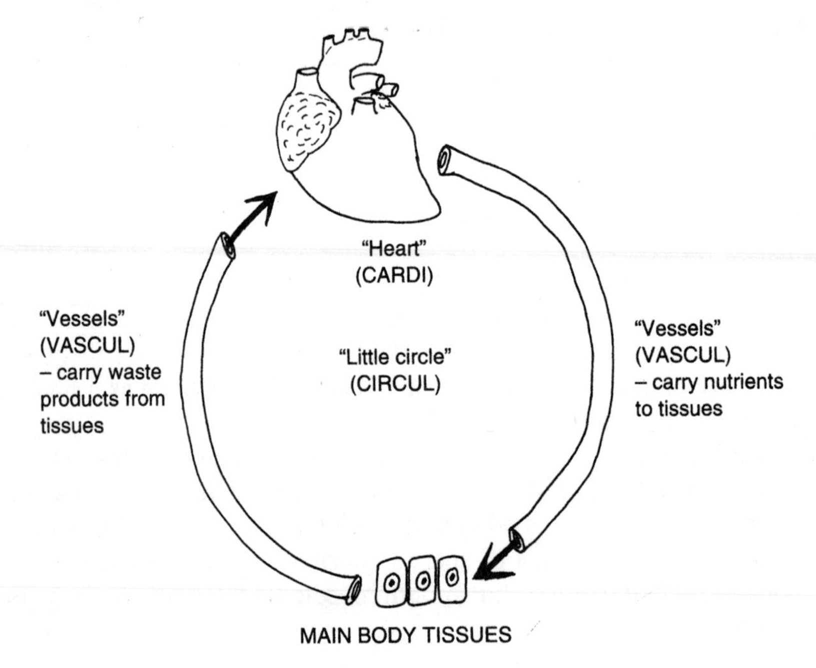

Fig. 8.1 An overview of the circulatory (cardiovascular) system.

connective tissue that indirectly ties most parts of the body together. The reason, of course, is that it circulates. Summarizing, we have:

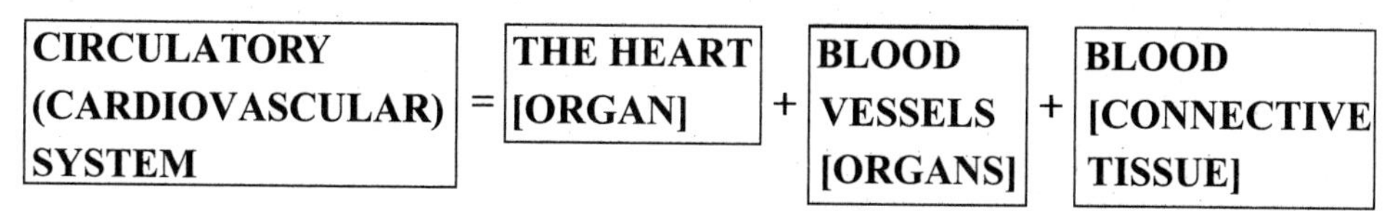

CIRCULATORY (CARDIOVASCULAR) SYSTEM	=	THE HEART [ORGAN]	+	BLOOD VESSELS [ORGANS]	+	BLOOD [CONNECTIVE TISSUE]

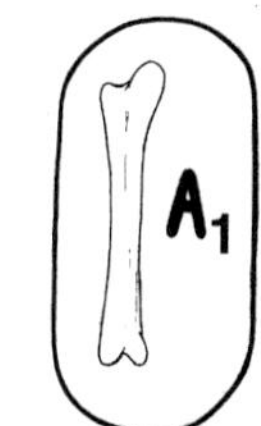

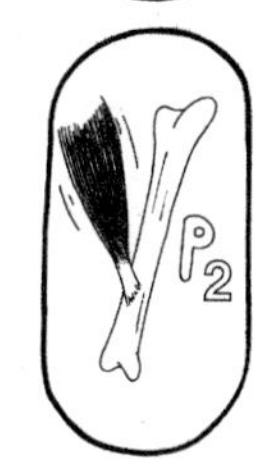

The complex function being carried out by this system is the temporary storage of blood within the heart, the pumping of nutrient-carrying blood out toward the rest of the body tissues, and finally the flowing of waste products from the tissues, back toward the heart.

GENERAL COMPONENTS OF THE VASCULAR NETWORK

"Can we be more specific about the particular *types* of blood vessels that are involved in this heart/vessel/main tissue/vessel/back to heart circulation?" an eager reader may ask. A quick answer is provided by a glance at Figure 8.2.

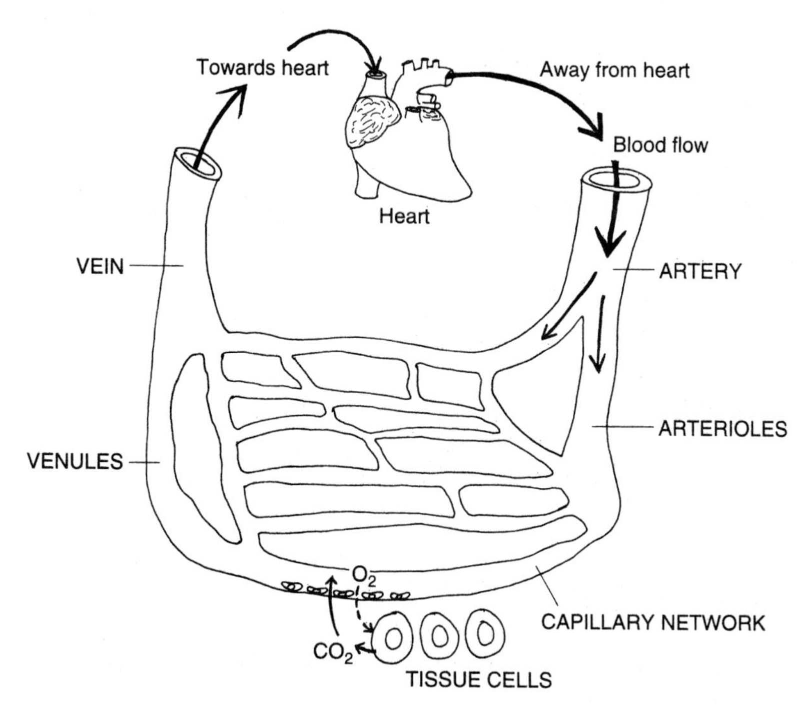

Fig. 8.2 The main types of vessels in the circulatory system.

Note that the *arteries* (**AR**-ter-**ees**) are the large-diameter vessels that always carry blood *away from* the heart. As they travel farther and farther away, they eventually split into many *arterioles* (ar-**TEER**-e-ohls). The arterioles are the "little (branches) of the arteries" (*arteriol*). When the arterioles finally reach the main body tissues, they branch even more extensively into a vast *capillary network*. The actual word, *capillary*, "refers to" (*-ary*) a "tiny hair" (*capill*). The term, *capillary*, thus reflects the fact that the lumen (light-space or open diameter) of these vessels is very narrow, like a hair! The blood within the capillary unloads its various nutrients, such as oxygen (O_2) and glucose (sugar), into the tissue cells. And the tissue cells, in turn, release the waste products of their aerobic metabolism, such as *carbon dioxide* (die-**AHKS**-eyed, abbreviated CO_2), into the bloodstream at the capillary level.

Finally, the waste-filled blood begins its return voyage. The *venules* (**VEN**-yools) start the journey back. Venules are literally the "tiny (branches of the) veins" (*venul*) "present" (*−e*) immediately *after* the capillary network. The blood in these venules soon flows into the *veins*. The veins are the large-diameter vessels that always carry blood back *toward* the heart.

In thumbnail sketch, we have:

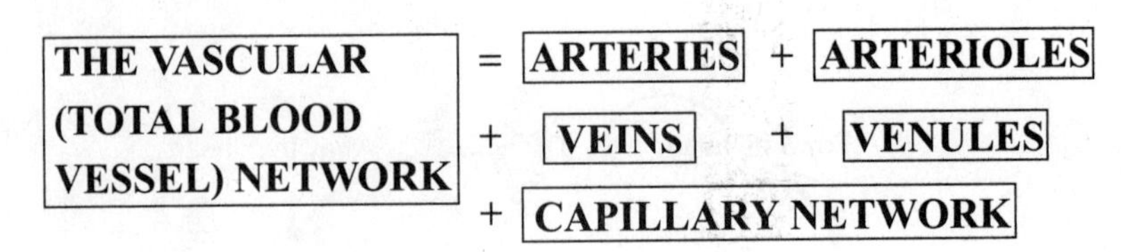

THE VASCULAR (TOTAL BLOOD VESSEL) NETWORK
= ARTERIES + ARTERIOLES
+ VEINS + VENULES
+ CAPILLARY NETWORK

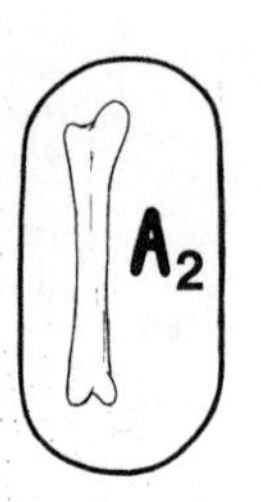

THE ONE-WAY CIRCULATION: VALVES TELL THE STORY

"Fine," the inquisitive student may persist, "but *how* do we know that the blood really *circulates* through these vessels in the first place?" The appropriate response to this question is, "Because of the pioneering work of *William Harvey*."

Before Harvey came Galen

William Harvey was an English physician who lived from 1578 to 1657. Before Harvey, the major understanding of how the blood circulates was largely false. The concept was based on the ancient teachings of Claudius Galen, a philosopher, a physician, and the very first physiologist. Review of Chapter 1 will help you recall that Galen is often called the Father of Experimental Physiology. [**Thinking probe:** Try to translate the word *physiologist* into its common

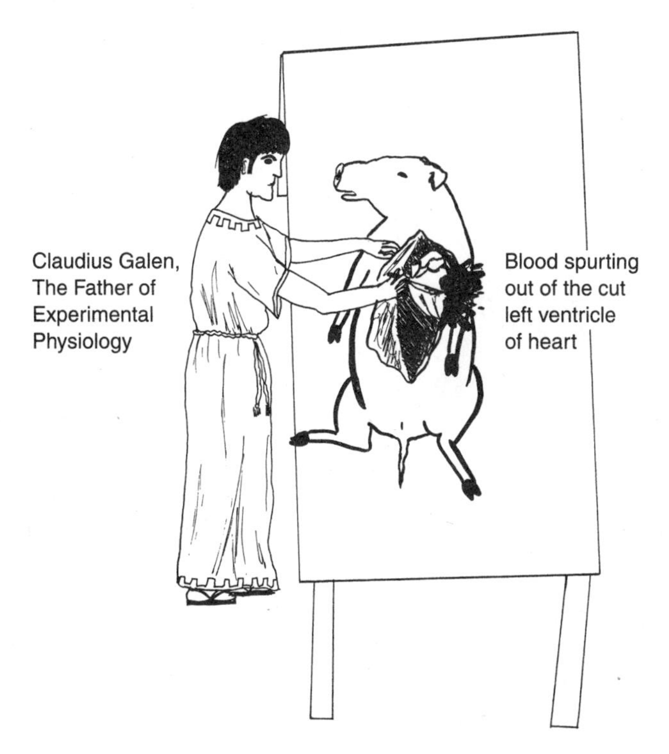

Fig. 8.3 Galen cuts open the left ventricle of the heart.

English meaning. The suffix is one that you have encountered several times!] And a quick look at Figure 8.3 will remind you that Galen carried out many dissections upon living animals. Very important among these living body functions is the pumping of blood by the heart. Galen thrust a knife into the left *ventricle* (**VEN**-trih-kul) of a pig lying on a dissection table. A ventricle is a "little belly"-like cavity at the bottom of the heart. The blood came strongly spurting out of this cut, thereby proving that blood was stored and pumped out of the heart under a great pushing force: the *blood pressure* (BP). Further, Galen showed that the arteries carry blood, not just air, as the earlier Greek scholars had mistakenly assumed. (The word, *artery*, originally meant "air-keeper" in Greek!)

The problem, though, was that Galen didn't think that the blood actually circulated through the body! Instead, he maintained that the blood pumped out of the left ventricle of the heart was *light arterial* (ar-**TEER**-e-al) *blood*, which was eventually absorbed and transformed into more body flesh! And the *dark venous* (**VEE**-nus)—"pertaining to" (*-ous*) "vein" (*ven*)—blood was part of a separate circulation that began in the liver.

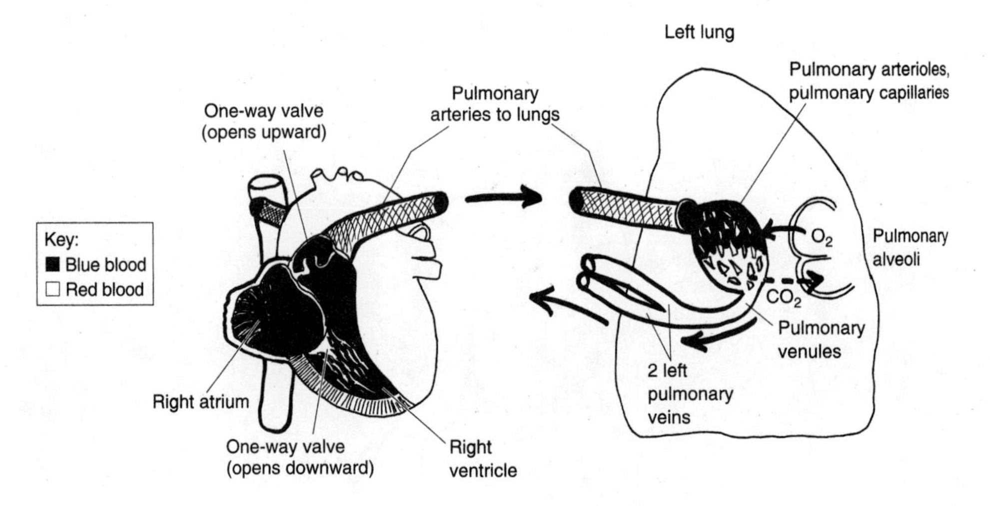

Fig. 8.4 An overview of the pulmonary (right heart) circulation.

Harvey makes a theory based upon one-way valves

For almost 2,000 years after Galen, no one seemed to seriously question his basic concepts of two separate, unconnected arterial and venous blood vessel systems that didn't circulate—No one, except William Harvey! Harvey learned from his anatomy teachers about the presence of one-way valves in the interior of the heart (Figures 8.4 and 8.5).

There are four chambers within the heart, and four one-way valves. At the top of the heart are the right and left *atria* (**A**-tree-ah). These serve as small "entrance rooms" for blood returning to the heart from veins. And at the bottom of the heart are the right and left *ventricles*. Figure 8.4 demonstrates that the entire *right* side of the heart is the pump for the *pulmonary* or "referring to" (*-ary*) "lungs" (*pulmon*) *circulation*. The one-way *valve* on this side opens and allows blood from the right atrium to be pushed down into the right ventricle. The blood from the right ventricle, in turn, is pumped out through a second one-way valve, up into an artery, and then on to the lungs. Here, the blood becomes oxygenated (filled with O_2).

Figure 8.5 reveals that the entire *left* side of the heart is a pump for the *systemic* or "referring to" (*-ic*) body "systems" (*system*) *circulation*. The one-way valve on this side opens and allows blood to pass from the left atrium down into the left ventricle. After the left ventricle contracts, it pushes blood up through a second one-way valve, up into a major artery, and eventually out to the tissues of various body organs (other than the lungs).

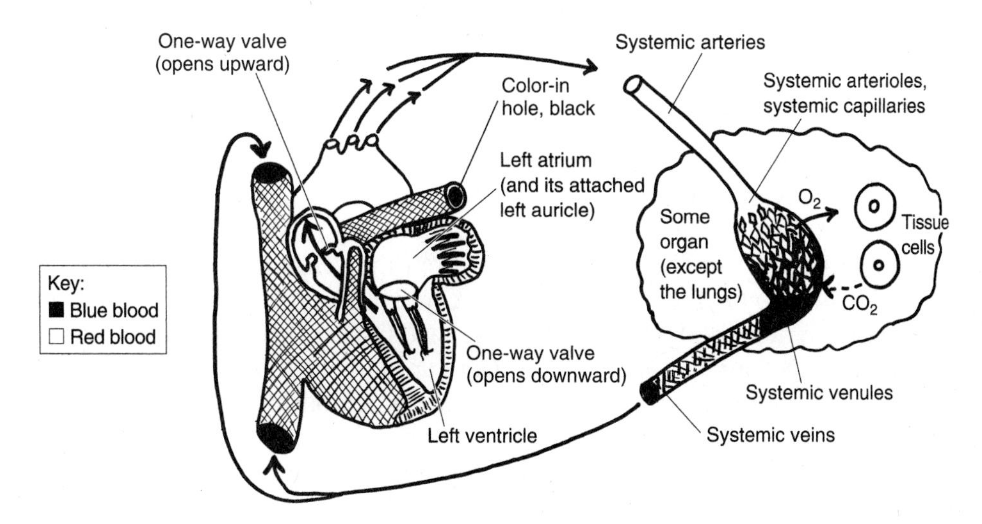

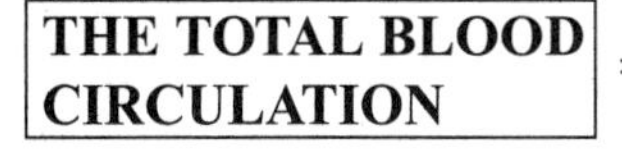

Fig. 8.5 An overview of the systemic (left heart) circulation.

Summarizing the total circulation, we have:

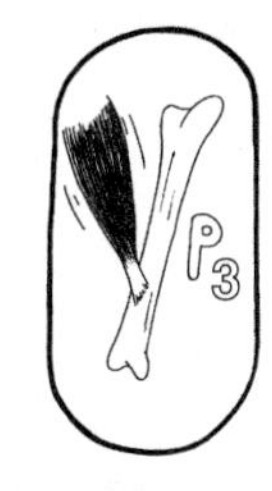

THE TOTAL BLOOD CIRCULATION	=	THE *PULMONARY* (RH) CIRCULATION	+	*THE SYSTEMIC* (LH) CIRCULATION
		(***circulation of blood to, through, and from both "lungs"***)		(***circulation of blood to, through, and from the organs of all body "systems" except for the lungs***)

Now, Harvey never fully identified the pulmonary (right heart) circulation, but he did make the very important point that the heart was the main blood pump. He also failed to realize that the capillaries actually connected the arterioles on one side with the venules on the other, thereby making one total blood circulation. (Look back at the basic plan of the circulatory system provided in Figure 8.2, if desired.) To quote his own words, "This organ [the heart] deserves to be styled the starting point of life and the sun of our microcosm, just as much as the sun deserves to be styled the heart of the world." **[Suggestion for extra reading:** The early Greek concepts of a *macrocosm* or "big universe" outside the body, plus a *microcosm* or "little universe" inside the human body, are discussed in more fascinating detail within the pages of *PHYSIOLOGY DEMYSTIFIED*.]

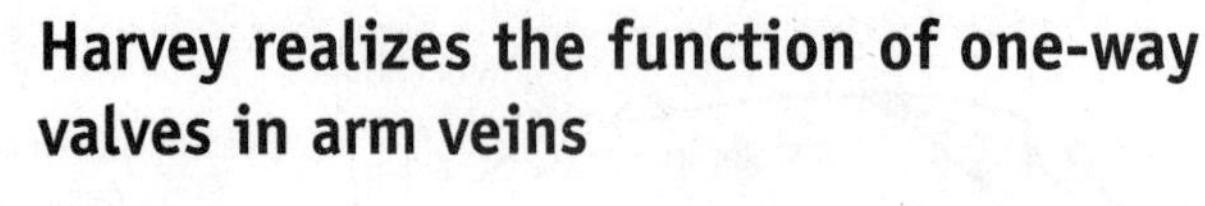

Harvey realizes the function of one-way valves in arm veins

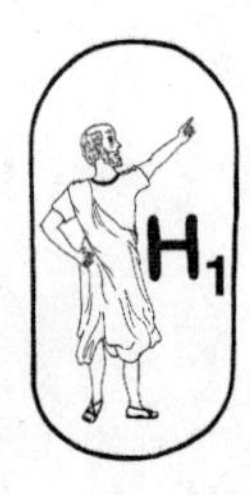

What sold Harvey on the one-way circulation of the blood (aside from the presence of four one-way valves in the heart) was the presence of one-way valves in many medium-sized veins.

Figure 8.6 (A) shows the internal anatomy of a medium-sized *peripheral* (puh-**RIF**-er-al) *vein*. This name comes from the vein's location on the outer "edge" (*periphery*) of the body. This vein could be in either the arm or leg. Note the presence of several *semilunar* (**sem**-ee-**LOO**-nar) *valves*. These valves are named for the "half" (*semi-*) "moon" (*lun*) appearance of their flaps.

Part of William Harvey's simple experiment is demonstrated in Figure 8.6 (B). Step #1: A ligature or "tie" (Chapter 2) was tightly wrapped around the lower arm, just above the elbow. This ligation ("process of tying off") stopped the one-way return flow of blood toward the heart from the veins in the lower arm. As a result, there was an obvious swelling of the veins in the lower arm with unreturned blood. In addition, their semilunar valves popped out and looked like swollen knots beneath the skin. Step #2: Using a finger, the experimenter pressed upon a vein at a point, *P*, that blocked return blood flow from the wrist area. The portion of the vein located right after the finger-blockage collapsed (sinking back into the skin). This collapsing was due to lack of return blood flow from the wrist. [**Thinking probe:** If the blood in these peripheral veins was flowing *away from* the heart, would the vein at point *P still* have collapsed? Why, or why not?]

LIGATION FOR CONTROL OF BLOOD LOSS

William Harvey used ligatures to help us understand the normal direction of blood flowing through healthy, undamaged blood vessels. But what happens if we get a cut and some of our blood vessels are torn open? The result is *hemorrhage* (**HEM**-or-uhj)—"bleeding." Uncontrolled and prolonged *hemorrhaging* (bleeding), of course, can be fatal! Why? Because people have a limited *total blood volume*. The total volume of blood in all of the vessels of an adult's body is about 5 to 6 *L* (*liters*). This number represents *normovolemia* (**nor**-moh-voh-**LEE**-me-ah). Somewhat similar to the word *normothermia*, *normovolemia* represents a "blood condition of" (*-emia*) "normal" (*normo-*) "volume" (*vol*). We can think of normovolemia as representing the maintenance of homeostasis (relative constancy) of our blood volume over time.

"Why is maintenance of normovolemia so important?" the questioner might probe. The answer is that normovolemia helps maintain a normal amount of *tissue perfusion* (per-**FYOO**-zhun). This term indicates the "process of" (*-ion*) "pouring [blood] over and through" (*perfus*) a tissue. This condition may

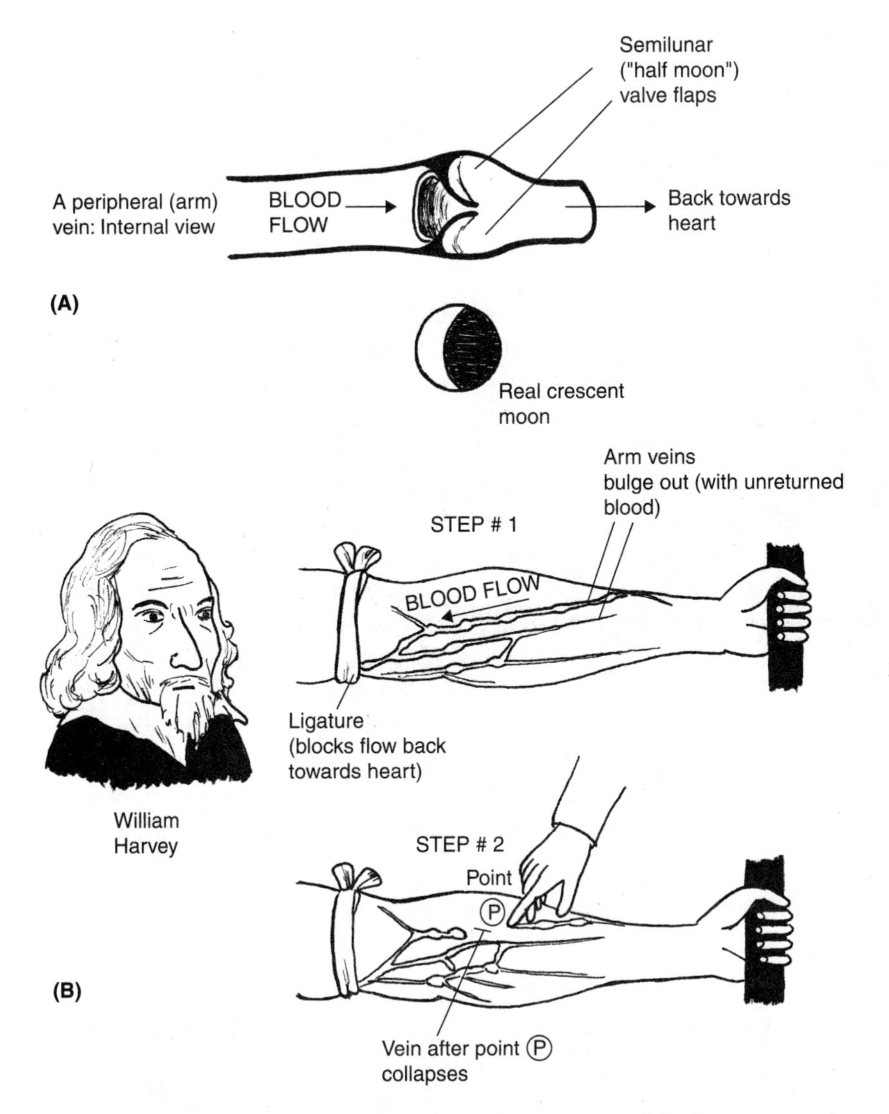

Fig. 8.6 William Harvey and his experiment with the valves of the lower arm veins. **(A)** Internal anatomy of a peripheral vein, showing a *semilunar* ("half-moon" shaped) *valve*. **(B)** Harvey demonstrates one-way valves in the lower arm veins with the help of a *ligature.*

alternately be called *normoperfusion* (**nor**-moh-per-**FYOO**-zhun). Adequate tissue perfusion (normoperfusion) supplies sufficient oxygen, glucose, and other nutrients to support the healthy metabolism of living tissue cells. The blood supply leaving the tissue also provides a medium for carrying away various metabolic waste products, such as CO_2.

Summarizing, we have:

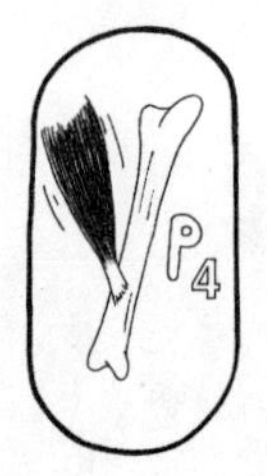

NORMOVOLEMIA (normal amount of circulating blood volume) → **NORMOPERFUSION** (normal amount of bathing of tissues with blood) → **ADEQUATE SUPPORT OF TISSUE METABOLISM**

If hemorrhaging or bleeding from a cut vessel goes on for too long, however, so much of the total blood volume will be lost that a state of *hypovolemia* (**high**-poh-voh-**LEE**-me-ah) results. [**Learning probe:** Quickly translate *hypovolemia* into common English. Check with the translation that follows.] Hypovolemia is a "blood condition of" (*-emia*) "deficient or below normal" (*hypo-*) "volume" (*vol*). In hypovolemia, not having enough total blood volume can result in a severe *tissue hypoperfusion* (**high**-poh-per-**FYOO**-zhun). This is literally a "below normal or deficient" (*hypo-*) "pouring [of blood] through" (*perfus*) the tissues. Such a hypoperfusion does *not* supply adequate nutrients to support normal tissue metabolism. The problem is especially severe in very oxygen-dependent organs, such as the brain and kidneys. If about one-fifth of the total blood volume is lost by hemorrhage (1 to 2 L in an adult), then the result is *hypovolemic* (**high**-poh-voh-**LEE**-mik) *shock*. This severe state of physiological shock can bring on *coma* (failure of the brain) as well as *renal* (**REE**-nal, "pertaining to kidney") *failure*! Coma and kidney failure, if not quickly compensated for by medical treatment, can lead to death. Putting all of this information together in sequence yields:

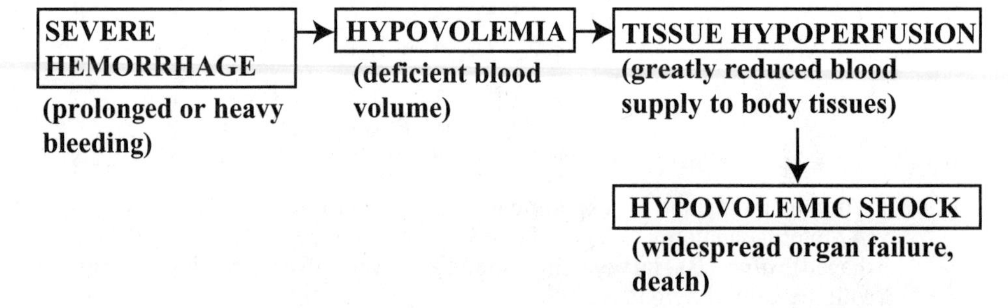

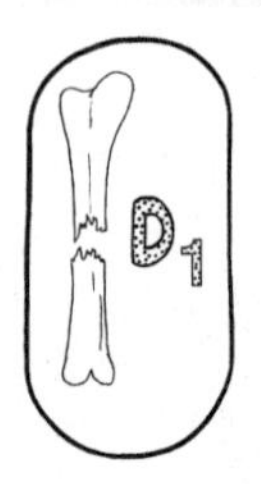

Enter Ambroise Paré

Let us talk about the days before modern surgical techniques and the routine transfusion of blood (giving of blood from a donor to a recipient). In these times, severe hemorrhaging from cut blood vessels was an especially

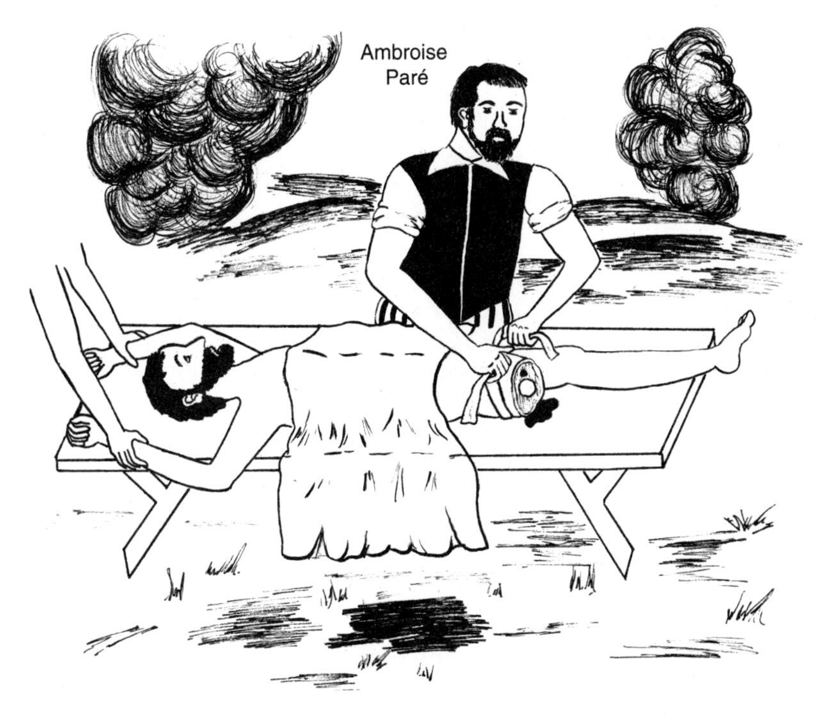

Fig. 8.7 Stopping blood loss on the battlefield. Ambroise Paré uses a ligature to control blood loss during leg amputation near the battlefield.

common casualty of war and battle. This was true in France during the mid-1500s (a few decades before the birth of the Englishman, William Harvey). *Ambroise* (Am-**bwah**) *Paré* (par-**AY**), a French army surgeon, wanted to treat wounded soldiers on the battlefield in a much kinder and more appropriate manner. During his lifetime, injured limbs of soldiers were often *amputated* (**am**-pyoo-**TAY**-ted) or "cut around" and removed right on the battlefield, with gunfire and cannons blazing overhead! (See Figure 8.7.)

The traditional practice was for army surgeons to pour boiling oil over the cut stump of the severed limb, thereby achieving *hemostasis* (**he**-mus-**TAY**-sis). This literally means a "control of" (*-stasis*) "bleeding" (*hemo*). But the pain of having boiling oil poured onto a cut limb stump must have been horrible! Being a kind person, Ambroise Paré discontinued the use of boiling oil, and reintroduced the use of ligatures to tie off cut stumps after amputation. Therefore, ligation (the process of tying off) gradually came to replace cauterization (the process of burning) with boiling oil, to the relief of thousands of soldiers!

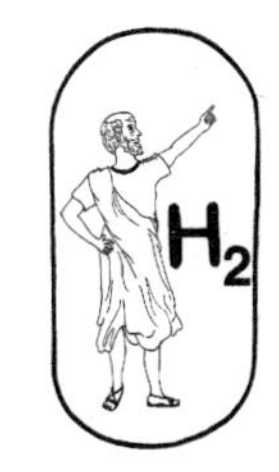

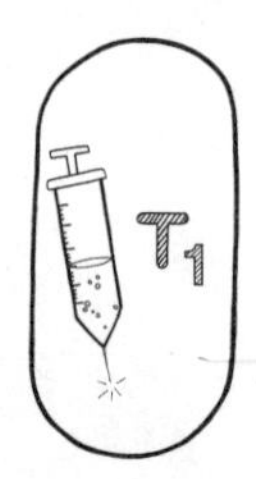

In conclusion, ligation of hemorrhaging blood vessels is one way to prevent severe hypovolemia and the resulting dangers of hypovolemic shock. Summarizing, we obtain:

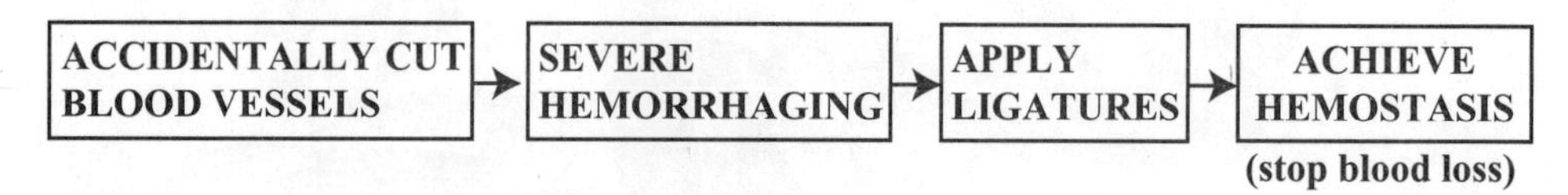

SUMMARY TABLE 8.1

Consult Summary Table 8.1 for a quick review of some important words and word parts.

Important Parameters of Cardiovascular Function

Now that we have a basic understanding of the normal anatomy of the heart and blood vessels, let us now discuss some of the related cardiovascular physiology. One of the important physiological parameters often measured in patients is *heart rate*, sometimes just called the *pulse* or *pulse* rate. The heart rate or pulse rate (abbreviated as HR) is usually measured in units of number of *heart beats per minute*. Most often, the *radial artery,* on the thumb side of the wrist, is the place where the HR or pulse is measured. (See Figure 8.8, A.) [**Thinking probe:** Can you name the particular lower arm *bone* along which this artery runs?] To measure the HR, a health care worker would place several fingers upon the radial artery (which runs along the radius), depressing it just enough to feel the blood pushing back against her fingertips. She would then count the number of pulsations (throbbing actions) of the pumped blood against her fingertips. This taking of the pulse with the fingertips is a good example of diagnosis by palpation ("touching"; see Chapter 5).

The results of palpating for the HR result in measurements that reflect different types of *cardia* (**KAR**-dee-ah)—"conditions" (*-ia*) of the "heart" (*card*) beat. *Normocardia* (**nor**-moh-**KAR**-dee-ah), therefore, denotes a "condition of normal heart" rate. In adults, the resting HR is about 72 beats per minute (bpm). This number, and the normal range around it (Figure 8.8, B), reflects a condition of normocardia. In contrast, *tachycardia* (**tak**-e-**KAR**-dee-ah) is a "condition of" (*-ia*) "fast" (*tachy-*) "heart" (*card*). Tachycardia is commonly defined as a resting HR exceeding 100 bpm (Figure 8.8, C). Finally, *bradycardia* (**brad**-e-**KAR**-dee-ah) is a condition of "slow" (*brady-*) HR. Bradycardia is

Summary Table 8.1 Words and Word Parts

Write in the *exact* meaning (literal English translation) for up to 10 key terms selected from the preceding block of text. After you are done, check your word meanings with the correct answers, which are given at the end of this chapter.

Key Terms	Prefixes	Roots	Suffixes	Exact Meanings
circulatory	(none)	circulat "little circle"	-ory "pertaining to"	1. ________
cardiovascular	(none)	cardi "heart"; vascul "little vessels"	-ar "relating to"	2. ________
capillary	(none)	capill "tiny hair"	-ary "referring to"	3. ________
venule	(none)	ven "vein"	-ule "tiny"	4. ________
arteriole	(none)	arteri "artery"	-ole "little"	5. ________
pulmonary	(none)	pulmon "lungs"	-ary "referring to"	6. ________
semilunar	semi- "half" or "partial"	lun "moon"	-ar "referring to"	7. ________
normovolemia	normo- "normal"	vol "volume"	-emia "blood condition of"	8. ________
hypovolemia	hypo- "below normal"	vol "volume"	-emia "blood condition of"	9. ________
hemostasis	(none)	hem "bleeding"	-stasis "control of"	10. ________

usually said to exist whenever the resting pulse is slower than about 60 bpm (Figure 8.8, D).

ASPECTS OF THE BLOOD PRESSURE

In addition to the pulse (HR), another very commonly assessed physiological parameter is the *blood pressure* (BP). It is formally called a type of *tension*.

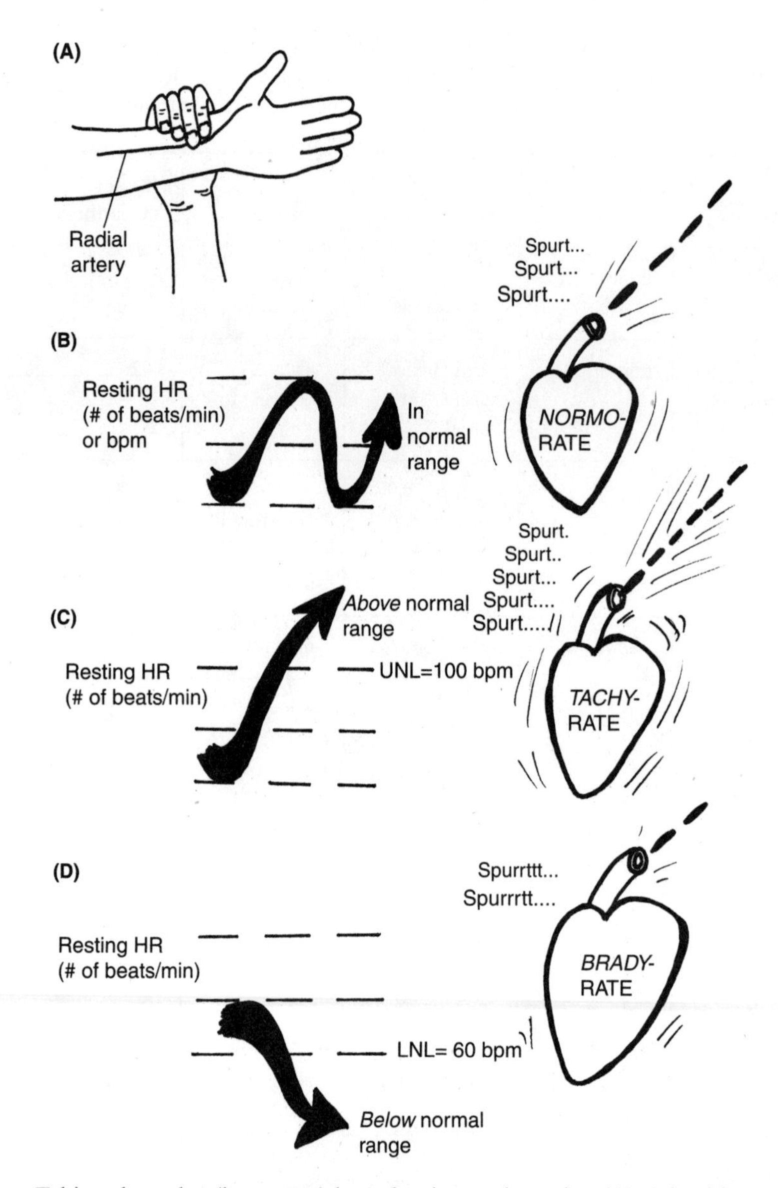

Fig. 8.8 Taking the pulse (heart rate) by palpation at the wrist. **(A)** A health care worker taking the pulse at the wrist by palpation of the *radial artery*. **(B)** *Normocardia* (heart rate or pulse rate *stays* in its *normal* range). **(C)** *Tachycardia* (heart rate or pulse rate rises *above* its upper normal limit [UNL] of 100 beats per minute). **(D)** *Bradycardia* (heart rate or pulse rate falls *below* its lower normal limit [LNL] of 60 beats per minute).

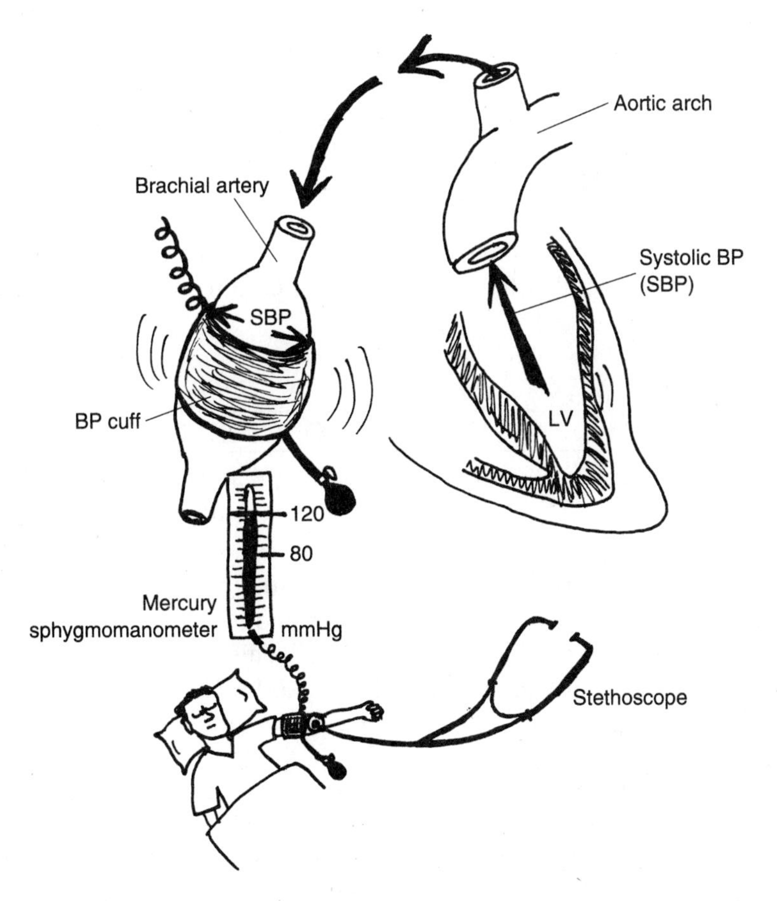

Fig. 8.9 Taking the blood pressure at the brachial artery. LV = left ventricle.

This is because the blood pressure is a type of pushing force, a pushing force created by the *systole* (**SIS**-toh-lee)—"contracting"—and emptying of the heart ventricles.

Figure 8.9 illustrates, for example, the effect of the systole (contraction) of the walls of the left ventricle. Whenever the left ventricle goes into systole and contracts, the pushing of its muscular heart wall creates the *systolic* (sis-**TAHL**-ik) *blood pressure* (*SBP*). The systolic BP, in turn, creates a pushing force upon the blood in the left ventricle. Blood flows up out of the left ventricle and into the *aortic* (**a-OR**-tik) *arch*, the major artery of the systemic circulation. After going through the aortic arch, the blood is pushed into the *brachial* (**BRAY**-kee-al) *artery*, which is present, as its name suggests, within the upper "arm" (*brachi*).

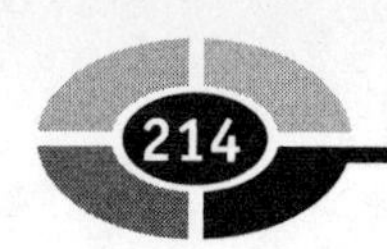

The brachial artery, in fact, is the usual site where the blood pressure is taken in a patient. The clinician inflates the cuff of a *sphygmomanometer* (**sfig**-moh-muh-**NAHM**-uh-ter) around the patient's forearm. The word, *sphygmomanometer*, is certainly a mouthful, isn't it? [**Learning suggestion:** Say the word, sphygmomanometer, three or four times to yourself, out loud. Practice makes perfect, you know!]

Sphygmomanometer is properly cut down into smaller pieces by word analysis as follows: (Remember that CV means "combining vowel" or "connecting vowel.")

Root	*CV*	*Root*	*CV*	*Suffix*
SPHYGM/	O/	MAN/	O/	METER
"throbbing pulse"		**"intervals"**		**"an instrument used to measure"**

Placing the rounded bell of a stethoscope over the brachial artery, the health care worker inflates the cuff of the sphygmomanometer and uses auscultation (listening skills) to hear the "throbbing pulse." This is the systolic BP, which creates a tension or "stretching" outward of the brachial artery every time a slug of blood is pumped out of the left ventricle. As the medical worker slowly lets the air out of the cuff, the point at which the throbbing can no longer be heard through the stethoscope is called the *diastolic* (die-ah-**STAHL**-ik) *blood pressure* (DBP). *Diastole* (die-**AH**-stoh-lee) literally means the "presence of" (*—e*) an "expansion" (*diastol*). Diastole is the resting and filling phase of each heart ventricle. The heart, no longer pumping, temporarily rests and fills with blood. This expands the heart in size (as the term, *diastole*, indicates). The diastolic BP is considerably lower than the systolic BP, because it represents the period when the heart is not contracting.

The entire period of contracting (systole) of all four heart chambers, followed by their resting and expansion with blood (diastole), is called one heartbeat or *cardiac cycle.* These, then, are the phases of one heartbeat (cardiac cycle) associated with the SBP and DBP:

ONE HEARTBEAT (CARDIAC CYCLE) = **SYSTOLE** **(ventricles "contract" and pump out blood)** + **DIASTOLE** **(ventricles relax, fill with blood, and "expand")**

and

BLOOD PRESSURE = **SYSTOLIC BP/DIASTOLIC BP**

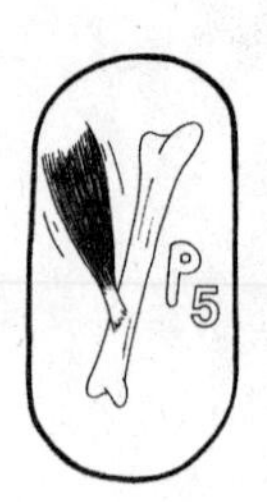

These BP readings are commonly measured in units of *millimeters of mercury*, abbreviated as *mmHg*.

Normal versus abnormal blood pressure

Thinking in terms of homeostasis and the normal range (as we did for both oral body temperature and HR), we get various kinds of *tension* (vessel "stretching" action resulting from BP). Specifically, we get the three terms *normotension*, *hypertension*, and *hypotension*. [**Learning activity:** Dissect the preceding three terms by inserting slash marks. Label the resulting word parts as prefix, root, and suffix. What do you get for the literal translation of each term? Check your translations with the homeostasis versus disruption-of-homeostasis pictures shown in Figure 8.10.]

As you probably suspect, normotension and its associated normal range of blood pressure (100/60 mmHg up to 140/90 mmHg) are generally associated with clinical health. Conversely, hypotension involving a BP significantly below 100/60 mmHg may be associated with hypoperfusion of body tissues. The reason is that the BP is the force pushing the blood through the organs and their tissues. Hence, with insufficient BP, there isn't enough blood flowing through the organs. In particular, the brain and kidneys may fail, and coma and death may follow!

Not any better, certainly, is hypertension (BP significantly beyond 140/90 mmHg). This excessive BP can overstretch the walls of arteries. Over time, this overstretching may cause the springy elastic fibers in the arterial wall

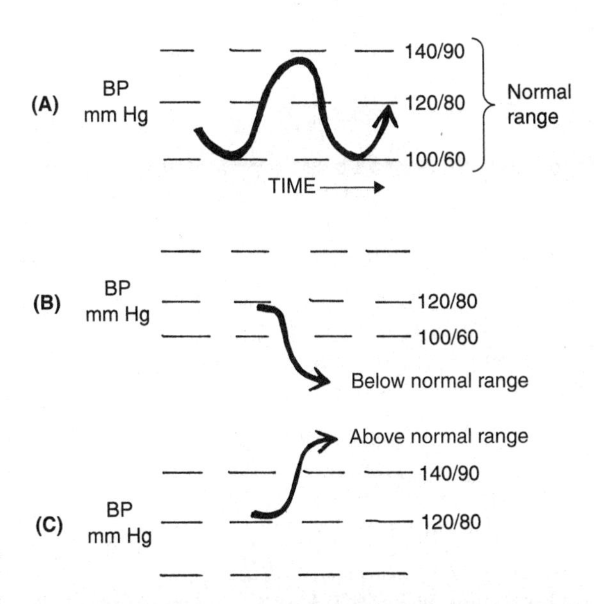

Fig. 8.10 The three possible states of blood pressure. **(A)** Normotension: BP *stays* in its normal range; **(B)** Hypotension: BP *falls below* its normal range; **(C)** Hypertension: BP *rises above* its normal range, often in association with *arteriosclerosis*.

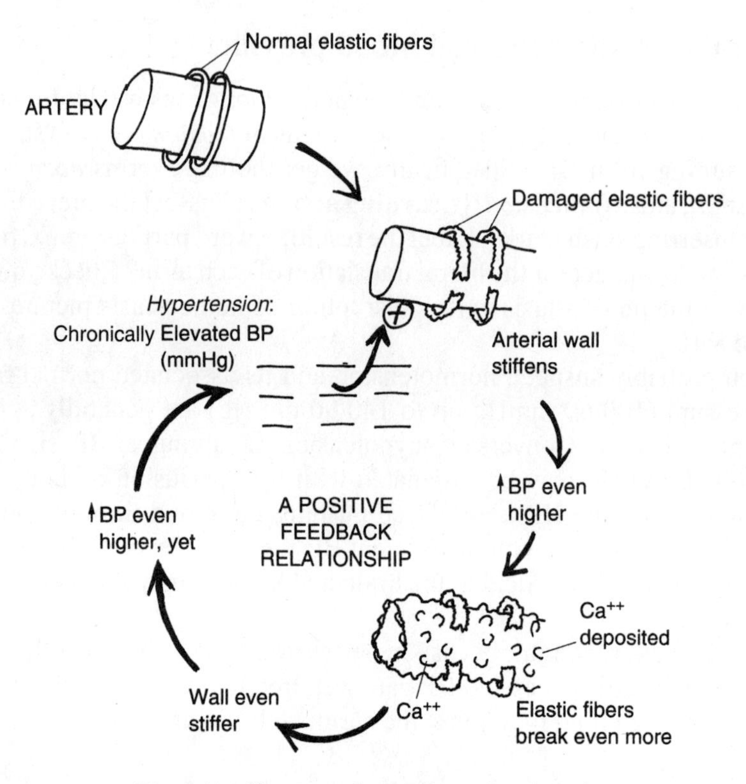

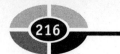

Fig. 8.11 Hypertension and arteriosclerosis.

to be damaged and broken. Such a condition may be associated with the disease called *arteriosclerosis* (ar-**TEER**-e-oh-sklair-**OH**-sis). This is literally "an abnormal condition of" (*-osis*) weakening, stiffening, and "hardening" (*scler*) of the "arteries" (*arteri*). This progressive hardening and stiffening of the wall occurs along with the depositing of *calcium* (Ca++) *ions*. [**Visualization exercise:** Imagine a steel pipe whose inner lumen is heavily limed up with calcium deposits from chronic exposure to hard water!] The arterial wall can get rock hard and brittle via a progressive *positive-feedback effect* or *vicious cycle*! (Study Figure 8.11.)

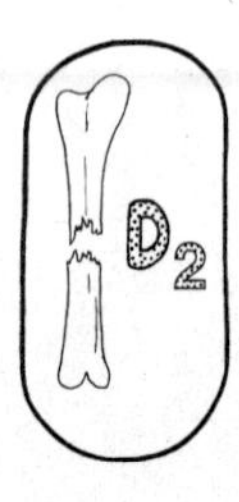

Closely associated with hypertension and arteriosclerosis is the occurrence of vessel *aneurysms* (**AN**-you-rizms). An *aneurysm* (*AN*-you-rizm) is a highly abnormal "widening" or ballooning out of the walls of an artery (Figure 8.12). If the aneurysm suddenly ruptures, then severe *internal bleeding* may occur. This situation is especially dire in cases involving a *ruptured cerebral* (seh-**REE**-bral) *aneurysm*. The *cerebrum* (seh-**REE**-brum) is, after all, the "main mass of the brain"! The patient suffers (in layman's lingo) a so-called *stroke*. A stroke is a sudden "strike" of some kind. In this case, it involves a sudden *cerebrovascular* (**suh-REE**-broh-**VAS**-kyoo-lar) *accident*, abbreviated as CVA. An artery within

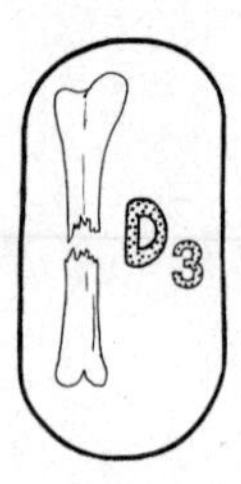

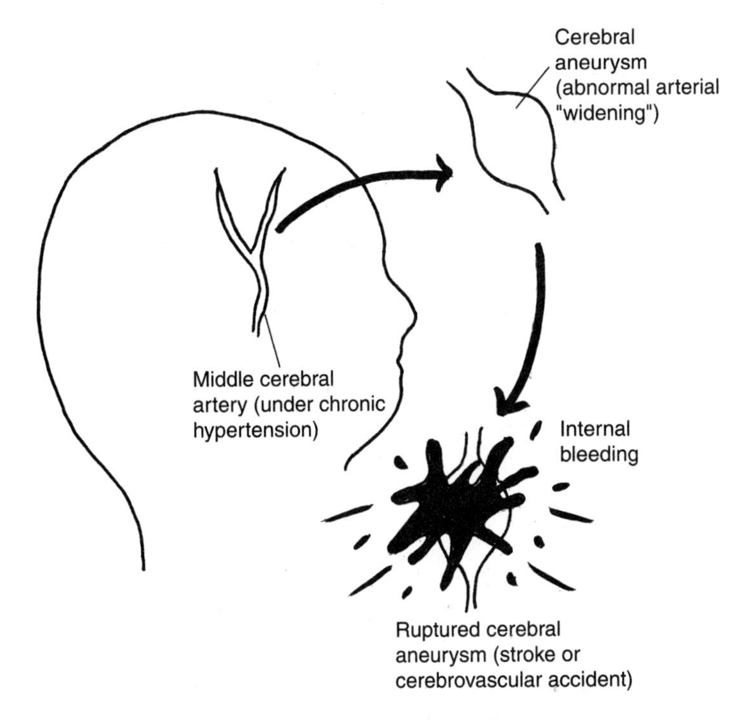

Fig. 8.12 Hypertension and a stroke or *cerebrovascular accident* (CVA).

the cerebrum has an aneurysm that suddenly breaks open, spilling blood over part or all of the brain! The consequences are usually loss of consciousness followed by paralysis (inability to move) of some part of the body.

The Coronary Arteries and "Heart Attacks"

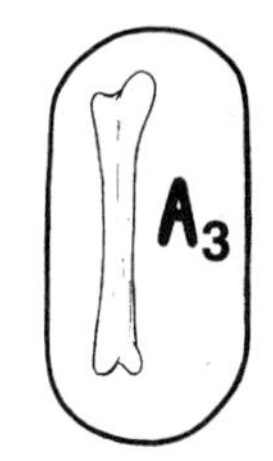

Along with strokes (cerebrovascular accidents), many people suddenly suffer death or disability from what is crudely called a "heart attack." To understand this major clinical disorder, we must first gain a basic familiarity with the *coronary* (**KOR**-uh-**nair**-ee) *circulation.*

Figure 8.13 does this job nicely for us. Here we see that the name *coronary* literally "refers to" (*-ary*) a "crown" (*coron*). In reality, what we mean is that there is a *right coronary artery* and a *left coronary artery*, both of which encircle the top of the heart like a "crown" (*coron*).

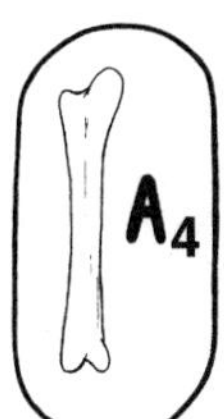

The coronary circulation is a so-called *special circulation* that serves the metabolic needs of the *myocardium* (my-oh-**KAR**-dee-um). The myocardium is the "muscular" (*my*) pumping tissue that is "present" (*-um*) within the "heart" (*cardi*) wall. A section of the myocardium is featured in Figure 8.14. It is the cardiac muscle fibers of the myocardium that contract (shorten) and pump the

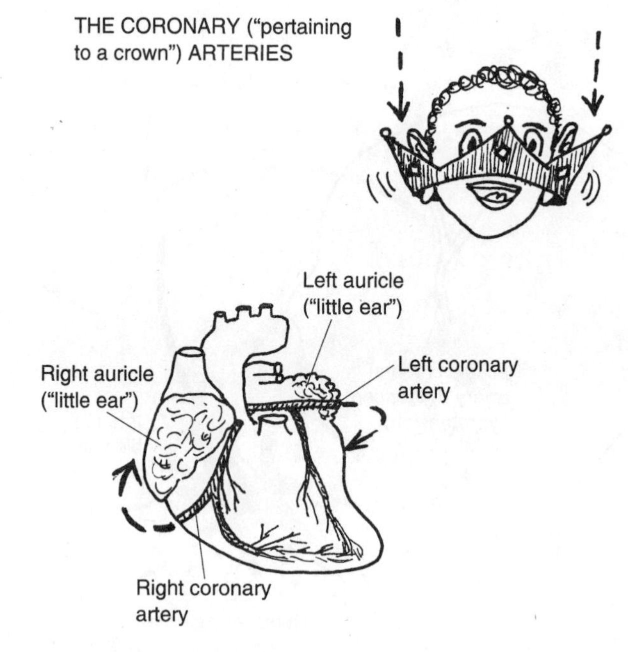

Fig. 8.13 The coronary circulation: A little prince gets "crowned."

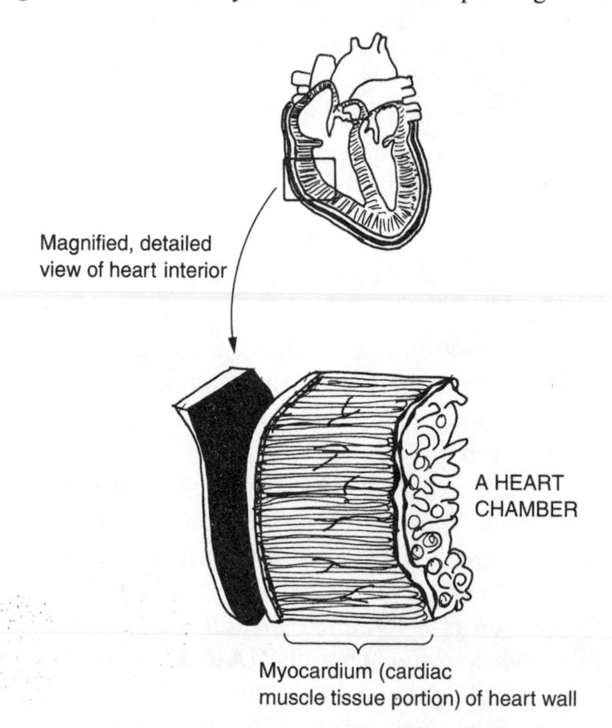

Fig. 8.14 The myocardium within the heart wall.

blood out of the ventricles during each cardiac cycle (heartbeat). Hence, the coronary circulation is the vital oxygen-supplying lifeline of the cardiac muscle fibers. Further, it is also the entire human body's critical lifeline! For without the minute-by-minute pumping action of the heart wall, we would soon fall prey to a deadly hypovolemic shock!

ATHEROSCLEROSIS AND CORONARY HEART DISEASE (CHD)

Most unfortunately, the lumens (inner passageways) of the vital coronary arteries are extremely narrow—only about as wide as a pencil lead. This simple fact makes them highly vulnerable to a total *occlusion* ("closing up"). The main culprits responsible for coronary artery occlusion are either *atheromas* (**ath**-er-**OH**-mahs) or *thrombi* (**THRAHM**-buy). An *atheroma* is literally a "fatty" (*ather*) "tumor" (*-oma*). The atheroma is not really a tumor *per se*, but rather a tumor-like bulge of *fatty plaque* (**PLAK**). The word, *plaque*, comes from the French and Dutch for "flat board" or "plate."

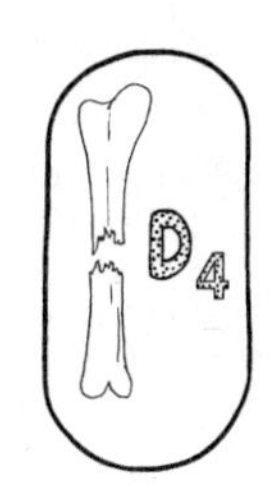

The principal component of fatty plaques (*atheromas*) is *cholesterol.* You surely have heard of cholesterol! It is a member of the *lipid* family of body chemicals, which include the blood fats. Cholesterol is synthesized naturally by the liver and plays an important role in stabilizing the plasma membranes of our body cells. Cholesterol itself, therefore, is not really the problem. Rather, it is *hypercholesterolemia* (**high**-per-koh-**les**-ter-awl-**EE**-me-ah) that's the problem! Technically speaking, we mean a "blood condition of" (*-emia*) "excessive" (*hyper-*) "cholesterol." When there is such an abnormally high level of circulating cholesterol, more of it tends to settle out of the bloodstream and onto the inner walls of the arteries. Over time, fatty plaques (atheromas) tend to build up, and the pathology of *atherosclerosis* (**ath**-er-**oh**-skluh-**ROH**-sis) results. [**Practice in word translation:** Go ahead and try to write the common English translation of *atherosclerosis*. It is quite similar to that for *arteriosclerosis*!]

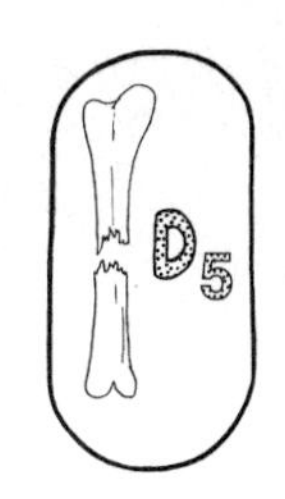

Eventually, atherosclerosis can become so severe within the coronary arteries that a large piece of atheroma suddenly occludes (closes up) the lumen. (Observe Figure 8.15.) Another possible outcome is that a *thrombus* (**THRAM**-bus)—stationary blood "clot" (*thromb*)—forms at the atheroma-narrowed lumen and blocks it.

Angina pectoris and coronary artery disease

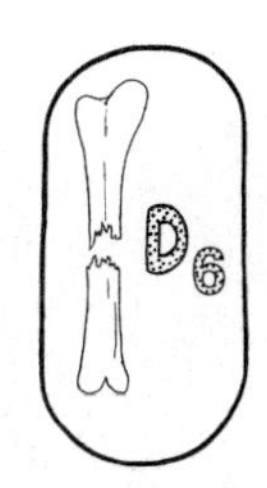

As the lumen of the coronary arteries becomes progressively blocked, there is a growing *ischemia* (is-**KEE**-me-uh)—"holding back of blood"—to the needy myocardium. This condition is technically called *myocardial*

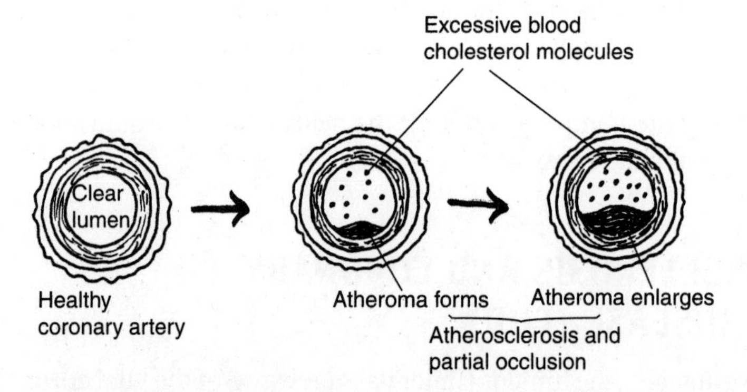

Fig. 8.15 Atherosclerosis and occlusion of the coronary arteries, as demonstrated in cross sections of healthy (*left*) and atheroma-affected (*center and right*) arteries.

(**my**-oh-**KAR**-dee-ul) *ischemia*. Such a blood-supply deficiency to the cardiac muscle eventually results in severe symptoms of *angina* (an-**JEYE**-nuh) *pectoris* (**PEK**-tor-is). This is a feeling of "strangling" (*angin*) in the "breast or chest" (*pector*). Figure 8.16 reveals the typical pattern of *anginal* (**AN**-jih-nal) pain. Such pain is frequently considered a "referred" type of pain, because it radiates outward from the heart and is "referred" (experienced) in other body areas.

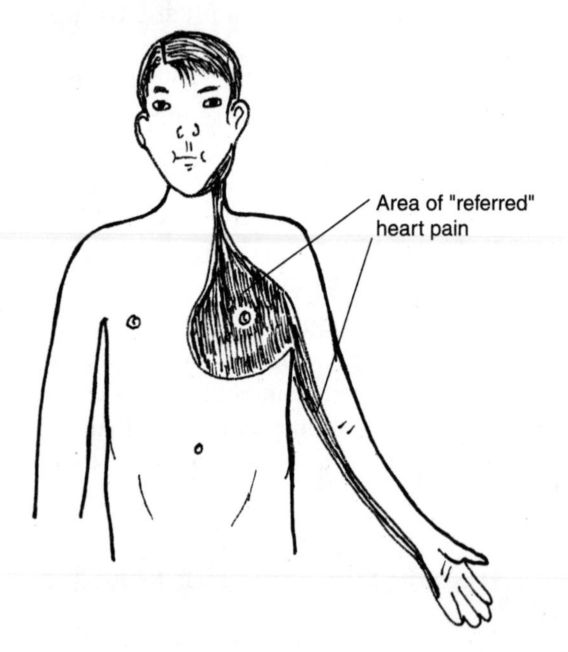

Fig. 8.16 Angina pectoris and its "referred" pain pattern.

When a person is having a so-called "heart attack," it really means that they are experiencing an episode of *severe acute myocardial ischemia*. This is a sudden (acute) deficiency of blood flow (ischemia) to the myocardium that results in severe angina pectoris. If the lumens of the coronary arteries are totally or nearly totally occluded, then *myocardial necrosis*—"an abnormal condition of heart muscle death"—may result. Another name for myocardial necrosis is *myocardial infarction* (**in-FARK**-shun), abbreviated as MI. An *infarct* (**IN**-farkt), in general, is a local area of necrosis or dead tissue present within an organ. The tissue necrosis (death) is the result of a blockage or "stuffing up" (*infarct*) of its blood supply.

The severe acute myocardial ischemia (*not* the myocardial infarction or MI) is most correctly considered the "heart attack." This is because the sudden "attack" upon the heart is one of severe ischemia resulting from blocked coronary arteries. In fact, a visible MI on the heart surface may not even form if the person dies immediately! If enough heart muscle dies, then the heart simply stops pumping the blood, and the other organs (like the brain and kidneys) quickly die as well. But if the person survives long enough (say, about a week to 10 days), then a visible myocardial infarct will appear as a reddish oval area on the heart wall, which later turns yellowish. Eventually, the myocardial infarct is healed by replacement with a patch of dense fibrous connective tissue. This patch is basically a whitish *cicatrix* (**SIK**-ah-triks) or "scar."

To summarize the preceding info:

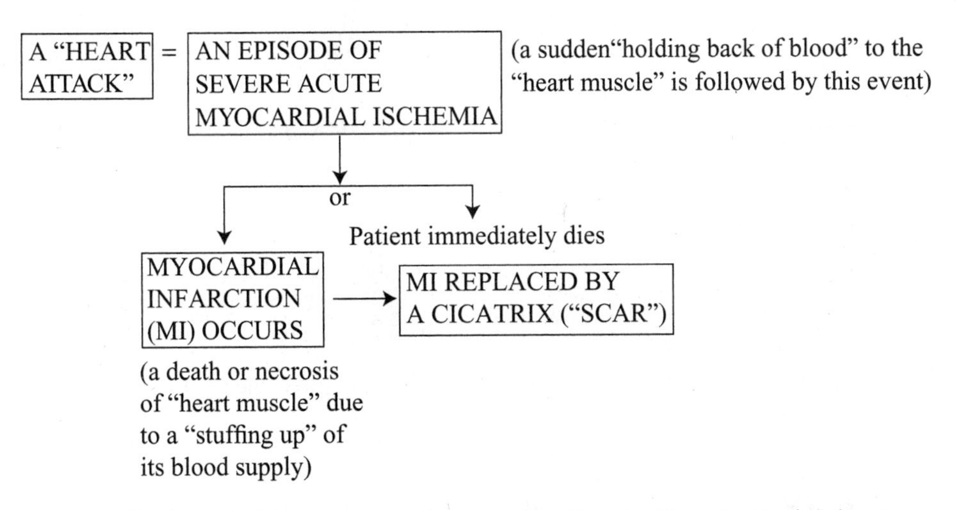

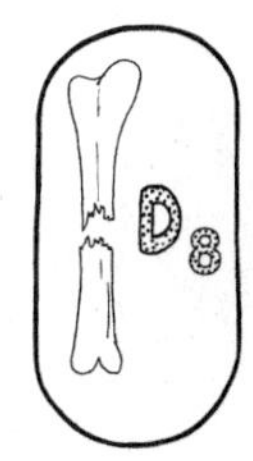

Overall, the whole sequence of events leading to "heart attack" (acute severe myocardial ischemia) is technically called either *coronary artery disease* (CAD) or *coronary heart disease* (CHD). The whole series of complex events in CAD/CHD is diagrammed and "demystified" within Figure 8.17.

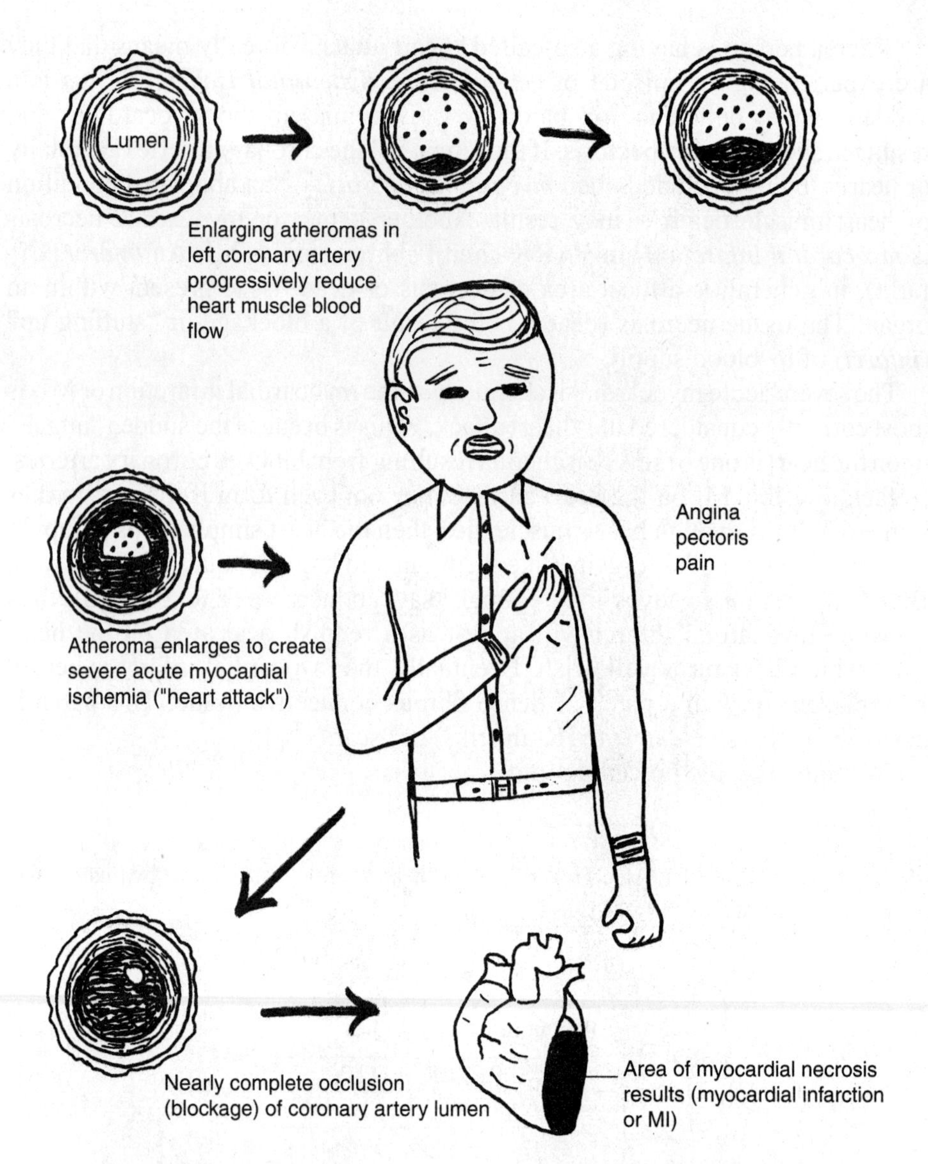

Fig. 8.17 The sequence of events in CAD leading to a "heart attack."

The Blood and Its Disorders

The last major part of the circulatory (cardiovascular system) is the blood connective tissue. Blood is a red, sticky connective tissue with a fluid intercellular substance called the *plasma*. It occupies about 4 to 6 liters of volume in the average-sized adult.

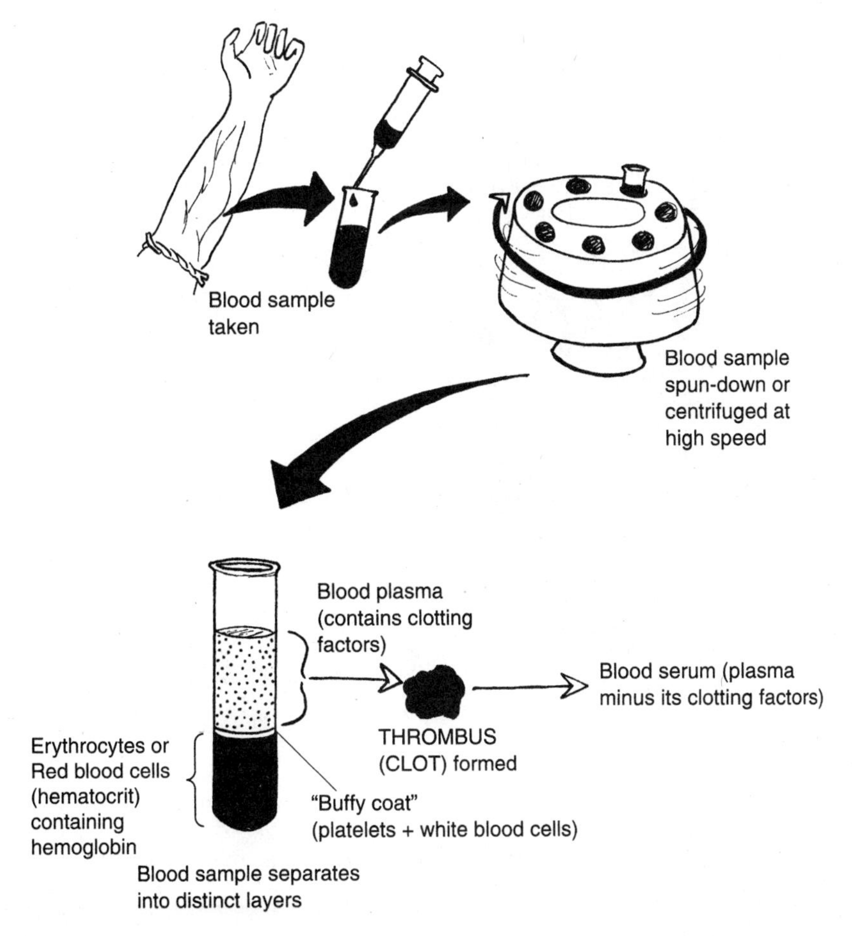

Fig. 8.18 General components of the blood when it is centrifuged.

THE HEMATOCRIT AND ERYTHROCYTES (RBCs)

Figure 8.18 shows how the blood separates when it is placed into a test tube and spun around by means of a *centrifuge* (**SEN**-trih-fyooj) machine. At the bottom of the test tube we find the heaviest component, called the *hematocrit* (he-**MAT**-oh-krit). The hematocrit consists of thousands of *erythrocytes* (air-**ITH**-roh-**sights**) or "red" (*erythr*) blood "cells" (*cytes*). The erythrocytes look red because of their high concentration of *hemoglobin* (**HEE**-moh-**glohb**-in). The hemoglobin molecule is a reddish-colored, "globe" (*glob*) -shaped "protein" (*-in*) present within red "blood" (*hem*) cells. Each hemoglobin molecule, in turn, can carry up to four oxygen molecules (O_2) through the bloodstream, and towards the oxygen-hungry tissue cells.

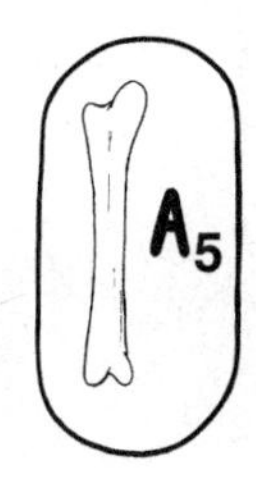

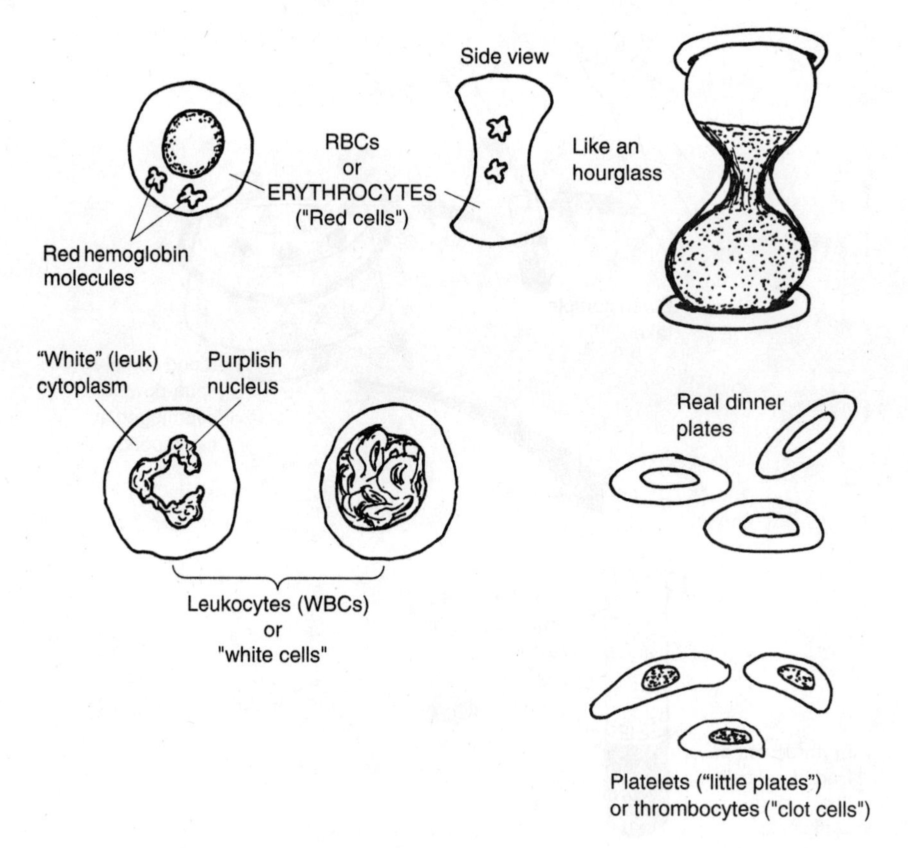

Fig. 8.19 The major types of formed elements in the blood.

"How about a closer look at the erythrocytes or RBCs (red blood cells), Noble Hippocrates?" the knowledge-thirsting modern reader may ask of our ancient host. This closer look is provided by Figure 8.19, which displays the so-called *formed elements* (cells and cell fragments) present within the blood. Observe that each RBC is indented on both sides, giving it an unusual hourglass shape.

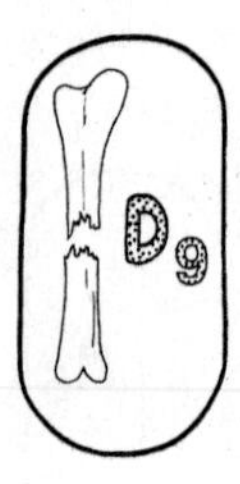

One major disorder of the erythrocytes is various types of *anemia* (ah-**NEEM**-e-uh). Taken literally, an anemia is a "condition" (*-ia*) "without" (*an-*) enough red "blood" (*em*) cells. One common type is *iron-deficiency anemia*. Each hemoglobin molecule contains four *iron atoms*, each of which can carry one oxygen molecule (O_2). One human RBC holds 200 to 300 million molecules of hemoglobin, so that's a lot of iron contained in the hemoglobin!

Therefore, when a person has a chronic bleeding, they lose thousands of RBCs—along with billions of hemoglobin molecules containing iron. The result is an iron deficiency within the bloodstream and a greatly reduced energy level. This weakness is caused by an inability to transport much oxygen through the bloodstream. In women, one type of excessive bleeding is a heavy *menstrual* (**MEN**-stroo-al) or "monthly" loss from the vagina. In both sexes, chronic *gastrointestinal* (**gas**-troh-in-**TES**-tih-nal) bleeding—from the "stomach" (*gastr*) and "intestines" (*intestin*)—can be due to a bleeding ulcer.

THE BUFFY COAT

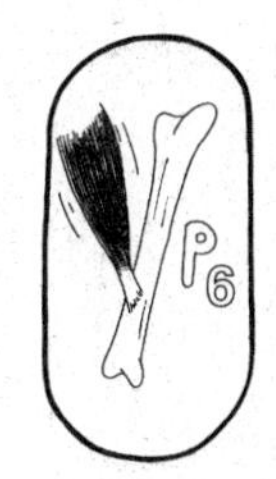

A look back at Figure 8.18 shows a thin, milky "buffy coat" in a centrifuged test tube. This layer contains the leukocytes and the *platelets* (**PLAY**-teh-**lets**) or *thrombocytes* (**THRAHM**-buh-**sights**). Review of Figure 8.19 reveals that the leukocytes are called "white" (*leuk*) blood cells because of the clear, whitish appearance of the cytoplasm around their purplish nuclei. The platelets get their name from their resemblance to "little plates" here and there within the bloodstream. The platelets carry the alternate physiological name of *thrombocytes* because their cell membranes are sticky and they collect together and help create thrombi (blood clots).

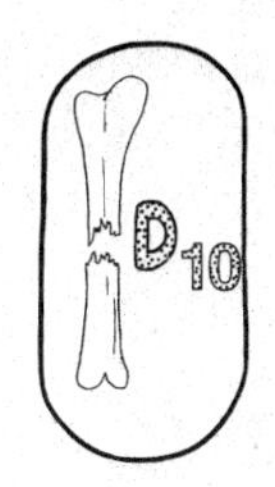

You may remember from our discussion of the immune-lymphatic system (Chapter 5) that the various types of leukocytes play important roles in body defense from foreign invaders (antigens). Hence, consider a clinical problem such as *leukocytopenia* (**loo**-koh-**sigh**-toh-**PEEN**-ee-ah). This is a "poverty of" (*-penia*) "white (blood) cells" (*leukocyt*) within the bloodstream. There should normally be about 10,000 leukocytes present in every cubic millimeter of blood. When there are fewer than half this number (5,000 leukocytes per cubic millimeter), then leukocytopenia exists. With so few leukocytes circulating, the body is much more prone to suffer various diseases and infections.

As far as platelets (thrombocytes) are concerned, they, too, must be present in sufficient numbers within the bloodstream. If they are greatly reduced in number, then blood clotting will be very show after a vessel is cut. As a result, the person may hemorrhage to death! (This stark fact explains why the platelets are alternately called thrombocytes or "clot"-making "cells.")

THE BLOOD PLASMA AND SERUM

A final peek back at the centrifuged blood in the test tube (Figure 8.18) shows the clear plasma, with its *clotting factors*, at the top. If the blood is allowed to sit, a thrombus (clot) soon forms. What is left of the plasma after the clot forms is called the *blood serum*. The clear, yellowish blood serum contains various proteins that play important roles in physiology. The *globulins* (**GLAHB**-yoo-lins), for instance, are a group of plasma proteins that include many antibodies (Chapter 5), which attack foreign invaders.

SUMMARY TABLE 8.2

Consult Summary Table 8.2 for a quick review of some important words and word parts.

Summary Table 8.2 Words and Word Parts

Write in the *exact* meaning (literal English translation) for up to 10 key terms selected from the preceding block of text. After you are done, check your word meanings with the correct answers, which are given at the end of this chapter.

Key Terms	**Prefixes**	**Roots**	**Suffixes**	**Exact Meanings**
normocardia	normo- "normal"	card "heart"	-ia "condition of"	1. ________
tachycardia	tachy- "fast"	card "heart"	-ia "condition of"	2. ________
bradycardia	brady- "slow"	card "heart"	-ia "condition of"	3. ________
arteriosclerosis	(none)	arteri "arteries"	-sclerosis "hardening of"	4. ________
myocardial	(none)	my "muscle"; cardi "heart"	-al "referring to"	5. ________
hypercholesterolemia	hyper- "excessive"	cholesterol	-emia "blood condition of"	6. ________
anginal	(none)	angin "strangling"	-al "relating to"	7. ________
thrombus	(none)	thromb "clot"	-us "presence of"	8. ________
ischemia	(none)	ischem "holding back of blood"	-ia "condition of"	9. ________
leukocytopenia	(none)	leuk "white"; cyt "cells"	-penia "a poverty of"	10. ________

Medical Case History: A Stubborn Dad Suffers Repeated "Small Heart Attacks"

Joe D., the father of two grown children, was stricken with severe angina pectoris on his way home from work. The pain started in his left jaw and then *radiated* (**RAY**-de-**ate**-ed) down into his whole left arm (Review Fig. 8.16, if desired.) "It feels like an elephant is sitting on my chest!" Joe exclaimed out loud to himself behind the steering wheel. His brow bathed in sweat, his pulse *tachycardic* (**tak**-ih-**KAR**-dik) and irregular, Joe finally pulled his car off to the side of the road. But his associated *dyspnea* (**DISP**-nee-ah)—"difficult" (*dys-*) "breathing" (*pnea*)—lasted for only a few minutes. Soon, the pain faded and Joe pulled back onto the road. When he finally arrived home, he never told his wife a thing! "Doctors and hospitals are for *babies*!" Joe said several times. "They're not for a *man*!"

Three weeks later, Joe suddenly grabbed his chest, grimaced with pain, and collapsed at work, right on the floor at the plant! The foreman gave him *CPR* or *cardiopulmonary* (**kar**-dee-oh-**PUL**-muh-**nair**-ee) *resuscitation* (re-**sus**-ih-**TAY**-shun).

When the *paramedics* (**pair**-uh-**MED**-iks) arrived, they put Joe onto a stretcher and whisked him away in an ambulance. In the hospital *ER* (*emergency room*), Joe was placed on artificial *ventilation* (**ven**-tih-**LAY**-shun) and given an *EKG* (or ECG)—that is, an *electrocardiogram* (e-**lek**-troh-**KAR**-dee-oh-gram). This a "record of" (*-gram*) the "electrical activity" (*electr*) of the "heart" (*cardi*). A number of *inverted* ("turned over") EKG waves suggested that one or more MIs were already present!

Joe was diagnosed with severe CAD on both sides of his heart. A *multiple coronary bypass operation* was carried out. Sections of several peripheral veins from his legs were extracted and surgically implanted around the *occluded* (ah-**KLOO**-ded) areas of the coronary arteries. Normal myocardial perfusion was re-established by this bypass procedure, and the patient eventually recovered and went home.

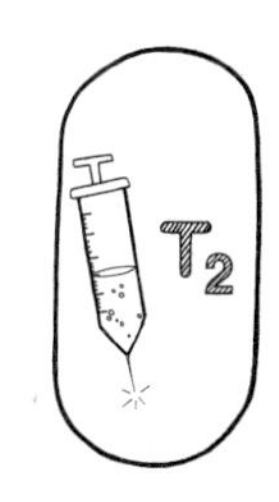

Probe of case history

(**A**) What two medical words would you use to label the severe pain that Joe was feeling before he had surgery? (**B**) When the case history said that veins were implanted around the "*occluded* areas" of the coronary arteries, what does this mean in regular English? [Check your short answers with the key near the end of this chapter.]

Quiz

Refer to the text in this chapter if necessary. A good score is at least 8 correct answers out of these 10 questions. The answers are listed in the back of this book.

1. By the lumen of a blood vessel, we mean its:
   (a) Amount of blood flow
   (b) Ability to withstand the force of blood pressure
   (c) "Light space" or opening channel
   (d) Relative weight
2. The two upper chambers of the heart are called the:
   (a) Atria
   (b) Arterioles
   (c) Ventricles
   (d) Myocardia
3. The portion of the total blood circulation controlled by the left side of the heart:
   (a) Systemic
   (b) Anginal
   (c) Pectoral
   (d) Pulmonary
4. "The patient is suffering from severe myocardial ischemia," means that:
   (a) The liver was bypassing the lungs
   (b) Perfusion of the heart muscle fibers was nearly totally blocked
   (c) Leukocytes increased vastly in both their numbers and size
   (d) The platelets just stopped sticking together!
5. William Harvey is noted for his contributions to:
   (a) Cancer research
   (b) Ligation of vessels to reduce severe hemorrhage
   (c) Thoroughly explaining the cell theory to interested laypeople
   (d) Clearly demonstrating the one-way circulation of the bloodstream
6. A patient in "hypovolemic shock" would have what key problem?
   (a) Choking and strangling on undigested food
   (b) Inadequate tissue perfusion due to an extremely low blood volume
   (c) Excessive pumping action of the heart, producing excessively high BP
   (d) Lack of hemoglobin in the leukocytes

7. The word, *hypocholesterolemia*, (**high**-poh-koh-**les**-ter-awl-**EE**-me-ah) is properly dissected with slash marks as:
   (a) Hyp/o/ch/olesterol/emia
   (b) H/ypo/cholestero/lemia
   (c) Hypo/cholesterol/emia
   (d) Hypo/choles/terole/mia

8. The word, *hypocholesterolemia*, is correctly translated to mean:
   (a) "A blood condition of above normal cholesterol"
   (b) "Inflammation of the veins"
   (c) "Removal of the cardia"
   (d) "A blood condition of deficient cholesterol"

9. The hematocrit portion of centrifuged blood mainly consists of:
   (a) Platelets
   (b) Leukocytes + thrombocytes
   (c) Erythrocytes
   (d) Wandering macrophages

10. A patient whose resting blood pressure was considerably higher than 140/90 mmHg would best be described as:
    (a) Leukemic
    (b) Anemic
    (c) Normotensive
    (d) Hypertensive

Memory Pillboxes for Chapter 8

Several key facts were tagged with numbered icons in the page margins of this chapter. Write a short summary of each of these key facts into a numbered cell or compartment within the appropriate type of *Memory Pillbox* that appears below.

Background and History **Pillboxes for Chapter 8:**

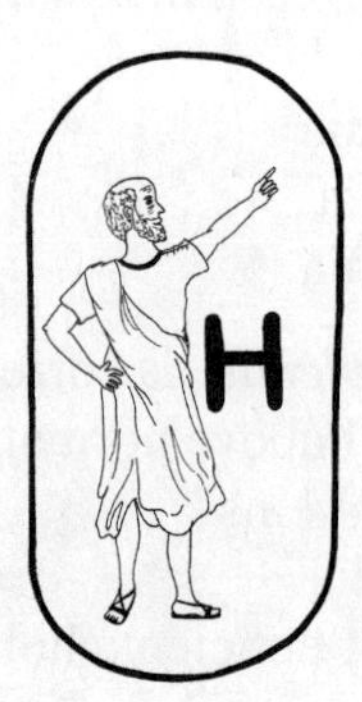

1	2

Anatomy **Pillboxes for Chapter 8:**

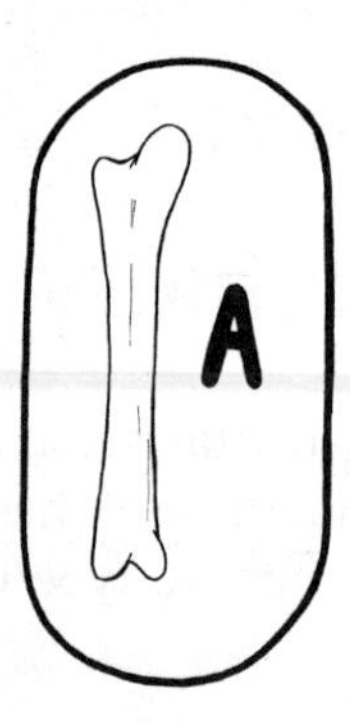

1	2

3	4

5

Physiology Pillboxes for Chapter 8:

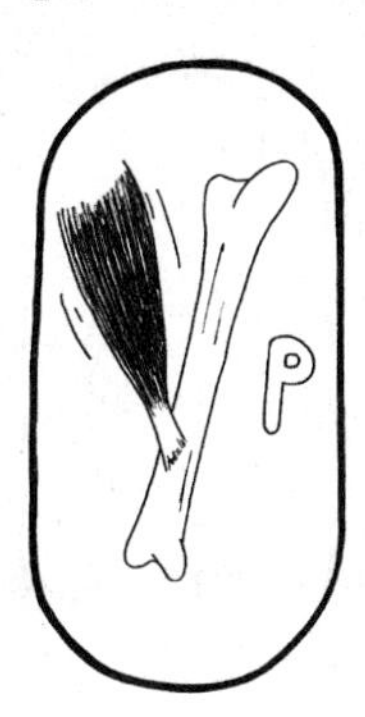

1	2

3	4

5	6

***Disease/Injury* Pillboxes for Chapter 8:**

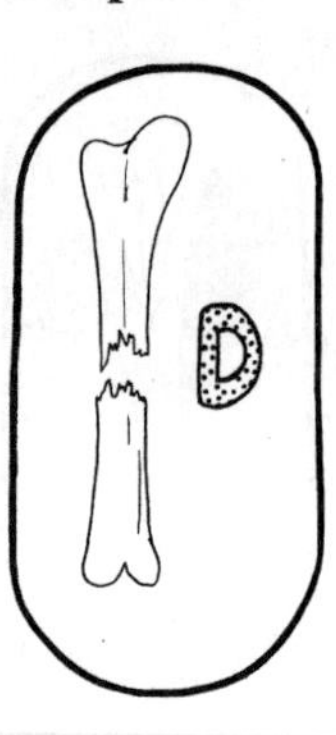

1	2

3	4
5	6
7	8
9	10

Treatment/Therapy **Pillboxes for Chapter 8:**

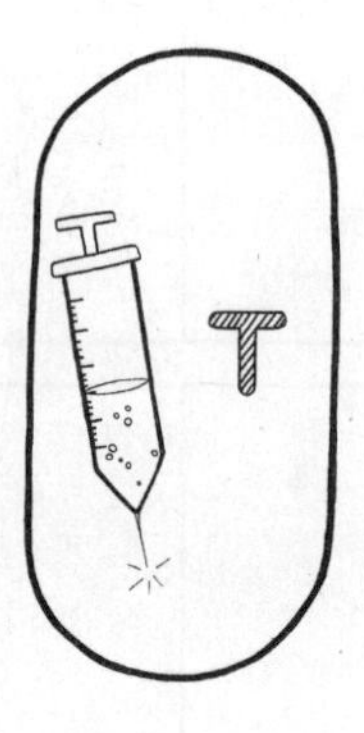

1	2

Answers for Chapter 8 Summary Tables

FOR SUMMARY TABLE 8.1

1. "pertaining to a little circle"
2. "relating to the heart and little vessels"
3. "referring to a tiny hair"
4. "tiny vein"
5. "little artery"
6. "referring to the lungs"
7. "referring to a half moon"
8. "a blood condition of normal volume"
9. "a blood condition of below normal volume"
10. "control of bleeding"

FOR SUMMARY TABLE 8.2

1. "a condition of normal heart"
2. "a condition of fast heart"
3. "a condition of slow heart"
4. "hardening of the arteries"
5. "referring to heart muscle"
6. "a blood condition of excessive cholesterol"
7. "relating to strangling"
8. "presence of a clot"
9. "a condition of holding back blood"
10. "a poverty of white cells"

Answers to Probe of Case History

(**A**) Angina pectoris. (**B**) The occluded areas of the coronary arteries had their blood flow "closed up."

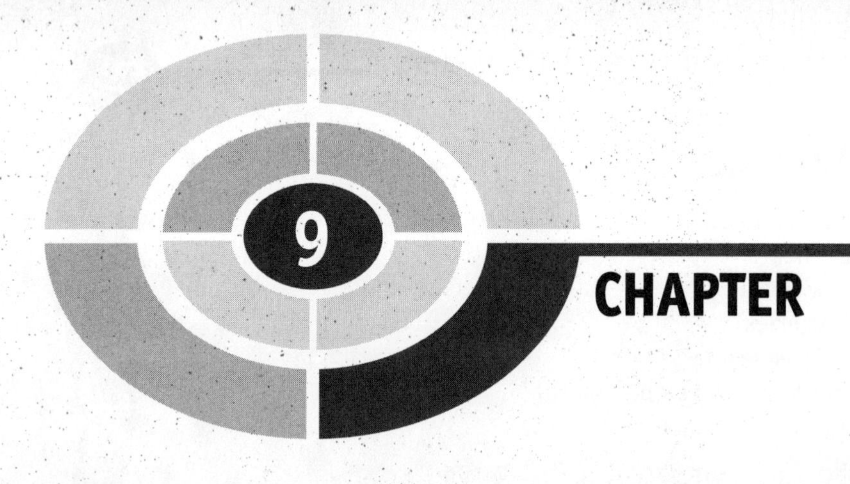

Terms Related to Disorders of the Respiratory System

Chapter 8 focused upon the circulatory (cardiovascular) system. This is the organ system whose basic job is moving the *blood*. Now, in Chapter 9, our emphasis is upon the *respiratory* (**RES**-pir-ah-**tor**-ee) system. The word *respiratory* literally "refers to" (*-ory*) "breathing" (*spirat*) "again" (*re-*). The respiratory system, therefore, is the organ system that allows us to breathe again and again. And in doing so, it is the organ system that moves *air* through body passageways.

Both the normal and some of the disease-related aspects of moving air through the respiratory system will be our chief focus in this chapter.

Background and History

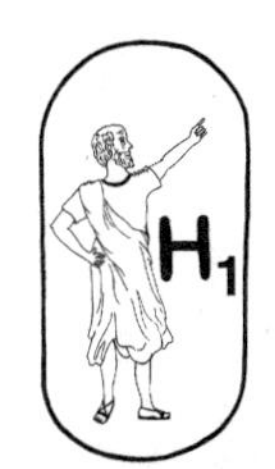

You may recall that Chapter 8 mentioned the two terms, *cardiopulmonary* (as in cardiopulmonary resuscitation) and *pulmonary* (as in the pulmonary or right-heart circulation). Thus, *pulmon/ary* literally "refers to the lungs." Another root for "lung" is *pneumon* (**NEW**-mun). Hence, a related term, *pneumonic* (**new-MAHN**-ik), also "pertains to the lungs."

AN OVERVIEW OF THE RESPIRATORY SYSTEM

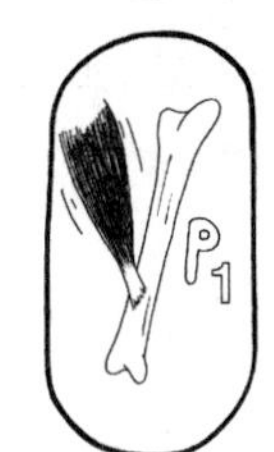

Whichever root we use, the "lungs" (pneumon or pulmon) are usually the first organs we think about whenever we hear the word, *respiration*. This word exactly translates to mean the "process of" (*-tion*) "breathing" (*spir*) "again" (*re-*).

But the lungs don't work alone in helping us to breathe! There are two main divisions of the respiratory pathway, also called the *respiratory tract*. The *upper respiratory tract* is situated at the superior end of the breathing pathway, while the *lower respiratory tract* lies at the inferior end. Further, because the lower respiratory tract branches extensively, it is sometimes called the *respiratory "tree."* [**Study suggestion:** Which division of the respiratory pathway do you think contains the lungs?]

THE RESPIRATORY (*"breathing again and again"*) SYSTEM = **THE UPPER RESPIRATORY TRACT** + **THE LOWER RESPIRATORY TRACT (*the respiratory "tree"*)**

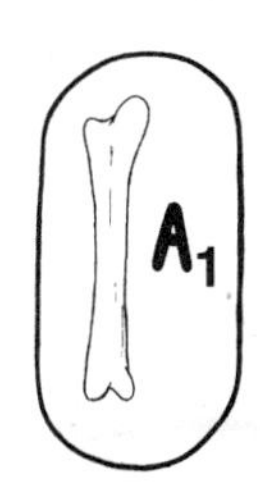

THE UPPER RESPIRATORY TRACT

The upper respiratory tract (Figure 9.1) is the superior portion of the respiratory system. Its specific components are the *nasal* (**NAY**-sal) *cavity*, the *oral cavity*, the *pharynx* (**FAIR**-inks), the *larynx* (**LAIR**-inks), and the *trachea* (**TRAY**-kee-ah).

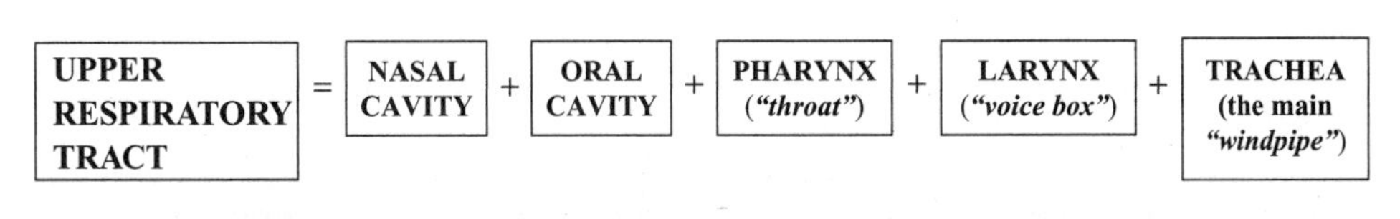
UPPER RESPIRATORY TRACT = **NASAL CAVITY** + **ORAL CAVITY** + **PHARYNX (*"throat"*)** + **LARYNX (*"voice box"*)** + **TRACHEA (the main *"windpipe"*)**

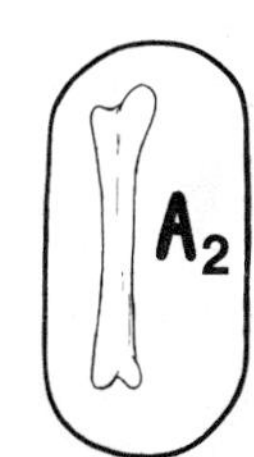

We usually inhale air through both our nasal cavity, which lies within the "nose" (*nas*), and our oral cavity, which sits inside the "mouth" (*or*). We also exhale

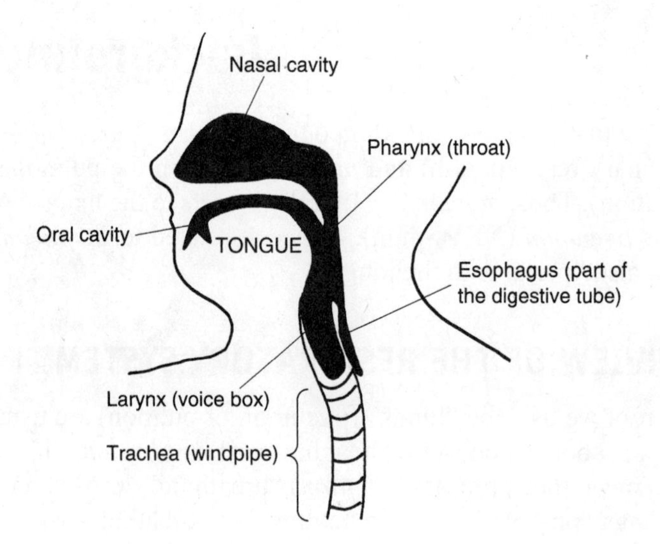

Fig. 9.1 The upper respiratory tract: Our airway down through the trachea.

through these two routes. Speaking much more medically, the nasal and oral cavities provide for two critically important physiological events. The first is *inspiration* (**in**-spih-**RAY**-shun)—the "process of" (*-tion*) "breathing" air (*spir*) "into" (in-) the body. The second event is *expiration* (**eks**-pih-**RAY**-shun). Expiration literally means the "process of" (*-tion*) "breathing" air (*pir*) "out of" (*ex-*) the body.

Adding both of these breathing processes together yields *pulmonary ventilation*. Now, the word *ventilation* exactly means "a process of fanning or blowing." [**Thinking probe:** Recall the last time you saw a *mechanical* ventilator in a building. What was it doing to refresh the air?] If we adapt this concept to include the lungs (*pulmon*), then we obtain the following summary relationship:

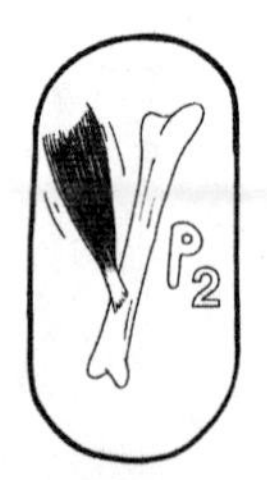

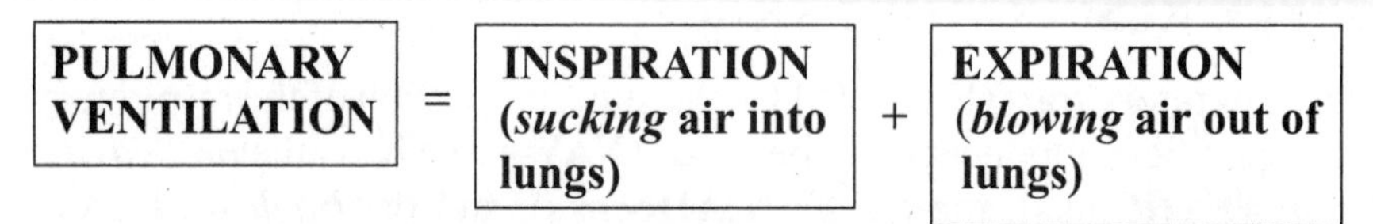

PULMONARY VENTILATION
=
INSPIRATION (*sucking* air into lungs)
+
EXPIRATION (*blowing* air out of lungs)

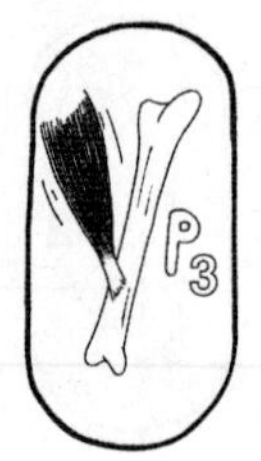

"Why aren't we talking about pulmonary *respiration*?" the clever reader may now be asking. "I thought we were talking about the *respiratory* system in this chapter!" The answer is: Even though respiration literally translates to mean "the process of breathing again," in modern usage it doesn't involve breathing at all! Instead, we have the *Respiration Rule:* Respiration is a process of gas exchange that occurs by a simple diffusion between two or more body compartments.

Within the upper respiratory tract, the walls of all the body structures are just too thick to permit diffusion of gases (such as O_2 and CO_2 molecules) across them. Hence, they do not permit respiration to occur! "Then what *do* they permit, old wise Hippocrates?" They permit pulmonary ventilation, which doesn't involve gas molecules moving across any walls!

Peeking back at Figure 9.1, we observe the pathway that inhaled gases like O_2 and CO_2 take during the inspiration phase of pulmonary ventilation. Both the nasal and oral cavities open into the *pharynx* (**FAIR**-inks), the anatomical name for the "throat." Observe that the pharynx (throat) is the common entryway into two other tubes. The *trachea* (**TRAY**-kee-ah) or main "windpipe" is the one more anterior or in front. And the *esophagus* or "gullet" is the entryway that is more dorsal (farther in the back). In this chapter, we will continue our travels down the trachea.

SOME DISORDERS OF THE UPPER RESPIRATORY TRACT

Many clinical problems of the upper respiratory tract involve the nasal cavity. During *rhinitis* ("inflammation of the nose") or acute coryza (the common cold; see Chapter 5), there is often a *catarrh* (kah-**TAR**). This is a "flowing down" of sticky *nasal mucus*, creating what is casually referred to as a "runny nose." The annoying catarrh, nasal congestion, and other bothersome symptoms of acute coryza can be relieved with various OTC ("over-the-counter") drugs. But the common cold itself has no cure! Why not? The chief difficulty is the nature of the culprit: a *rhinovirus* (**rye**-noh-**VEYE**-rus)! Antibiotics like penicillin are useless against such a rhinovirus, because it's not even alive, so it can't be "killed"!

"What if I get the *flu*, Hippocrates?" What we actually mean by "the flu" is really a case of *respiratory influenza* (in-floo-**EN**-zuh). It derives from the Italian for "influence." "Does that mean a person with the flu is drunk, because he's 'under the influence'? HA! HA!" Originally, it was thought that terrible epidemics of the flu (influenza) were a result of the harmful "influence of the stars" upon human affairs! Capsulizing some flu information yields:

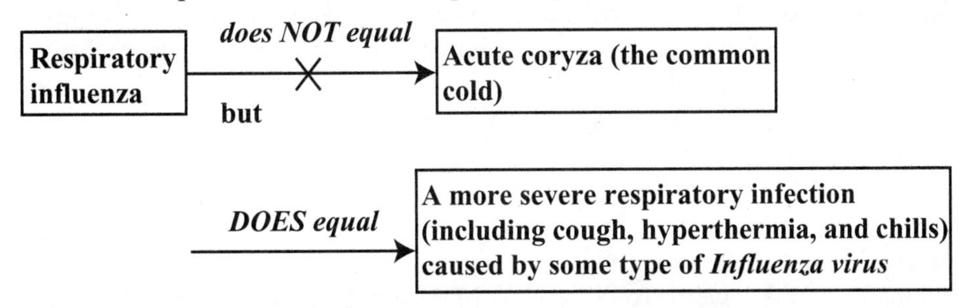

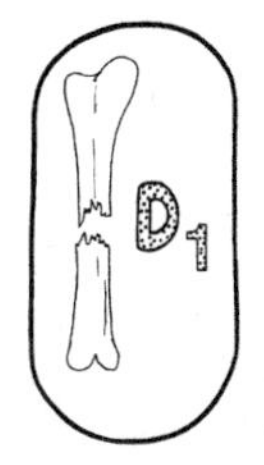

Much more alarming than catarrh is *epistaxis* (**ep**-is-**TAX**-is) or "nose-bleed." Epistaxis is usually the result of ruptured capillaries in the nasal *mucosa*

(myew-**KOH**-sah), the nose's lining "mucous" membrane. But the really frightening stuff includes *hemoptysis* (he-**MAHP**-tih-sis). This is literally a "spitting up" (*-ptysis*) of "blood" (*hem*). Such a horrible clinical symptom may be caused by cancer of the lung!

"What if I just have a sore throat, Hippocrates? What do we call *that*?" Well, Dear Reader, sore throat or "painful" (*-algia*) "throat" (*pharyng*) is correctly called ________/_______. [**Word dissection practice**: Try to write the correct medical term in the preceding blank, inserting a slash mark between its root and suffix.] Such *pharyng/algia* (**fair**-in-**GAL**-jee-ah) usually reflects a case of *pharyngitis* (***fair***-in-***JEYE***-tis) –an "inflammation of the throat."

WHAT COMES AFTER THE TRACHEA? THE LOWER RESPIRATORY TRACT!

The lower respiratory tract (bottom half of Figure 9.2) is the inferior portion of the respiratory system. Specifically, it is the highly branched, treelike portion lying below the trachea. Hence, it is sometimes called *the respiratory "tree"*:

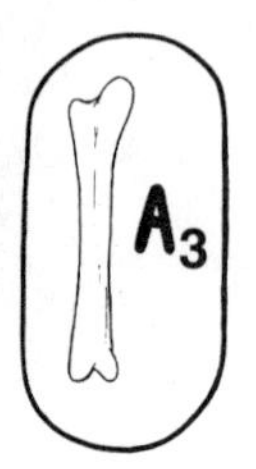

LOWER RESPIRATORY TRACT	=	*THE RESPIRATORY "TREE":* R & L PRIMARY BRONCHI + SMALLER BRONCHI + BRONCHIOLES + ALVEOLAR DUCTS + PULMONARY ALVEOLI

At its bottom end, the trachea forks into the *right and left primary bronchi*. Each *primary bronchus* (**BRAHNK**-us) is a "first-order" (*primary*) "windpipe"—branch (*bronch*). Like the trachea, each primary bronchus has rigid walls and a noncollapsible lumen. This permits a steady and continuous flow of air into and out of the lungs.

After entering the medial (middle or inner) border of a lung, each primary bronchus successively forks into a series of smaller and smaller hollow branches. Indeed, Figure 9.2 makes the visual metaphor of an inverted (upside down) olive tree. The trunk of this respiratory tree, of course, is the trachea. Its two major forked branches are the right and left primary bronchi. Once inside a lung, each primary bronchus splits into a series of smaller bronchi. These, in turn, eventually subdivide into a series of *bronchioles* (**BRAHNK**-ee-ohls)—"little" (*-oles*) "bronchi." Once their lumens narrow down to less than half a millimeter in diameter, the bronchioles are called the *terminal* ("pertaining to the end") *bronchioles*.

Finally, as the lower boxed picture in Figure 9.2 shows, several *respiratory bronchioles* branch off the tip of each terminal bronchiole. The respiratory bronchioles hook into a group of *pulmonary alveoli* (al-**VEE**-oh-lie). Each

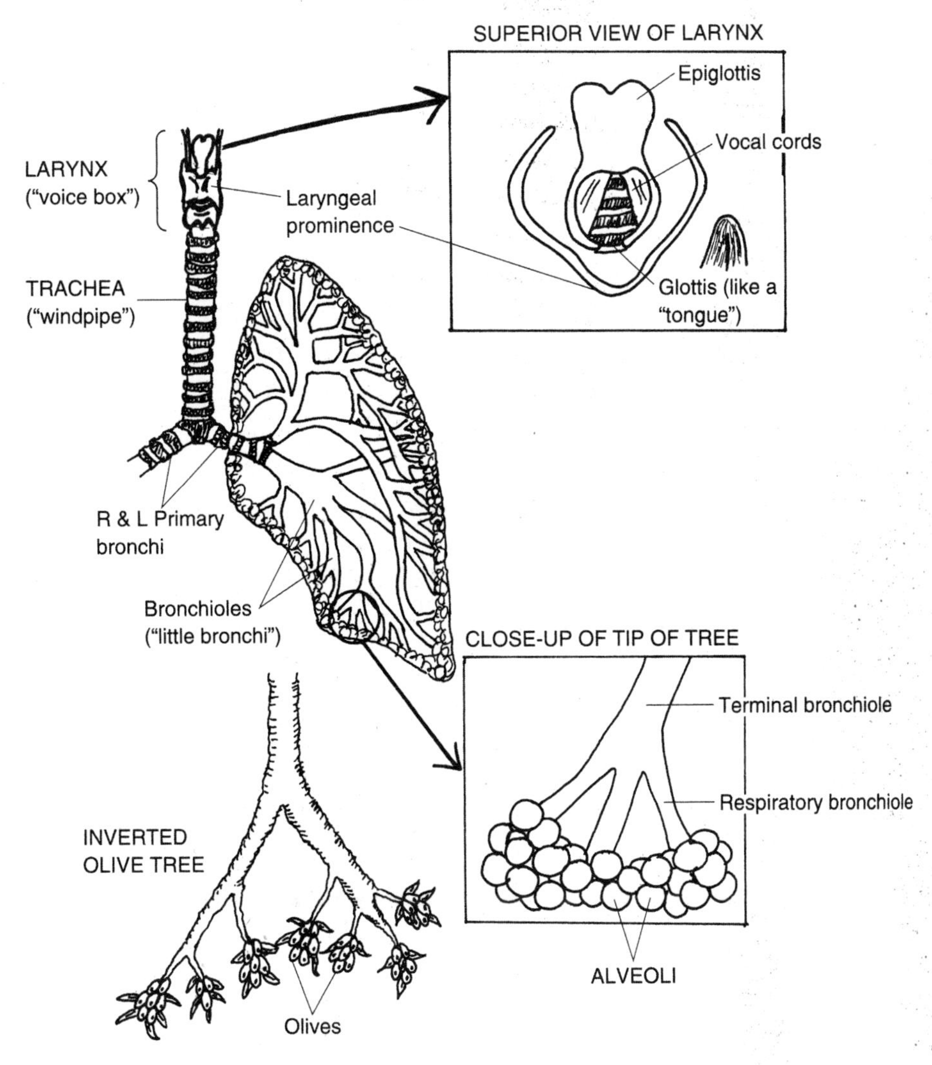

Fig. 9.2 The larynx, trachea, and lower respiratory tract (respiratory "tree").

pulmonary alveolus (al-**VEE**-oh-lus) is literally a "little cavity" (*alveol*) within the "lung" (*pulmon*). Doesn't each alveolus look somewhat like a hollow grape or olive attached to a hollow stem? Each lung is a spongy, highly vascular (blood vessel–rich) organ that contains about 150 million alveoli!

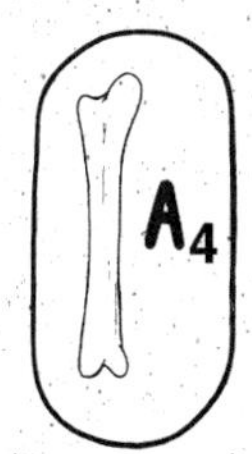

"Wow! That's very impressive, Noble Hippocrates! And considering both of our lungs, that's 300 million pulmonary alveoli 'doing their own thing' within our chest! But, just *what* is the *'thing'* that they're *doing*?"

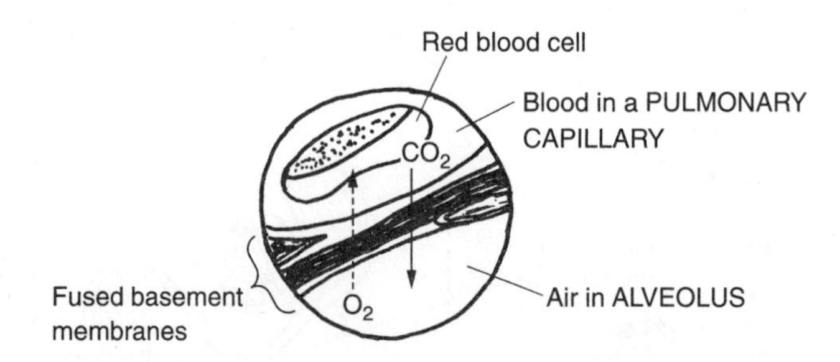

Fig. 9.3 Respiration (gas exchange) between the air in an alveolus and the blood in a pulmonary capillary.

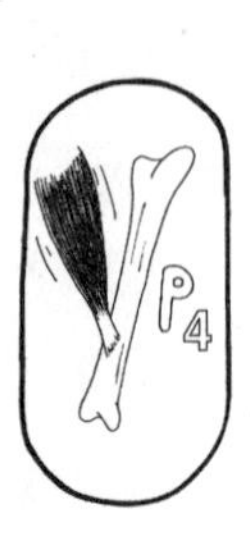

Well, my Curious Friend, what all those millions of pulmonary alveoli are doing is called *respiration!* That is, they are key body structures that permit gas exchange between the respiratory system and the bloodstream. (Consult Figure 9.3.) The alveoli are thin-walled, so they allow the easy diffusion of oxygen (O_2) molecules from their interior into the blood of adjacent *pulmonary capillaries*. This oxygenates the blood, turning it a bright cherry-red. And carbon dioxide (CO_2) molecules in the bloodstream easily diffuse in the opposite direction—across the walls of the pulmonary capillaries and into the nearby alveoli. Once the CO_2 molecules diffuse into the pulmonary alveoli, they are eventually exhaled from the oral or nasal cavity by the process of expiration.

In summary, remember that the only part of the entire respiratory system that actually participates in respiration are the 300 million pulmonary alveoli! All the rest of the system is involved in one main function: ventilation!

NORMAL VERSUS ABNORMAL TYPES OF PULMONARY VENTILATION

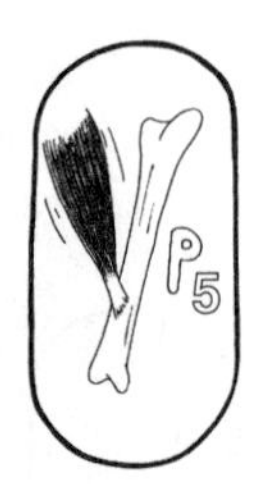

Quite frequently, a nurse will take the *vital* (**VEYE**-tal), or "pertaining to" (*-al*) "life" (*vit*) *signs* of a patient. Such vital signs typically include the pulse (heart rate), body temperature, and *respiratory rate* (RR). The RR is customarily measured in units of number of breaths per minute. [**Thinking probe:** Is RR in breaths per minute an anatomical parameter or a physiological one? Try to explain your reasoning.]

Now, because the nurse is generally counting the number of times that the patient's chest rises per minute, he or she is really counting the number of inspirations taken every minute. In short, the nurse is really measuring the patient's *ventilatory* (**VEN**-tih-lah-**tor**-ee) *rate*. Therefore, the respiratory rate (ventilatory rate) can be described using medical terms involving ventilation. Specifically, these are *normoventilation* (**nor**-moh-ven-tih-**LAY**-shun),

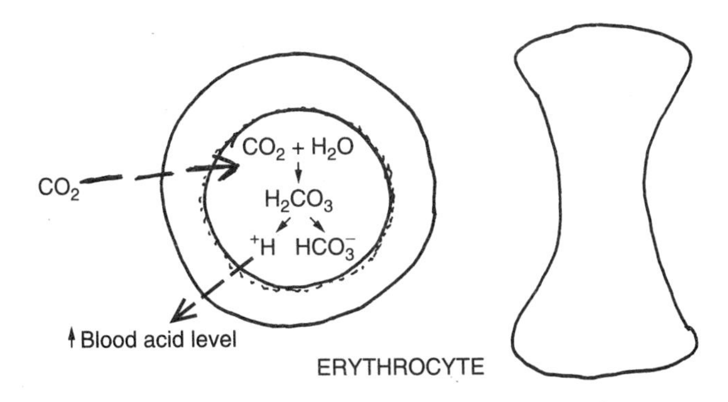

Fig. 9.4 Body acid (H+ ion) creation from CO_2 within RBCs.

hyperventilation (**high**-per-ven-tih-**LAY**-shun), and *hypoventilation* (**high**-poh-ven-tih-**LAY**-shun).

Connection of ventilation to acid-base balance and oxygenation

Acid-base balance represents the proper or optimal state of balance between various *acids* and *bases* or *alkali* (**AL**-kah-**lie**) within the bloodstream. "But why should we be worrying about acids and bases or alkali in this chapter, Good Hippocrates? I thought we were just dealing with various respiratory gases, like oxygen (O_2) and carbon dioxide (CO_2)!"

Yes, we are dealing with respiratory gases like carbon dioxide, so the answer to your question lies in the chemical reactions that happen once CO_2 molecules diffuse into an erythrocyte (RBC). Figure 9.4 reveals that CO_2 reacts with water (H2O) inside of an RBC to eventually produce *hydrogen* (*H+*) *ions*. These H+ ions are *acids*, since an acid is defined as a hydrogen ion donor, that is, a giver of H+ ions. Therefore, every time there is an accumulation of extra CO_2 molecules within our bloodstream, there is an increase in blood *acidity* or acid level.

Now, normoventilation is breathing at an appropriate rate and depth for current body conditions. This helps maintain acid-base balance, since just the right amount of CO_2 is exhaled. It also results in *normoxia* (norm-**AHKS**-ee-ah)—a "normal condition of oxygen" in the bloodstream. Summarizing, we have:

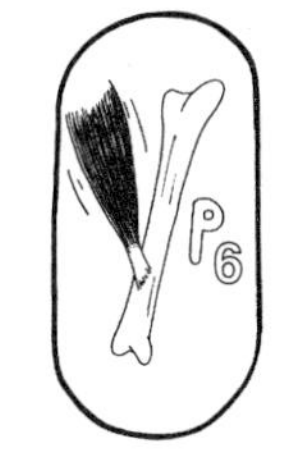

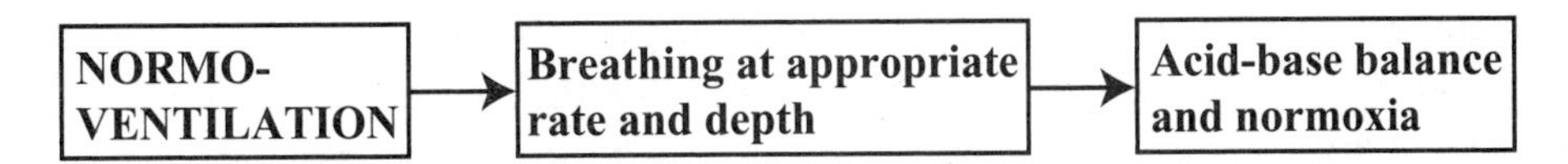

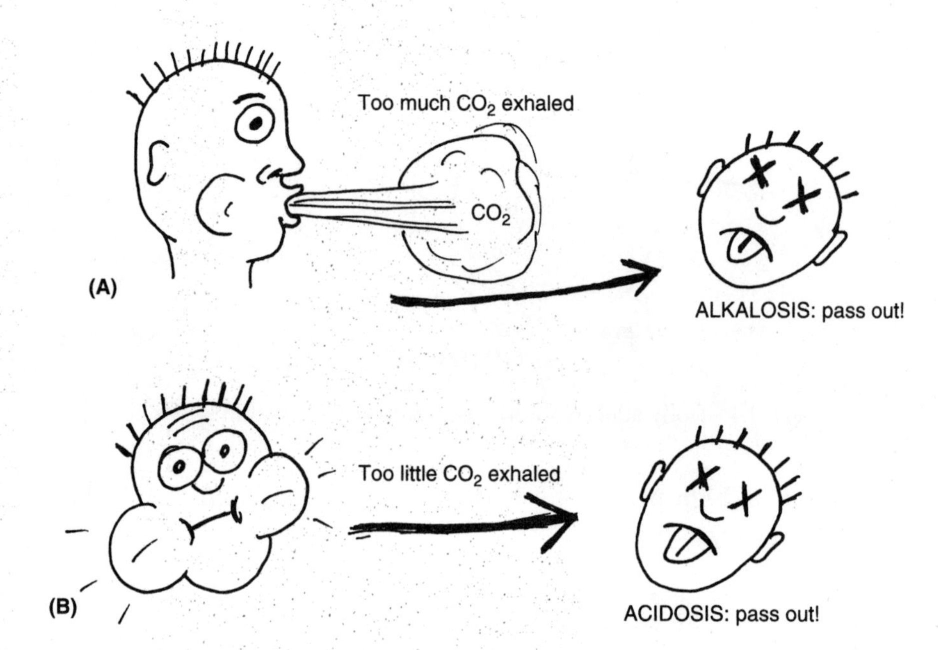

Fig. 9.5 Upsets in body acid-base balance. **(A)** Hyperventilation and ALKALOSIS; **(B)** Hypoventilation and ACIDOSIS.

Hyperventilation, in contrast, is a "condition of" (*-tion*) "excessive" (*hyper-*) "fanning or blowing" (*ventil*). (Study Figure 9.5, A.) Too much CO_2 is lost during excessive amounts of expiration, so that not enough body acid (H+ ions) are produced. The base/alkali levels in the person's bloodstream are pushed out of balance. Thus, a state of *alkalosis* (**al**-kuh-**LOH**-sis)—an "abnormal condition of" (*-osis*) too much body base or "alkali" (*alkal*) results. The *hyperventilating* (**high**-per-**VEN**-tih-**lay**-ting) person's brain reacts to this alkalosis by experiencing dizziness, which may progress to *syncope* (**SIN**-kuh-**pea**) or "fainting." In most clinical cases, *hysterical hyperventilation* is the main cause. (Think, for example, of a parent crying hysterically over a severely hurt child in a hospital emergency room.) Summarizing:

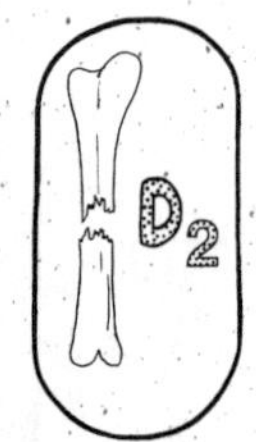

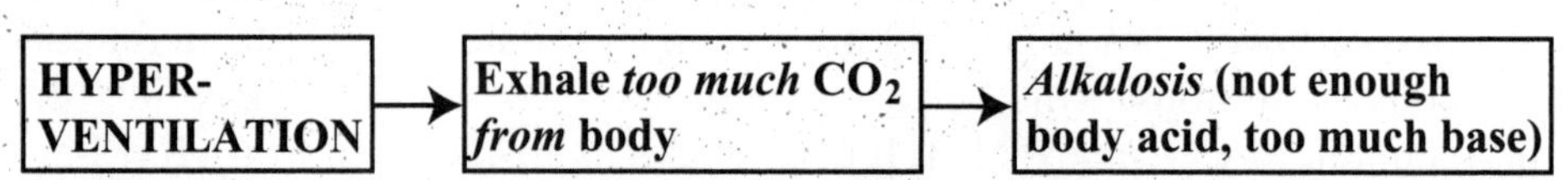

Hypoventilation, the exact opposite of hyperventilation, is a "condition of deficient (*hypo-*) fanning or blowing." (Examine Figure 9.5, B.) Now, our tissue cells are constantly producing more CO_2 as a by-product of their aerobic metabolism (see Chapter 6). If we *hypoventilate* (**high**-poh-**VEN**-tih-layt), then we do *not* exhale this tissue-produced CO_2 in sufficient amounts. More body

acid (H+ ions) are created within our RBCs. As a result, *acidosis* (**ass**-ih-**DOH**-sis) may occur. This is an "abnormal condition of" (*-osis*) too much body "acid." Too many H+ ions around the brain can lead to unconsciousness and even coma!

Now during hypoventilation, the accumulation of excess H+ ions (acid) within the bloodstream is only half of the problem! Because the person is breathing at a deficient rate and/or depth, they are also not taking in enough fresh air via inspiration. Hence, there is a strong danger of suffering *hypoxia* (high-**PAHKS**-ee-ah). This is a "condition of" (*-ia*) "deficient or below normal" (*hypo-*) body "oxygen" (*oxy*). Profiling this info, we have:

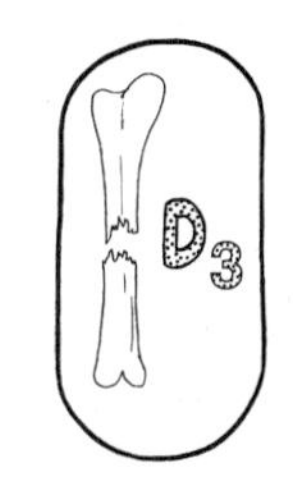

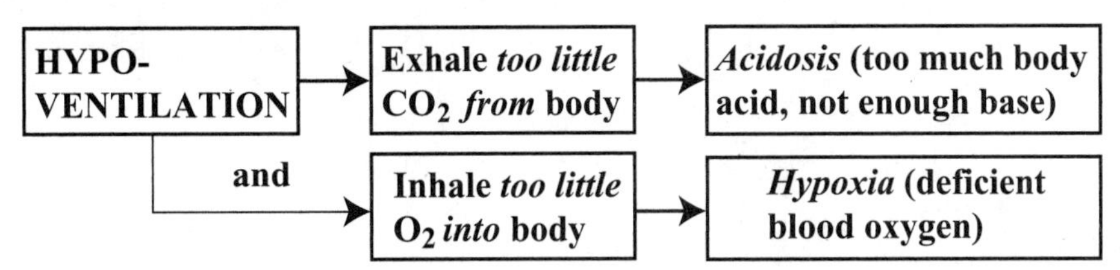

Potential causes of hypoventilation

Hypoventilation leading to hypoxia is very dangerous, because it provides far too little O_2 to allow our oxygen-consuming tissue cells to function normally. As a result, such hypoxia may lead to widespread tissue necrosis (death).

"Gee, Hippocrates! This hypoventilation stuff leading to hypoxia sounds really dangerous! What are some medical problems that could cause this condition?"

Let us discuss two potential causes: *pneumococcal* (**new**-moh-**KAHK**-al) *pneumonia* (**new**-**MOAN**-yuh) and *emphysema* (**em**-fih-**SEE**-muh). First, pneumonia is alternately called *pneumonitis* (**new**-mun-**EYE**-tis). [**Memory probe:** *Pneumon* is a root with the same meaning as *pulmon*. See if you can translate this root, along with the suffix, *-itis*. What do you get?] Pneumonitis (pneumonia) is literally an "inflammation of" (*-itis*) the "lungs" (*pneumon*).

The most common type of pneumonia caused by bacteria is pneumococcal in origin. This means that it "pertains to" (*-al*) "lung" (*pneum*) "berries" (*cocc*). The *pneumococci* (**new**-moh-**KAHK**-see) are oval or berry-shaped bacteria of the cocci (Chapter 3) type. Pneumococcal pneumonia often occurs when a *URI* (upper respiratory infection) caused by pneumococci spreads downward into the lungs. A frequent URI example is *acute sinusitis* (**sigh**-nus-**EYE**-tis). A sinusitis is usually an "*inflammation of*" (*-itis*) some particular bony *sinus* (**SIGH**-nus)—a hollow "curved bay" (*sin*) within a bone. *Frontal sinusitis*, for instance, is a painful inflammation of the *frontal sinus* within the frontal bone of the forehead. The affected person can suffer severe *cephalalgia* (headache).

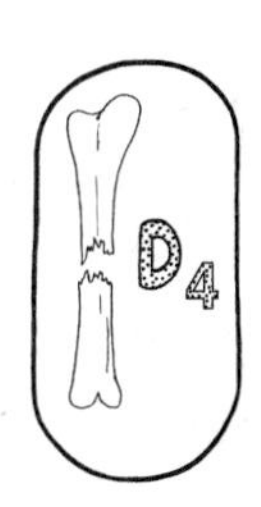

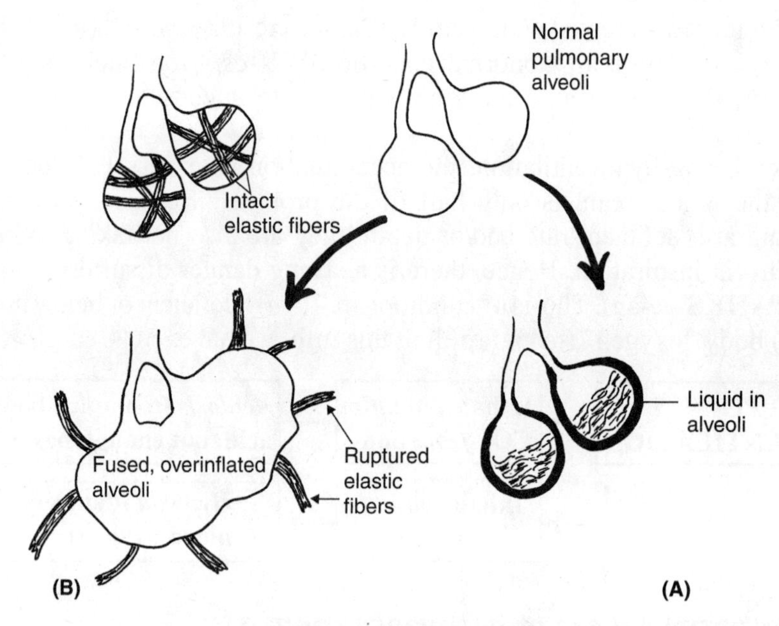

Fig. 9.6 Two potential causes of hypoventilation: Pneumococcal pneumonia and pulmonary emphysema. **(A)** Pneumonia (pneumonitis): The alveoli are partially filled with fluid. **(B)** Pulmonary emphysema: The alveoli are overinflated, and the surrounding elastic fibers have been destroyed.

When, say, the pneumococci causing a frontal sinusitis travel down into the pulmonary alveoli, they set up a secondary infection (pneumonitis or pneumonia) within the lungs. As a result of this inflammation, large amounts of a protein-rich fluid may accumulate within the alveoli. This is very dangerous, because it begins to fill the alveoli with liquid! The person struggles to breathe (having dyspnea), but with each breath, the patient hypoventilates, because the fluid-filled alveoli don't have much room for air! (See Figure 9.6, A.)

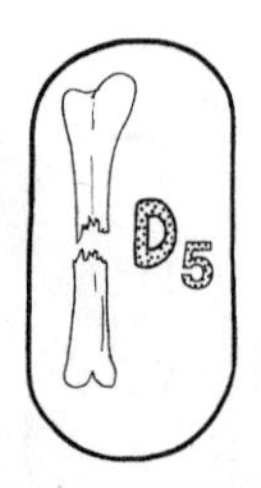

In addition to pneumonia, another frequent cause of hypoventilation is *pulmonary emphysema*, which comes from the ancient Greek for "blowing up" (*emphysem*) of the "lungs" (*pulmon*). Chronic exposure to cigarette smoke, for instance, which contains dangerous toxins (poisons), can cause destructive changes in the elastic fibers around the walls of the alveoli (Figure 9.6, B). As the elastic fibers break, the alveoli become overinflated and flabby. The *emphysematous* (**em**-fih-**SEEM**-ah-tus) patient often develops a big "barrel chest." The reason for the barrel chest is that the overstretched pulmonary alveoli do not snap back to a smaller position during expiration. As a result, the person hypoventilates, unable to deflate the alveoli or exhale enough stale CO_2 from the body.

Hence, the hypoventilation may be accompanied by acidosis. (Again, acidosis is the result of too many H+ ions or acid produced from accumulated CO_2.)

SUMMARY TABLE 9.1

Consult Summary Table 9.1 for a quick review of some important words and word parts.

Summary Table 9.1 Words and Word Parts

Write in the *exact* meaning (literal English equivalent) for up to 10 key terms selected from the preceding block of text. After you are done, check your word meanings with the correct answers, which are given at the end of this chapter.

Key Terms	Prefixes	Roots	Suffixes	Exact Meanings
pneumonic	(none)	pneumon "lungs"	-ic "pertaining to"	1. ________
respiratory	re- "again"	spirat "breathing"	-ory "refers to"	2. ________
inspiration	in-"into"	spir "breathing"	-tion "process of"	3. ________
ventilation	(none)	ventil "fanning or blowing"	-tion "act of"	4. ________
hemoptysis	(none)	hem "blood"	-ptysis "spitting up"	5. ________
bronchiole	(none)	bronchi "bronchi/windpipes"	-ole "little"	6. ________
normo-ventilation	normo- "normal"	ventil "fanning or blowing"	-tion "act of"	7. ________
normoxia	norm- "normal"	ox "oxygen"	-ia "condition of"	8. ________
hyper-ventilation	hyper- "excessive"	ventil "fanning or blowing"	-tion "act of"	9. ________
hypoxia	hyp- "deficient"	ox "oxygen"	-ia "condition of"	10. ________

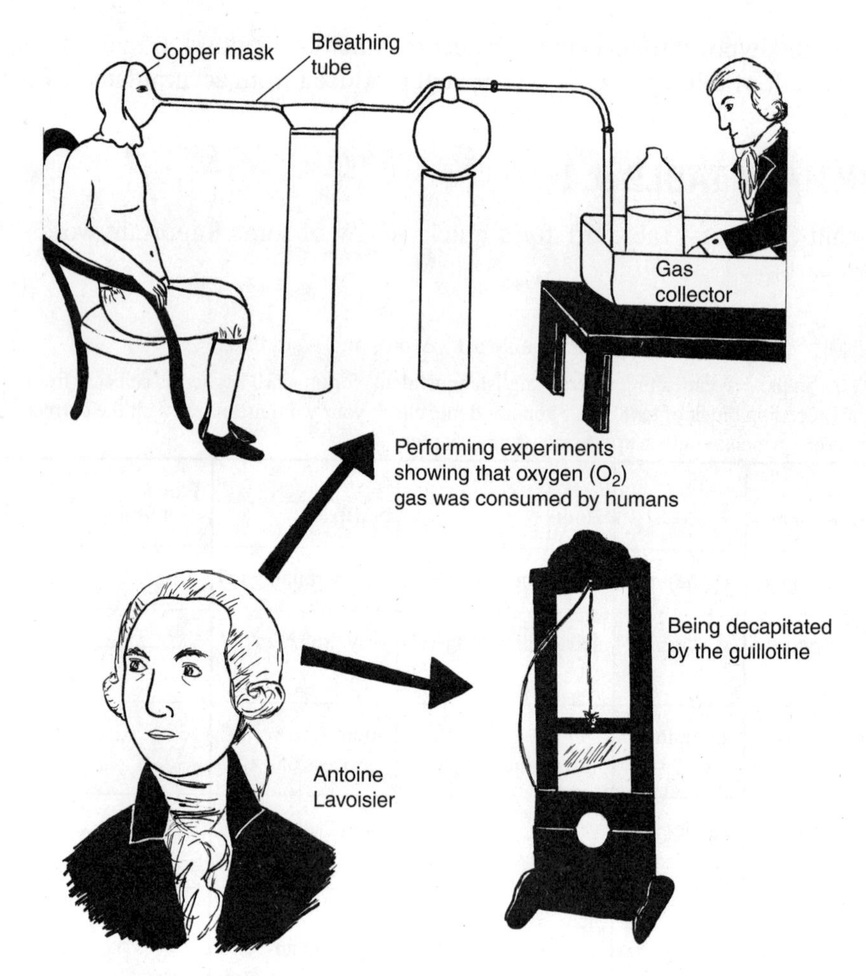

Fig. 9.7 Gas and the guillotine: The saga of Antoine Lavoisier.

GAS AND THE GUILLOTINE: THE SAGA OF ANTOINE LAVOISIER

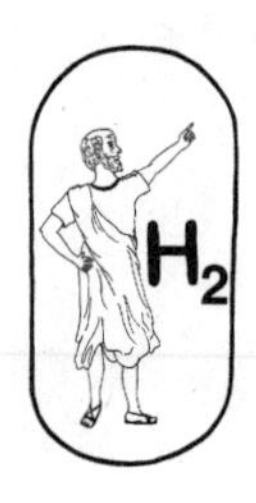

"If we are now, in the early 21st century, so concerned with maintaining tissue normoxia, O Wise Hippocrates, then *who* was it who taught us this important fact in the first place?" It was a French scientist and chemist who lived from 1743 to 1794. His name was *Antoine* (an-**TWAN**) *Lavoisier* (lah-**VWAH**-see-**ay**). He carried out experiments using a copper mask to show that oxygen gas was consumed by humans (Figure 9.7). Lavoisier showed that O_2 consumption, pulse rate, and respiratory rate increased during exercise. He even named the element oxygen, which means "acid-former." He is often considered the Father of Modern Chemistry. But because of his former ties to the hated monarchy, this noble scientist was *decapitated* (deh-**CAP**-ih-**tay**-ted) during the Reign of Terror of the French Revolution. Poor Antoine had his "head" (*capit*) cut "off" (*de-*) by the dreaded *guillotine* (**GIL**-uh-**teen**)! "The Republic has no need of geniuses!" the judge cruelly declared when an appeal was made to save Lavoisier's life. There is a strange legend that Lavoisier arranged a final experiment at his death. He supposedly told an assistant to count the number of times that he blinked after he had his head cut off! (The legend says he blinked 15 to 20 times, but this is very doubtful!)

Medical Case History: An Emergency Tracheotomy to Treat Airway Obstruction

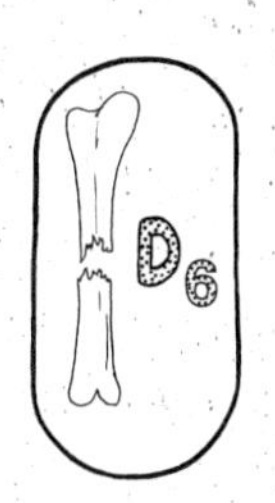

We have talked about the importance of inhaling adequate oxygen during inspiration and of the grave dangers we face during tissue hypoxia. If hypoventilation tends to result in hypoxia, then *apnea* (**AP**-nee-ah)—total "lack" (*a-*) of "breathing" (*pnea*)—is even worse! If a state of apnea lasts for just a few minutes, a "condition of" (-ia) severe tissue *anoxia* (an-**AHK**-see-ah) results. This is a complete "lack" (*an-*) of tissue "oxygen" (*ox*). Loss of consciousness and irreversible brain damage are the terrible consequences of this deadly duo (apnea leading to anoxia)!

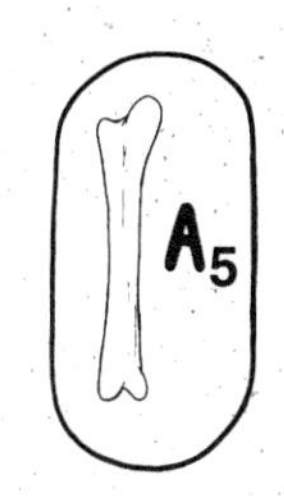

In the present clinical case, George B. was gulping down big pieces of steak during a business lunch. He had a few drinks, and he was busy talking and laughing with a customer while he ate. The clinical problem George suffered involved his *epiglottis*—a small flap of cartilage that forms a lid "upon" (*epi-*) the *glottis* (**GLAHT**-is) (see Figure 9.8, A, and review Figure 9.2.) The glottis is a small "tongue" (*glott*) -shaped opening between the *vocal cords* of the larynx.

Normally, when a person swallows a food *bolus* (**BOH**-lus), it's just a small, soft "ball" (*bol*) of food that is "present" (*-us*). After the person flips the bolus back into the pharynx, the bolus falls down and pushes the epiglottis shut from above (Figure 9.8, B). This small flap closes snugly over the top of the glottis. Such closure prevents *pathologic* (**path**-oh-**LAJ**-ik) *respiratory aspiration* (**as**-pih-**RAY**-shun). This is the potentially deadly "breathing in" (*aspir*) of food, liquid, or other foreign objects into the larynx and airways. Under normal conditions, the food bolus just slides down into the esophagus, and finally enters the stomach.

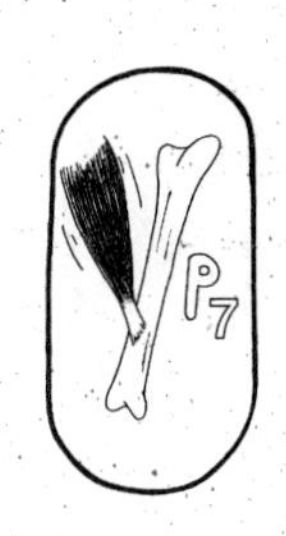

But George B. just wasn't paying attention. He was doing too much laughing and talking while he bolted down huge chunks of partially chewed steak. Suddenly, a big piece of steak became wedged in between the epiglottis and the glottis, thereby completely occluding the opening into his larynx! (Study Figure 9.8, C.)

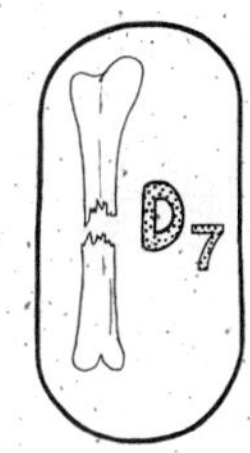

Almost immediately, poor George made the *Heimlich* (*HIGHM*-lik) *sign*, also called the *universal choking signal*. (This sign was first described by

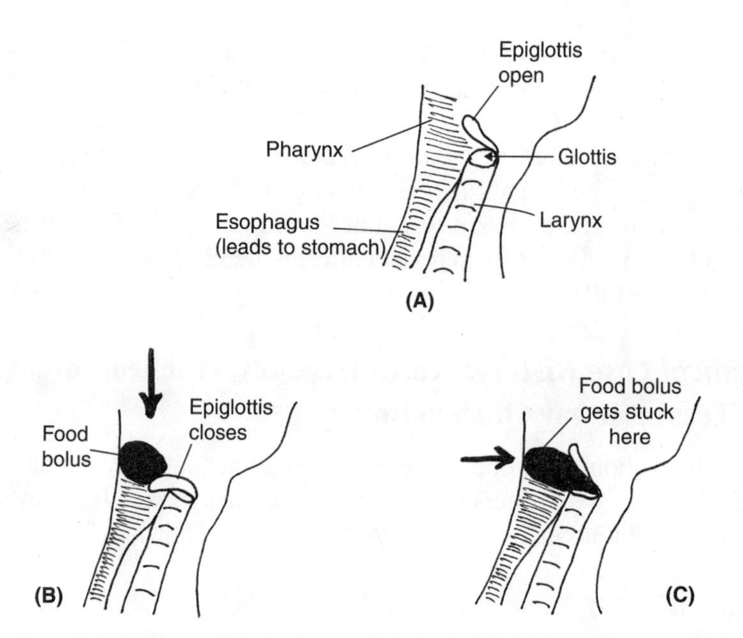

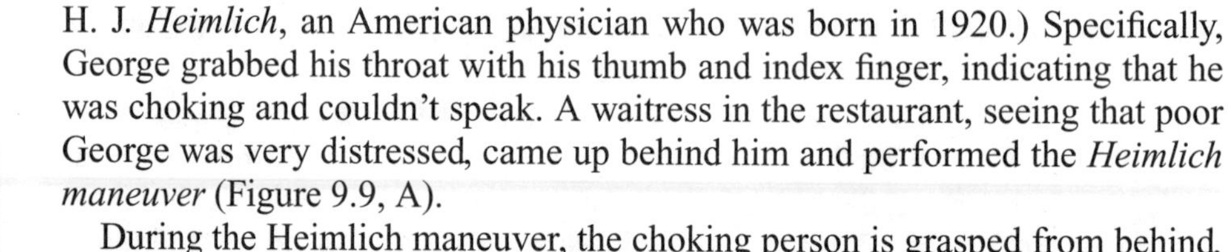

Fig. 9.8 Normal versus abnormal closing of the epiglottis. **(A)** Anatomic position of epiglottis as a lid "upon" the "glottis" (tongue-shaped opening in top of larynx). **(B)** Normally, a small food bolus pushes the epiglottis shut during swallowing. **(C)** During choking, a large bolus (chunk of steak) gets wedged between the epiglottis and the glottis, occluding the larynx.

H. J. *Heimlich*, an American physician who was born in 1920.) Specifically, George grabbed his throat with his thumb and index finger, indicating that he was choking and couldn't speak. A waitress in the restaurant, seeing that poor George was very distressed, came up behind him and performed the *Heimlich maneuver* (Figure 9.9, A).

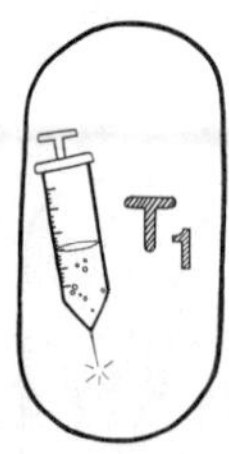

During the Heimlich maneuver, the choking person is grasped from behind, with the rescuer pressing one fist into the *substernal* (sub-**STER**-nal) area of the victim's thorax (chest). The rescuer places her other hand firmly over her fist. The rescuer then pulls her fist firmly and sharply into the *epigastric* (**ep**-ih-**GAS**-trik) *region* of the thorax. As the phrase indicates, this is the region lying "upon" (*epi-*) the "stomach" (*gastr*). The pressing fist greatly increases the *intra-abdominal* (**in**-trah-ahb-**DAHM**-ih-nal) *pressure.* The greater pressure forces the wedged-in food bolus out of the choking person's larynx. If successful in dislodging the food bolus, the Heimlich maneuver prevents death by *asphyxiation* (as-**fik**-see-**AY**-shun). Asphyxiation exactly means the "process of" (*-tion*) "stopping the pulse" (*asphyx*).

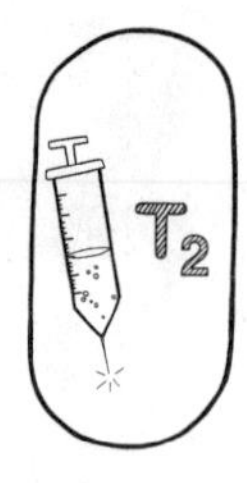

In this instance, most unfortunately, the Heimlich maneuver was unsuccessful. A physician sitting at another table suddenly rose to his feet and offered

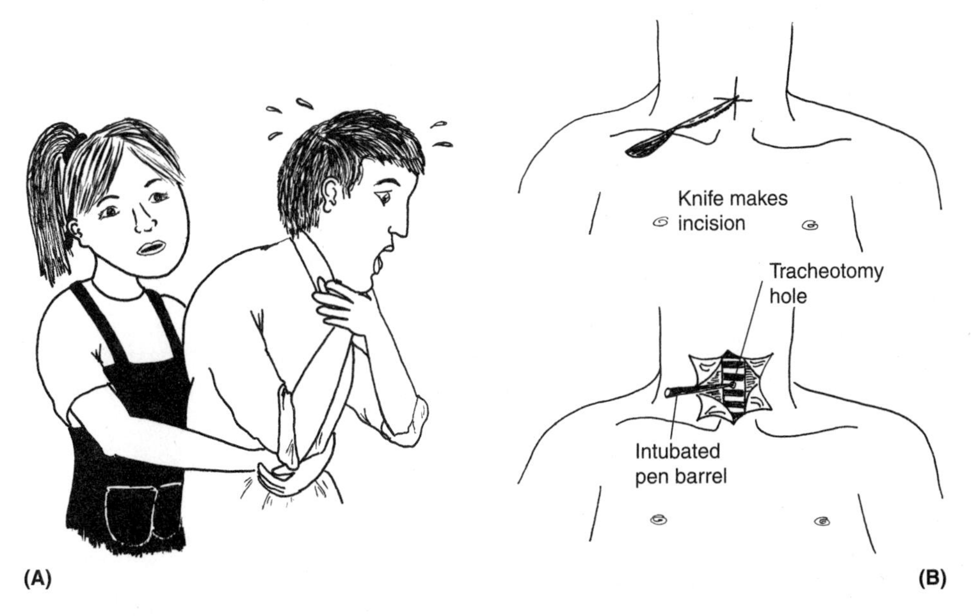

Fig. 9.9 The Heimlich maneuver and an emergency tracheotomy. **(A)** George makes the *universal choking signal*, prompting a nearby waitress to perform the *Heimlich maneuver*. **(B)** A doctor makes an incision into the neck with a steak knife, then inserts his pen into the resulting *tracheotomy* hole. The hollow pen barrel intubates the hole, thereby establishing a new airway below the *laryngeal* steak obstruction.

assistance. Grabbing the sharp steak knife from George's dinner plate, the doctor slammed George onto his back and performed an emergency *tracheotomy* (**trayk**-ee-**AHT**-oh-me) (Examine Figure 9.9, B.). This involves "the process of making a cut or incision" (*-otomy*) into the front of the "windpipe" (*trache*). This small, temporary opening let just enough air into poor George's lungs to prevent a deadly state of tissue anoxia, unconsciousness, and quick death by asphyxiation (suffocation)!

To maintain a *patent* (**PAT**-ent) or "open" airway, the doctor took a pen out of his shirt pocket and removed the ink cartridge. He then used the empty barrel to *intubate* (**IN**-too-bait) George's trachea. After the pen "tube" (*tub*) had been inserted "into" (*in-*) the windpipe, any accidental closing of the tracheotomy opening was prevented. This allowed poor George to *ventilate* (**VEN**-tih-**layt**) normally until the paramedics and ambulance arrived.

Probe of case history

(**A**) Extract the root and suffix from the word, *apnea*. Now, combine them with the prefix in *tachycardia* (Chapter 8). Write down the resulting medical term.

What is its common English translation? (**B**) During the description of the Heimlich maneuver, the rescuer's fist was placed against the choking victim's "substernal area." What is the literal meaning of *substernal*? To which specific bone does it refer? [Check your short answers with the key near the end of this chapter.]

Quiz

Refer to the text in this chapter if necessary. A good score is at least 8 correct answers out of these 10 questions. The answers are listed in the back of this book.

1. Respiration differs from ventilation in that:
   (a) Respiration is actually a process of gas exchange
   (b) Ventilation involves the exchange of CO_2 for O_2
   (c) Respiration requires conscious effort
   (d) Ventilation in humans occurs by a mechanical, nonliving process
2. The upper respiratory tract includes the:
   (a) Trachea, bronchi, and lungs
   (b) Pharynx, larynx, and trachea
   (c) Oral cavity, nasal cavity, and gonads
   (d) Nasal cavity, pharynx, and esophagus
3. The exact opposite of inspiration is:
   (a) Aspiration
   (b) Respiration
   (c) Inhalation
   (d) Expiration
4. Catarrh represents:
   (a) A musical instrument related to the guitar
   (b) Severe coughing spells
   (c) Runny nose
   (d) Fainting episodes
5. Respiratory influenza is:
   (a) Just another name for the "stomach flu"
   (b) Basically identical to acute coryza/rhinitis
   (c) An incurable carcinoma of the respiratory tree
   (d) Infection with a non-cold virus that results in cough, hyperthermia, and chills

6. The very end-part of the respiratory "tree":
   (a) Bronchiole
   (b) Pulmonary alveolus
   (c) Primary bronchi
   (d) Epiglottis

7. Named the element, oxygen, and discovered its role in human metabolism:
   (a) Shen Nung
   (b) Henry Cabot Lodge
   (c) Antoine Lavoisier
   (d) William Shepherd

8. The only part of the so-called respiratory system that actually participates in the respiratory process:
   (a) Bronchioles
   (b) Pulmonary alveoli
   (c) Laryngeal prominence
   (d) Vocal cords

9. Hyperventilation is properly dissected with slash marks as:
   (a) Hy/perv/entil/ation
   (b) H/yper/ventila/tion
   (c) Hyper/venti/la/tion
   (d) Hyper/ventil/a/tion

10. The word, *hypoxia*, indicates what specific body condition?
    (a) Insufficient tissue O_2 concentration
    (b) An excessive amount of carbon dioxide in the trachea
    (c) Extremely high alveolar nitrogen content
    (d) A complete absence of breathing

Memory Pillboxes for Chapter 9

Several key facts were tagged with numbered icons in the page margins of this chapter. Write a short summary of each of these key facts into a numbered cell or compartment within the appropriate type of *Memory Pillbox* that appears below.

***Background and History* Pillboxes for Chapter 9:**

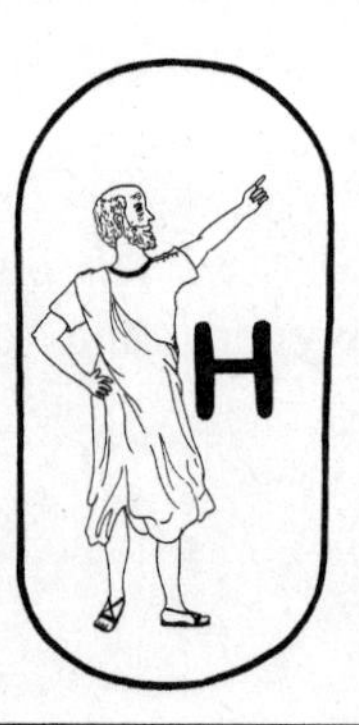

1	2

***Anatomy* Pillboxes for Chapter 9:**

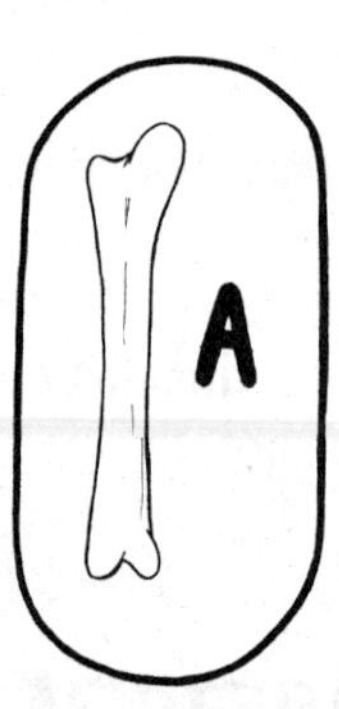

1	2

3	4

5

***Physiology* Pillboxes for Chapter 9:**

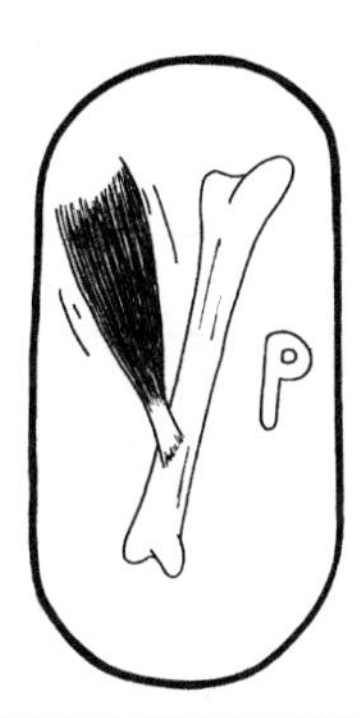

1	2

3	4

5	6

7

Disease/Injury **Pillboxes for Chapter 9:**

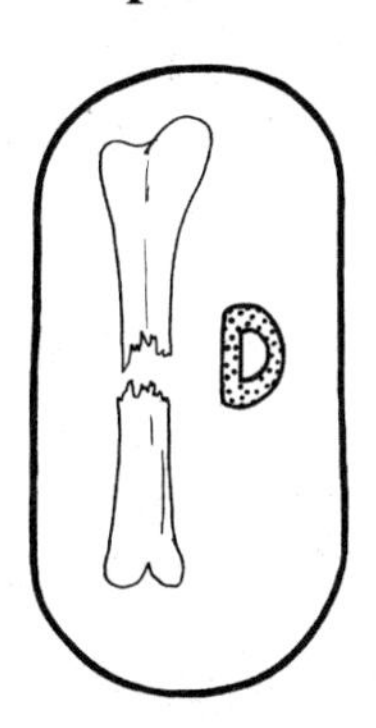

1	2
3	4
5	6

7

Treatment/Therapy **Pillboxes for Chapter 9:**

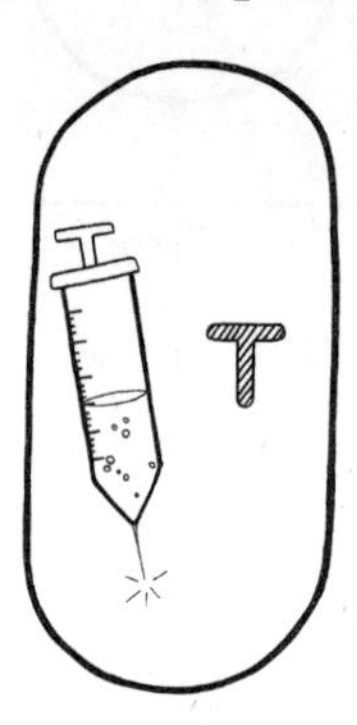

1	2

3

Answers for Chapter 9 Summary Table

FOR SUMMARY TABLE 9.1

1. "pertaining to lungs"
2. "referring to breathing again"
3. "process of breathing into"
4. "act of fanning/blowing"
5. "spitting up blood"
6. "little bronchi/windpipes"
7. "act of normal fanning or blowing"
8. "condition of normal oxygen"
9. "act of excessive fanning/blowing"
10. "condition of deficient oxygen"

Answers to Probe of Case History

(**A**) Tachypnea = "condition of fast breathing" (**B**) Substernal = "pertaining to (something) below the sternum (breastbone)."

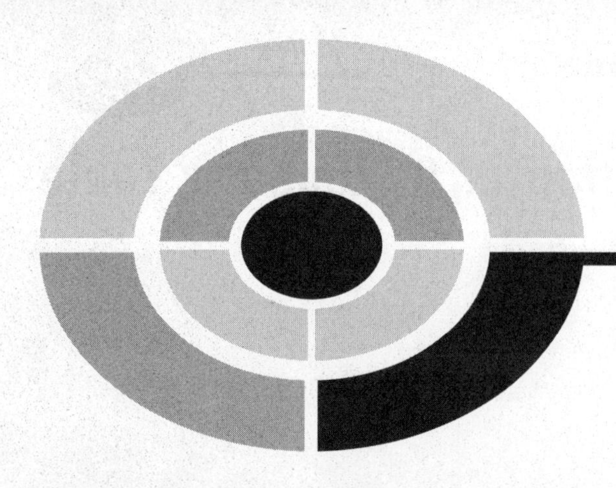

Test: Part 4

DO NOT REFER TO THE TEXT WHEN TAKING THIS TEST. A good score is at least 18 (out of 25 questions) correct. The answers are in the back of the book. It's best to have a friend check your score the first time so you won't memorize the answers if you want to take the test again.

1. The chief pump for the systemic portion of the circulatory system:
   (a) Right atrium
   (b) Left ventricle
   (c) Aorta
   (d) Right ventricle
   (e) Right atrium

2. *Systol/ic* translates to mean:
   (a) "Referring to my good ol' sister"
   (b) "Presence of heart muscle"
   (c) "Relating to contracting"
   (d) "Presence of a (heart) contraction"
   (e) "Relaxation phase of the heart"

3. If a surgeon *ligates* a vessel, what is done to the vessel?
   (a) It is removed from body
   (b) It is repaired and relined
   (c) It is put on red alert!
   (d) The lumen is tied off
   (e) The vessel becomes inflamed

4. Vessels that are located immediately after the capillary networks:
   (a) Large veins
   (b) Major arteries
   (c) Arterioles
   (d) Middle-sized arteries
   (e) Venules

5. *Capillary* is correctly dissected as:
   (a) Capill/ary
   (b) Cap/il/lar/y
   (c) Ca/pill/ary
   (d) Capi/llary
   (e) C/apill/ar/y

6. Capillary literally translates to mean "_________" in regular English.
   (a) "Two rivers"
   (b) "Referring to a reefer"
   (c) "Pertaining to a tiny hair"
   (d) "A huge cavity that is present"
   (e) "Too many hairs (on someone's head)"

7. The blood picks up oxygen in this portion of the total blood circulation:
   (a) Heart valve
   (b) Peripheral systemic arteries
   (c) Coronary circulation
   (d) Pulmonary capillaries
   (e) Lymphatic capillaries

8. Means "red (blood) cell present":
   (a) Erythr/o/blast
   (b) Lymph/o/cyte
   (c) Erythr/o/cyt/e
   (d) Rubrocyt/osis
   (e) Leuk/o/cyt/ic

9. A new term built to mean "pertaining to (something) within the heart":
   (a) Epicardial

(b) Myocarditis
(c) Intravascular
(d) Endocardic
(e) Extracorporeal

10. BP = ________:
(a) EKG + STP
(b) PDQ + QUIP
(c) SBP – DBP
(d) SBP/DBP
(e) DBP + SBP – ATP

11. The pulse rate is a physiological parameter that indicates:
(a) Number of cardiac cycles/minute
(b) Electrical rhythm of the heart
(c) Liters of blood pumped/hour
(d) Temperature of the venous blood in degrees Celsius
(e) Homeostasis of hematocrit concentration in grams

12. "Hardening of the arteries":
(a) Atherosclerosis
(b) Coronary plaque
(c) Arteriosclerosis
(d) Hemocytopenia
(e) Acute coronary thrombosis

13. Blood pressure is frequently measured at this particular vessel:
(a) Brachial artery
(b) Internal carotid artery
(c) Aortic arch
(d) Femoral vein
(e) Middle cerebral artery

14. Someone with a large aneurysm is in great danger of experiencing:
(a) Sleep apnea
(b) Skin cancer
(c) Arterial hypotension
(d) Severe internal hemorrhaging
(e) Premature blood clotting

15. Hemostasis is most closely related to which of the following processes?
(a) Blood platelets sticking together
(b) WBCs wandering through vessel walls
(c) Erythrocytes swelling up with H_2O

(d) Homeostasis of blood volume in milliliters
(e) Effective antigen-antibody reactions

16. *Somnolent* (**SAHM**-noh-**lent**) means "referring to" (*-ent*) "sleep" (*somn*). Suppose a patient is diagnosed as having *somnolent apnea*. In layman's language, this suggests that:
(a) They are "living" in a "sleepy" little village
(b) The concentration of "red" cells in their bloodstream is "deficient"
(c) Their "sleeping" period contains moments when their "breathing stops"
(d) The patient can "not sleep," due to "difficult breathing"
(e) Special "little berries" (pills) are needed to "produce sleep"

17. Disease often caused by chronic "hyperexposure" to cigarette smoke:
(a) Carcinoma of the skin
(b) "Blowing up" (*emphysem*) of the alveoli
(c) Postural hypotension
(d) Chronic irritability and depression
(e) Asphyxiation

18. What is meant by a *bolus*?
(a) A "thirsty" sensation
(b) Soft "ball" of partially digested food
(c) Rounded, "berry-shaped" bacteria
(d) A hard knob on the front of the larynx
(e) Some interference with normal respiration

19. An abnormal condition of too much body base:
(a) Alkalosis
(b) Hypercapnia
(c) Aerobic metabolosis
(d) Acidosis
(e) Hyperglycemia

20. "A spitting of blood":
(a) Hemosiderosis
(b) Hematogenesis
(c) Lymphocytosis
(d) Hemoptysis
(e) Lung hyperinflation

21. Both respiratory influenza and acute coryza have this in common:
(a) Caused by a viral infection
(b) Result from mutation of once-normal tracheal bacteria

(c) Diarrhea and vomiting as customary symptoms
(d) Hyperthermia
(e) Atrial fibrillation

22. The throat is technically named the:
(a) Oral cavity
(b) Nares
(c) Esophagus
(d) Larynx
(e) Pharynx

23. A cardiorespiratory type of disorder would literally involve problems in:
(a) Both the respiratory tree and the general blood circulation
(b) Neither the lungs nor the heart
(c) The brain and thorax, but not include the lungs
(d) The heart and "breathing again" organ system
(e) Only the lower respiratory tract

24. Contains millions of hemoglobin molecules:
(a) Erythrocyte
(b) Pneumococcus
(c) Thrombocyte
(d) Platelet
(e) Cardiac muscle fiber

25. The medical phrase for having a "heart attack" is:
(a) Experiencing an episode of anemia
(b) Severe acute myocardial ischemia
(c) Chronic CAD
(d) Essential hypertension
(e) Formation of a myocardial infarct (MI)

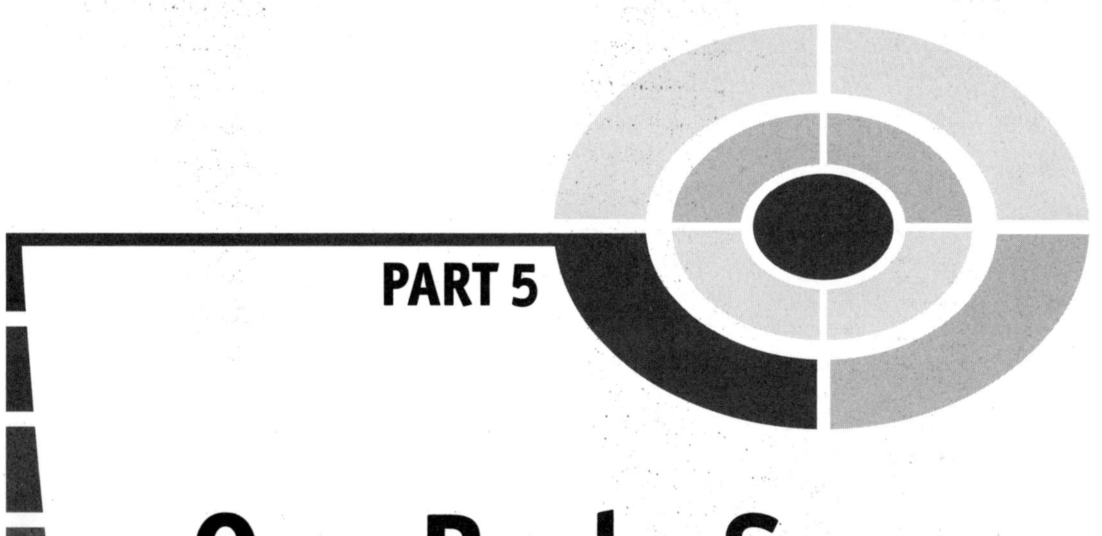

PART 5

Our Body Senses

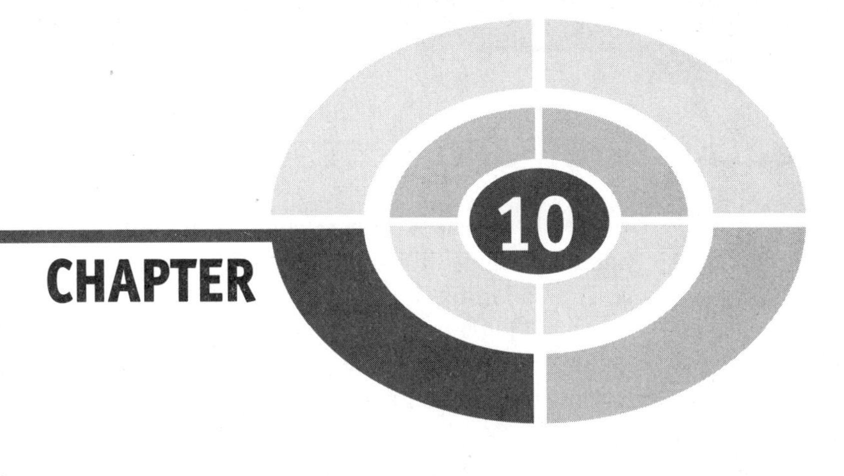

Terms Related to Disorders of the Glands and Skin

In the last few chapters, we have been looking at the cardiovascular (circulatory) and respiratory systems. These are organ systems that push fluids (blood or air) through pipes or vessels deep within the body interior. Now, in Part 5, we will consider the ways in which our body *senses* detect, integrate, and communicate information about the environment. And by environment, we are referring to both the *external environment* "outside" of the body and the *internal environment* that lies "within."

This discussion of environmental impacts will begin with the glands and our covering: the skin.

Background and History

Chapter 10 considers our *integumentary* (**in**-teg-you-**MEN**-tary) *system*. This system "pertains to" (*-ary*) our body "covering" or *integument* (in-**TEG**-you-ment). In addition, it discusses the *glandular* (**GLAN**-dyoo-lar) *system*, which "refers to" (*-ar*) our body's "little acorns" (*glandul*). In simpler language, the integumentary system involves our skin and its various components. And the glandular system is the organ system composed of all our *glands*.

OVERVIEW OF THE INTEGUMENTARY SYSTEM (SKIN)

The skin (integument) is the largest organ in the human organism. It is named for its basic function of covering the body surface. Included within the skin are a number of *accessory* (**ak-SESS**-or-ee) or "added" *structures*, such as the hairs, nails, and various glands.

In overview, then:

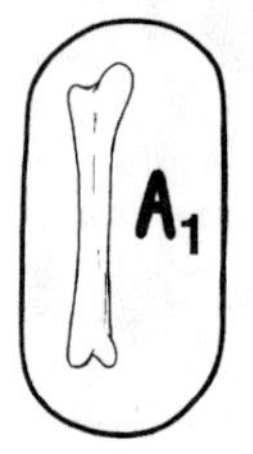

INTEGUMENTARY SYSTEM = **SKIN** + **ACCESSORY STRUCTURES**

or

= **SKIN** + **HAIRS** + **NAILS** + **GLANDS**

THE SKIN AND ITS DISORDERS

Two roots for "skin" are *derm* and *dermat* (**DER**-mat). Using the suffix, *-is*, we can use the first root to build *dermis* (**DUR**-mis). This means "presence of the skin." The fundamental anatomy of the human skin is pictured in Figure 10.1. Note that the figure makes an imaginative connection to the skin of a peach, which covers the soft, wet fruit as an integument. [**Thinking probe:** How is this situation of the peach integument similar to the role of the human integument?]

The integuments of both human skins and fruity peaches have the name of their outermost layer in common. It is called the *epidermis* (**ep**-ih-**DER**-mis). The epidermis is a thin, tough, relatively waterproof layer "present" (*-is*) "upon" (*epi-*) the "skin" (*derm*) surface. Go out and work in the hot sun. Beads of sweat (salty water) will form on your epidermis, but won't pass through it. Likewise, wash off a peach under running water. On its epidermis, too, the water collects and beads, rather than penetrates. The same valuable waterproofing function occurs in the opposite direction as well. In both cases, *dehydration* (**dee**-high-**DRAY**-shun) is prevented. Dehydration is literally the "process of" (*-tion*) losing "water" (*hydr*) "from" (*de-*) the body interior.

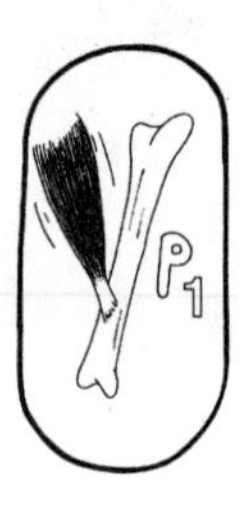

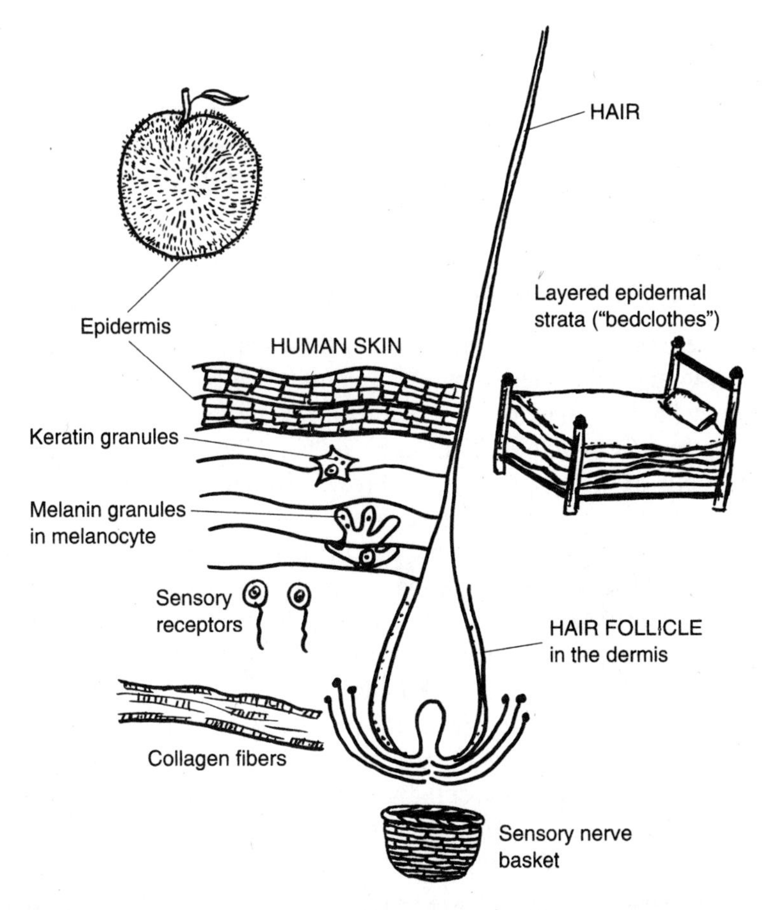

Fig. 10.1 The human skin: A "peachy" integument.

If we change the analogy to one of a bed covered with sheets and blankets, we can also consider the epidermis to consist of a series of *epidermal* (**ep**-ih-**DER**-mal) *strata* (**STRAT**-uh). These are thin sheets of epithelial cells that occur in many "layers or bed covers" (*strat*).

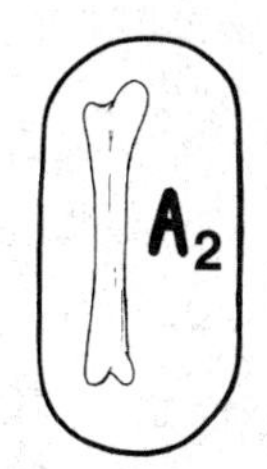

EPIDERMIS = Thin sheets or strata of epithelial cells that have an important body waterproofing function

Figure 10.1 also features the dermis, which is the tough, fibrous (fiber-rich) connective tissue layer of the skin. The many *collagen* (**KAHL**-uh-jen) fibers within the dermis act like "glue" (*colla*) "producers" (*gen*), making the skin hard to stretch.

Taking the dermis together with the epidermis, gives us the *true skin*:

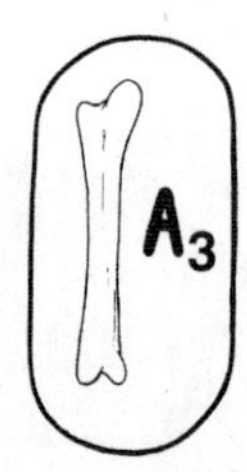

THE TRUE SKIN	=	DERMIS	+	EPIDERMIS
		(Deep connective tissue layer)		**(Superficial epithelial strata)**

Melanocytes and related disorders

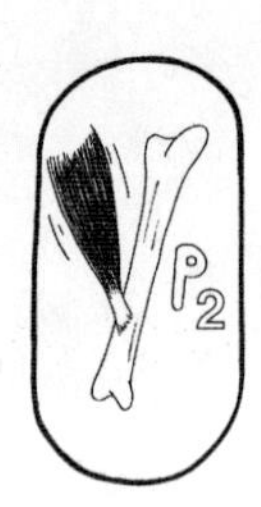

Near the base of the dermis (Figure 10.1) lie a great number of *melanocytes* (**MEL**-uh-nuh-**sights**). These "black" (*melan*) "cells" (*cytes*) are large and shaped somewhat like an octopus. The long arms of the melanocyte's cytoplasm are used to inject *melanin* (**MEL**-uh-nin), a "black" (*melan*) "substance" (*-in*), into nearby cells of the epidermis. The brownish-black melanin granules make our skin pigmented. In addition, these granules help absorb harmful *ultraviolet* (UV) *rays* in the sunlight that strike the skin surface.

It is thought that chronic overexposure to the UV rays from sunlight cross-links the *dermal* collagen fibers, creating wrinkles. But much worse, these rays may trigger mutations in skin cell DNA molecules (Chapter 6). Such mutations can result in *melanoma* (mel-uh-**NOH**-muh).

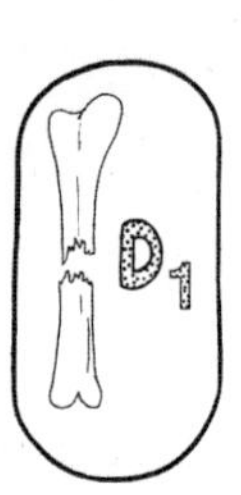

Such "black tumors" (*-omas*), unfortunately, frequently become malignant. A diagnosis of *malignant melanoma* is therefore a frightening one! Most malignant melanomas arise from abnormal cell division in the melanocytes of normal skin. They are typically *asymptomatic* (**AY**-sim-tom-**AT**-ik), or "without symptoms," in their early stages. A sudden increase in the size of dark moles, especially moles with irregular margins, should be checked by a *dermatologist* (dur-muh-**TAHL**-uh-jist). A dermatologist is "one who specializes in the study of" (*-ologist*) the "skin" (*dermat*).

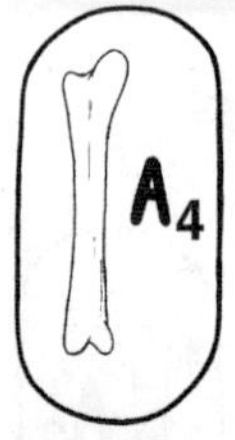

Hair follicles, sensory receptors, and sebaceous glands

Observe back in Figure 10.1 that a *hair follicle* (**FAHL**-uh-kul) is shown in the dermis, along with a number of *sensory receptors*. A hair follicle is a "little bag" surrounded by a membrane and containing a hair. The hair, like the epidermis, is colored by melanin granules. "What is the main function of our hairs, Noble Hippocrates?" Well, let's find out for ourselves! Now, gently brush your fingertips across the hairs of your leg or forearm, without actually touching the skin surface. Don't you feel a tingling sensation? The function of our hair is mainly assisting our sense of touch, since a *sensory nerve basket* lies at the base of the hair follicle. When you bend the hair within its follicle, you activate this sensory nerve basket. [**Thinking probe:** Why do mice, and the cats who chase

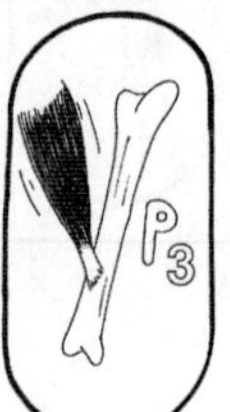

them into little holes in walls, have such long whiskers on their faces? What is the likely function of these long whiskers?]

Other sensory receptors (not connected to the hair follicles) act as "ones that" (*-or*) "receive" (*recept*) information about various body senses. These senses include those of touch, pain, cold, heat, vibration, and pressure. (The associated nervous system activities will be discussed in Chapter 11.)

When a person is going bald, they are said to suffer from *alopecia* (**al**-oh-**PEA**-she-ah) or "fox mange"! In reality, the hair follicles do not totally lose their hairs. Rather, the large hairs are periodically shed, and very thin hairs replace them. So a supposedly bald person really does still have hair!

Sometimes our hairs (like our skin) feel greasy. This is due to *sebum* (**SEE**-bum) or "grease" (*seb*). Sebum is secreted by one or more *sebaceous* (seh-**BAY**-shus) *glands*. These glands are attached to the sides of a hair follicle (Figure 10.2, A). The sebum helps lubricate the skin surface. The problems occur when there is a *hypersecretion* (**high**-per-see-**KREE**-shun) or "excessive" (*hyper-*) secretion of sebum. Usually this is accompanied by an abnormal accumulation of *keratin* (**KAIR**-uh-tin), or "horn substance," as well. The excessive amount of sebum and keratin building up within the hair follicle can eventually block its opening onto the skin surface (Figure 10.2, B).

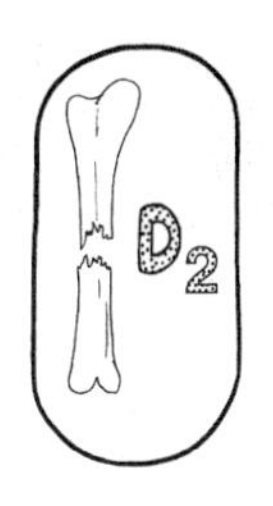

The result is a *comedo* (**KAHM**-eh-doh) or blackhead. The word, *comedo*, comes from the Latin for "eat up." This strange name comes from the action of skin bacteria, which actively "eat up" the sebum and keratin plug of the blackhead. The blackhead's dark color is not the result of dirt, but rather the effect of oxygen upon the sebum plug. A type of *dermatitis*—"inflammation of" (*-itis*) the "skin" (*dermat*)—often follows.

The action of bacilli feeding upon sebum releases *fatty acids*, which are extremely irritating to the surrounding tissue. Leukocytes enter the hair follicle and die, creating a white pimple with pus. *Acne* (**AK**-nee) *vulgaris* (vul-**GAIR**-is) often results. This is a disease of "the common people" (*vulgar*) which involves the creation of raised red "points" (*acne*) on the skin surface. These acne lesions (places of damage) are technically called *papules* (**PAP**-yools) or "pimples." If the pimples become filled with liquid pus, then they are properly called *pustules* (**PUS**-chools)—"little" (*-ules*) sacs of "pus" (*pust*).

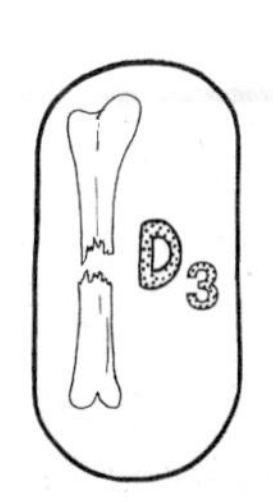

"What causes these awful pimples and pustules of acne vulgaris, Hippocrates?" Well, they were common even in my day, long ago. The fact that acne often begins during *adolescence* (**ad**-uh-**LES**-ens), the time when we start to "grow up" (*adolesc*), provides a strong clue. This is the time in life when the *androgens* (**AN**-droh-**jens**) or "male" (*andr*) "producing" (*-gens*) hormones, begin to rise to high levels within the bloodstream. It is thought that these androgens stimulate the hypersecretion of sebum that gives rise to acne vulgaris.

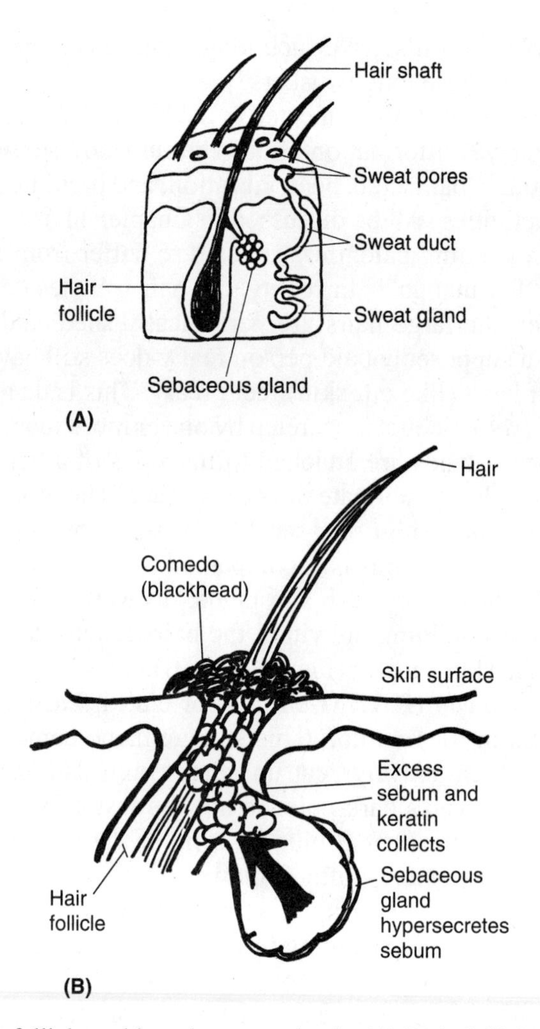

Fig. 10.2 The hair follicle and its sebaceous glands. **(A)** Hair follicle with sebaceous glands attached **(B)** Excess sebum and keratin plug the opening of the hair follicle, creating a *comedo* (blackhead).

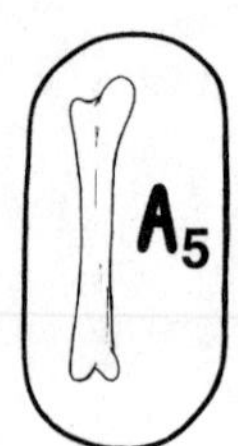

Sweating and the sweat glands

Sebum-secreting sebaceous glands are not the only glands found in human skin. There are millions of *sweat glands* as well. A look at Figure 10.2 (A) allows you to see a sweat gland, along with its *sweat duct*, which carries the sweat out onto the skin surface through a *sweat pore*. Most interesting, sweating is technically called *perspiring* (per-**SPIR**-ing). And *perspiration* (**per**-spir-**AY**-shun) is literally the "process of" (*-tion*) "breathing" (*spir*) "through" (*per*). Doesn't the sweat pore in Figure 10.2 (A) look somewhat

like a little oval mouth on the skin surface, which seems to be "breathing" out sweat?

Sweat is a weak saline (saltwater) solution whose major job is assisting with *thermoregulation* (**ther**-moh-reg-you-**LAY**-shun)—the "regulation" of body "heat or temperature" (*therm*). The hot body essentially boils H_2O molecules in the sweat off the skin surface, thereby losing heat to the surrounding air by *evaporation* (eh-**vap**-or-**AY**-shun). This is the "process of" (*-tion*) making water "vapor."

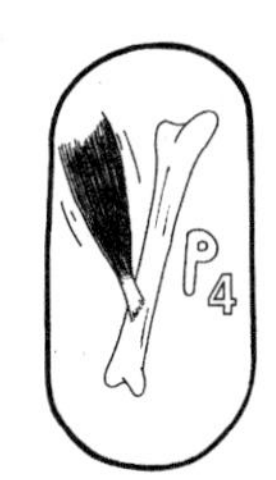

We know that the root for "water" is *hydr*. It makes good sense, then, that the root for "sweat" (which contains lots of water) is *hidr*—with a difference in spelling of just one letter! *Hidrosis* (high-**DROH**-sis) is a term meaning a "condition of" (*-osis*) "sweating" (*hidr*). And *hyperhidrosis* (**high**-per-high-**DROH**-sis) logically, is a "condition of excessive" (*hyper-*) "sweating." Hyperhidrosis, if continued long enough, can result in serious dehydration. Therefore, various chemical *antiperspirants* (**an**-tih-**PER**-spir-ants)—"substances that" (*-ant*) act "against" (*anti-*) "sweating"—may be prescribed.

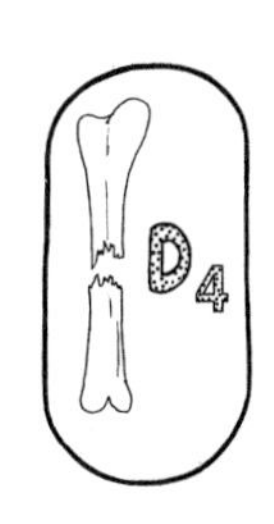

A synonym (similar word) for hyperhidrosis is *diaphoresis* (**die**-uh-for-**EE**-sis). Recall that perspiration literally means "a process of breathing through," with *per-* being the prefix for "through." We have seen the prefix, *dia-*, used to mean "through" a number of times in this book. Thus, not surprisingly, diaphoresis literally means "a process of" (*-esis*) "carrying" (*phor*) "through" (*dia-*). What is being "carried through" the pores, of course, is sweat. A summary of the preceding info on sweating yields:

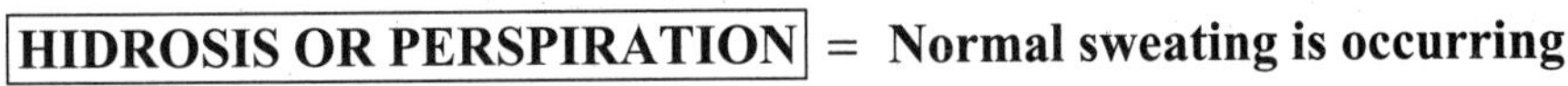
HIDROSIS OR PERSPIRATION = **Normal sweating is occurring**

while

HYPERHIDROSIS OR DIAPHORESIS = **Excessive sweating is occurring**

SUMMARY TABLE 10.1

Consult Summary Table 10.1 for a quick review of some important words and word parts.

GLANDS AND HORMONES

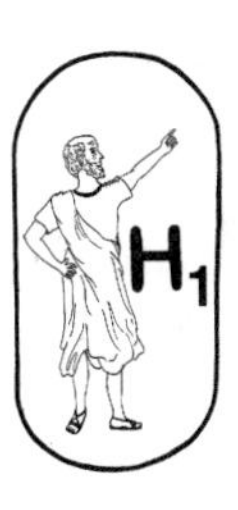

Very closely related to the skin are the various types of glands. It is fascinating to learn that the word *gland* actually means "acorn" in Latin! This probably arises from the ancient observations (made since Hippocrates' time) that many glands are small and rounded—much like real acorns! Consider, for example,

Summary Table 10.1 Words and Word Parts
Write in the *exact* meaning (literal English equivalent) for up to 10 key terms selected from the preceding block of text. After you are done, check your word meanings with the correct answers, which are given at the end of this chapter.

Key Terms	Prefixes	Roots	Suffixes	Exact Meanings
integumentary	(none)	integument "covering"	-ary "referring to"	1. ________
glandular	(none)	glandul "little acorns"	-ar "relating to"	2. ________
dermis	(none)	derm "skin"	-is "presence of"	3. ________
epidermis	epi- "upon"	derm "skin"	-is "presence of"	4. ________
dehydration	de- "from"	hydr "water"	-tion "process of"	5. ________
melanoma	(none)	melan "black"	-oma "tumor"	6. ________
asymptomatic	a- "without"	symptomat "symptoms"	-ic "pertaining to"	7. ________
dermatologist	(none)	dermat "skin"	-ologist "one who specializes in studying"	8. ________
perspiration	per- "through"	spir "breathing"	-tion "process of"	9. ________
hyperhidrosis	hyper- "excessive"	hidr "sweating"	-osis "abnormal condition of"	10. ________

the acorn-like *pituitary* (pih-**TOO**-ih-**tair**-ee) *body* (Figure 10.3). It is attached to the base of the brain by a hollow *pituitary stalk.* This makes it look quite a bit like a real acorn with its stem, doesn't it? And the nearby *pineal* (**PIN**-ee-al) *gland* does, indeed, seem to "refer to" (*-al*) the shape of a "pine" (*pine*) cone.

Both the pituitary gland and pineal gland secrete *hormones* into the bloodstream. These are chemical messengers that travel throughout the body and

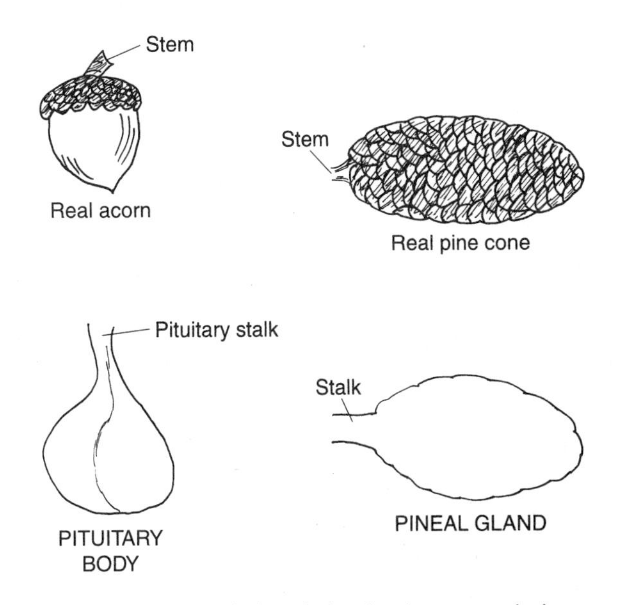

Fig. 10.3 Pituitary and pineal glands: Acorns and pinecones.

"arouse" (*hormon*) or stimulate a great many different physiological actions. Somewhat like an acorn taking root in the ground or the seeds of a pinecone scattered widely by the wind, these hormones (chemical messengers) can move far from their original sources.

The different types of glands

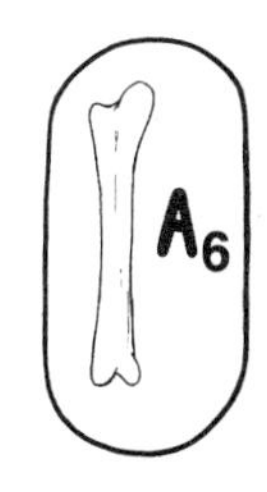

In general, a gland is defined as one or more epithelial cells specialized for the function of *secretion*—the release of some useful product. Consider, for instance, the two types of glands we have talked about in the skin: the sebaceous glands and sweat glands. [**Learning & memory probe:** What is the useful product secreted by the sebaceous glands, and what does it do? How about the secretion of the sweat glands?]

The sebaceous and sweat glands are classified as *exocrine* (**EKS**-uh-krin) *glands*. An exocrine gland is a gland that "secretes" (*crin*) some useful product "out" (*exo-*) into a duct (a slender passageway), which then carries the secretion to some body surface. (View Figure 10.4, A.) A peek back at Figure 10.2 reinforces the truth that both the sebaceous and sweat glands secrete their useful products into ducts.

The pituitary and pineal glands, in dramatic contrast, are classified as *endocrine* (**EN**-duh-**krin**) *glands*. The endocrine glands are ductless glands that "secrete" (*crin*) hormones directly "into" (*endo-*) the bloodstream, within the gland itself. As Figure 10.4 (B) displays, once the hormone molecules enter the

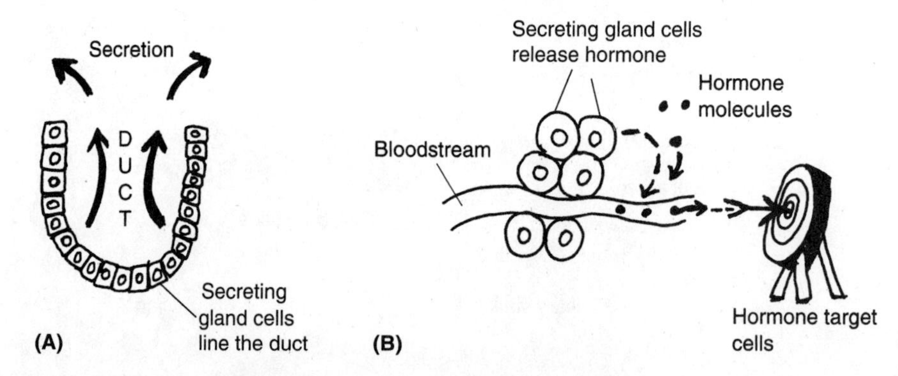

Fig. 10.4 Exocrine versus endocrine glands. **(A)** Simplified view of exocrine gland and its duct. **(B)** Endocrine gland cells secreting hormone.

bloodstream, they are eventually carried to a number of specific *hormone target cells*. They are called target cells because these specific cells (and not other kinds of cells) are sensitive to the hormone's presence and respond dramatically to it.

Contemplate, for instance, the well-known hormone, *insulin* (**IN**-suh-lin). The word, *insulin*, comes from the Latin for a "neutral substance or protein" (*-in*) that is secreted by "little islands" (*insul*). A careful study of Figure 10.5 demonstrates the reason for the "little island" connection. Another Latin term for "little island" or "island" is *islet* (**EYE**-let). The *pancreatic* (**pan**-kree-**AT**-ik) *islets* are also called the *Islets of Langerhans* (**LAHNG**-ur-hahns). These are "little islands" of endocrine gland cells scattered here and there throughout the *pancreas*. The pancreas is soft, without bones, and therefore consists of "all" (*pan-*) "flesh" (*creas*). Langerhans was the last name of the German anatomist who first described the islets (little islands) in the pancreas. Note from the detailed sketches of Figure 10.5 that the pancreatic islets (Islets of Langerhans) contain two populations of cells: the *alpha* (**AL**-fuh) cells and the *beta* (**BAY**-tuh) cells. The alpha cells secrete a hormone called *glucagon* (**GLOO**-kah-gahn) into the bloodstream. Glucagon circulates throughout the body and acts to *increase* the blood glucose concentration. The beta cells, in comparison, secrete insulin. Insulin acts to help move glucose out of the bloodstream and into its target cells. This glucose-moving action of insulin causes a *decrease* in the blood glucose concentration. Summarizing the above info, we have:

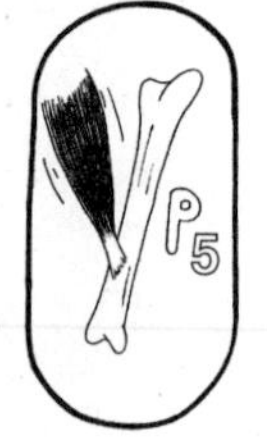

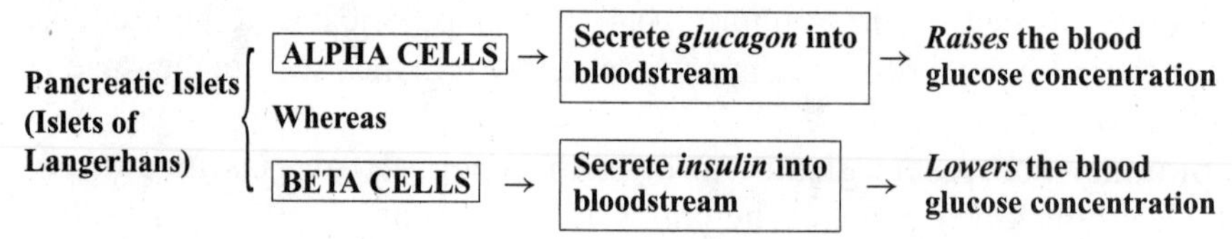

Another strange thing about the pancreas is the presence of a *pancreatic* (**pan**-kree-**AT**-ik) *duct*. The pancreatic duct is a long passageway that runs all

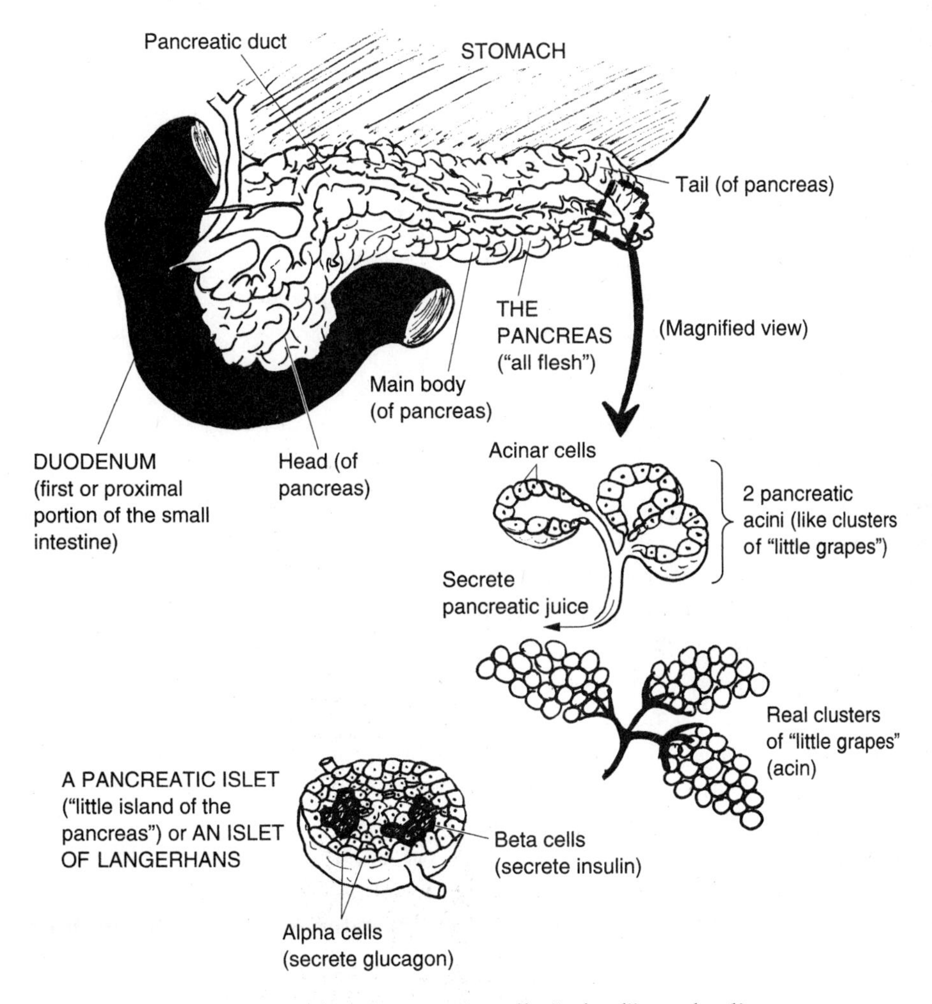

Fig. 10.5 The pancreas: A really "mixed" up gland!

the way through the main body of the pancreas. The middle of Figure 10.5 (magnified views) teaches us that thousands of *pancreatic acini* (**AS**-uh-neye) are arranged like clusters of "little grapes" (*acin*) around the sides of the pancreatic duct. The *pancreatic acinar* (**AS**-uh-nar) *cells* within these grape-like clusters secrete *pancreatic juice*. The pancreatic juice, which is rich in *digestive enzymes*, leaves the pancreatic acini and enters the pancreatic duct. The pancreatic duct carries its juice all the way into the *duodenum* (dew-**AHD**-eh-num), which is the first or *proximal* (**PRAHKS**-ih-mal) portion of the *small intestine*. It is located "near" (*proxim*) the pancreas.

From the preceding information, we can conclude that the pancreas is a *mixed gland* because it contains both an endocrine portion (the pancreatic islets) as well as an exocrine portion (the pancreatic acini and pancreatic duct). Let us put all of this knowledge together into a simple word equation for the entire glandular system. The result is:

THE GLANDULAR SYSTEM	=	ENDOCRINE GLANDS	+	EXOCRINE GLANDS	+	MIXED GLANDS
		(internal secretion of hormones directly into the bloodstream)		***(external secretion of useful products into ducts)***		***(contain both endocrine and exocrine components)***

Endocrine diseases

Using our basic overview of the glands, we can discuss a few representative examples of *endocrine* diseases. (The important and complex subject of the endocrine glands is covered in much greater depth in *ANATOMY DEMYSTIFIED* and *PHYSIOLOGY DEMYSTIFIED*.)

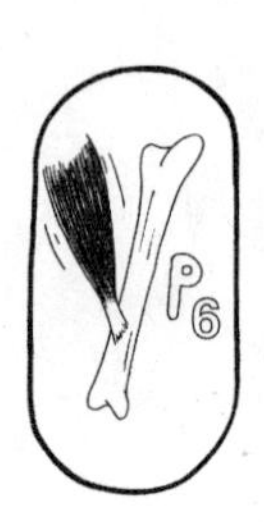

Let us talk now about giants and dwarfs! And when we do such an intriguing thing, we are *not* talking about the *normosecretion* (**nor**-moh-see-**KREE**-shun)—"normal secretion"—of certain hormones. Normosecretion, like the normotension and normothermia mentioned in earlier chapters, is generally associated with biological order and clinical health. [**Anticipation probe:** Based on your prior reading, what do you anticipate are the general categories of secretion associated with morbidity?]

In general, endocrine diseases are of two broad kinds: (*1*) diseases of hormone *hypersecretion* (**high**-per-see-**KREE**-shun), which is an "above normal or excessive" secretion; or (*2*) diseases of hormone *hyposecretion* (**high**-poh-see-**KREE**-shun), which is a "below normal or deficient" amount of secretion. Bringing everything together yields:

HORMONE *NORMO*SECRETION = **Biological order and clinical health of associated body parameters**

while

HORMONE *HYPER*SECRETION = **Biological disorder and endocrine diseases of hormone *"excess"***

and

HORMONE *HYPO*SECRETION = **Biological disorder and endocrine diseases of hormone *"deficiency"***

Giants and dwarfs

We could go through dozens of different endocrine diseases. But any particular disease that we chose to study would either be a disease of hormone excess or one of hormone deficiency. Keeping this simple statement in mind should help you "demystify" this complex field for yourself!

Perhaps the most clear (and physically startling!) contrasts between endocrine diseases having these two exactly opposite hormone conditions are provided by the pituitary body. This oval body includes the *anterior pituitary* (pih-**TOO**-ih-**tair**-ee) *gland*, which sits toward the "front" (*anteri*). Among the many hormones that the anterior pituitary secretes, *growth hormone* (*GH*) provides us with a fine example.

Growth hormone (GH) is secreted into the bloodstream by the anterior pituitary gland and then circulates throughout the body. Quite unusual among the hormones, its targets are almost every cell within the human organism! Growth hormone stimulates such very basic cellular functions as protein synthesis, growth, and cell division. As you might expect, GH levels are usually highest in the bloodstream during the early years of life, when our bodies are still growing and adding billions of new cells. Its rate of secretion then tapers off as the body matures over time.

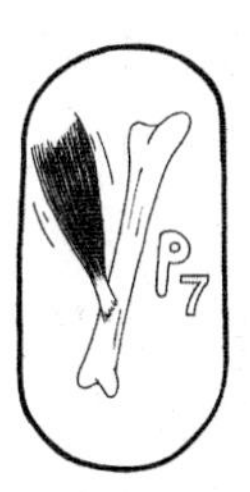

"What happens if a young child's secretion of GH is abnormally *low*, Noble Hippocrates?" In this case, we have a *hyposecretion* of GH and a depressed level of protein synthesis, body growth, and cell division. The endocrine disease that may result is called *pituitary dwarfism* (**DWARF**-izm). There is a severe retardation of growth during childhood, so that the adult is unusually short. But in a *pituitary dwarf* (unlike some other kinds of dwarfs), the body limbs and parts are only slightly out of their normal proportion. (See Figure 10.6 [A] *right*).

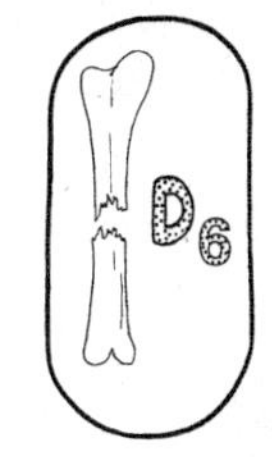

"What about the exactly opposite problem of a young child with an abnormally *high* secretion of GH?" If the GH *hypersecretion* is chronic, so that the "excess" (*hyper-*) amount lasts for several years during early childhood, then *pituitary gigantism* (jeye-**GANT**-izm) may result. Gigantism is literally a "condition of" (*-ism*) being a "giant" (*gigant*). (Study Figure 10.6 [B] *left*.) In such cases of gigantism that are the result of hypersecretion of GH, the affected person has an extremely tall stature, but the body limbs usually remain in their normal proportions.

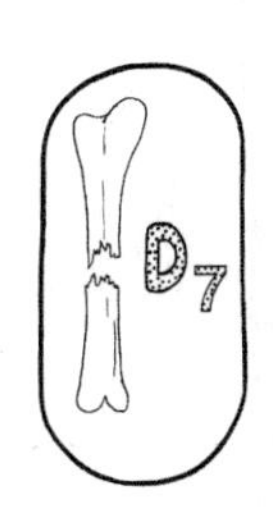

"What if the person is *already* an adult and they have a large hypersecretion of GH?" In this situation, the person can't get any taller, of course, because the *growth plates* in their long bones have already fully *ossified* (**AHS**-ih-**feyed**)—turned to "bone" (*ossi*). So instead of the bones getting longer, they get thicker and heavier! The official medical term for this problem is *acromegaly* (**AK**-roh-**meg**-ah-lee). (Examine part (C) near the top of Figure 10.6.) There is

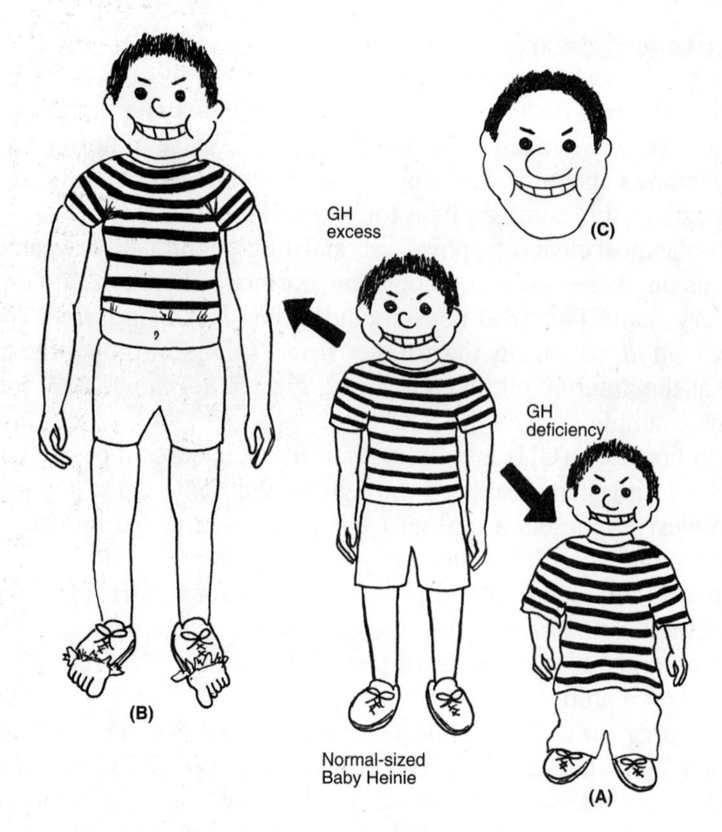

Fig. 10.6 The effects of normal versus abnormal secretion of growth hormone (GH). **(A)** At right is Baby Heinie as a *pituitary dwarf* (a result of *hyposecretion* of GH during childhood). **(B)** On the left is Baby Heinie as a *Pituitary Giant* (a result of *hypersecretion* of GH during childhood). **(C)** The inset shows the facial features of Baby Heinie with *acromegaly* (a result of *hypersecretion* of GH during adulthood).

a dramatic "enlargement of" (*-megaly*) the jawbones, nose, fingers, and other parts of the body "extremities" (*acr*). The massive jawbones tend to give the face a coarse appearance.

SUMMARY TABLE 10.2

Consult Summary Table 10.2 for a quick review of some important words and word parts.

Medical Case History: Diabetes Mellitus and Insulin Shock

Any "demystifying" of the endocrine glands must include some discussion about the most important endocrine disease of them all. We are referring to

Summary Table 10.2 Words and Word Parts

Write in the *exact* meaning (literal English equivalent) for up to 10 key terms selected from the preceding block of text. After you are done, check your word meanings with the correct answers, which are given at the end of this chapter.

Key Terms	Prefixes	Roots	Suffixes	Exact Meanings
pineal	(none)	pine "pine"	-al "relating to"	1. ________
exocrine	exo- "out of"	crin "secreting"	-e "presence of"	2. ________
endocrine	endo- "into"	crin "secreting"	-e "presence of"	3. ________
insulin	(none)	insul "little islands"	-in "neutral substance/ protein"	4. ________
pancreatic	pan- "all"	creat "flesh"	-ic "pertaining to"	5. ________
normosecretion	normo- "normal"	secret "secreting"	-ion "condition of"	6. ________
hyposecretion	hypo- "deficient"	secret "secreting"	-ion "condition of"	7. ________
hypersecretion	hyper- "excess"	secret "secreting"	-ion "condition of"	8. ________

diabetes (**die**-uh-**BEE**-teez) *mellitus* (**MEL**-ih-**tus**), of course! The name of this common disease reflects one of its major signs—*glycosuria* (**gleye**-koh-**SUR**-ee-ah)—and one of its major symptoms—*diuresis* (**die**-your-**EE**-sis). The word, *diabetes*, means "a passer-through" or "siphon" (*diabet*). This is because of the fact that any type of *diabetic* (**die**-uh-**BET**-ik) disease involves a marked diuresis. This is literally a "process of" (*-esis*) too much "urine" (*ur*) passing out "through" (*dia-*) the body. (Consult Figure 10.7.) The word, *mellitus*, denotes the "presence of" (*-us*) something that is "honey-sweet" (*mellit*). The major clinical sign of glycosuria reflects this mellitus name. Glycosuria exactly translates as "a condition of" (*-ia*) "sweet" (*glyc*) "urine" (*ur*).

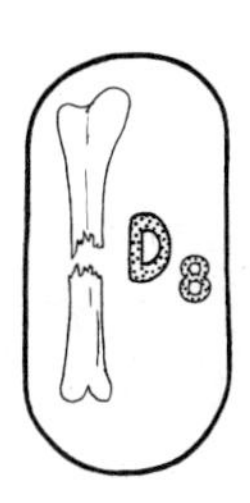

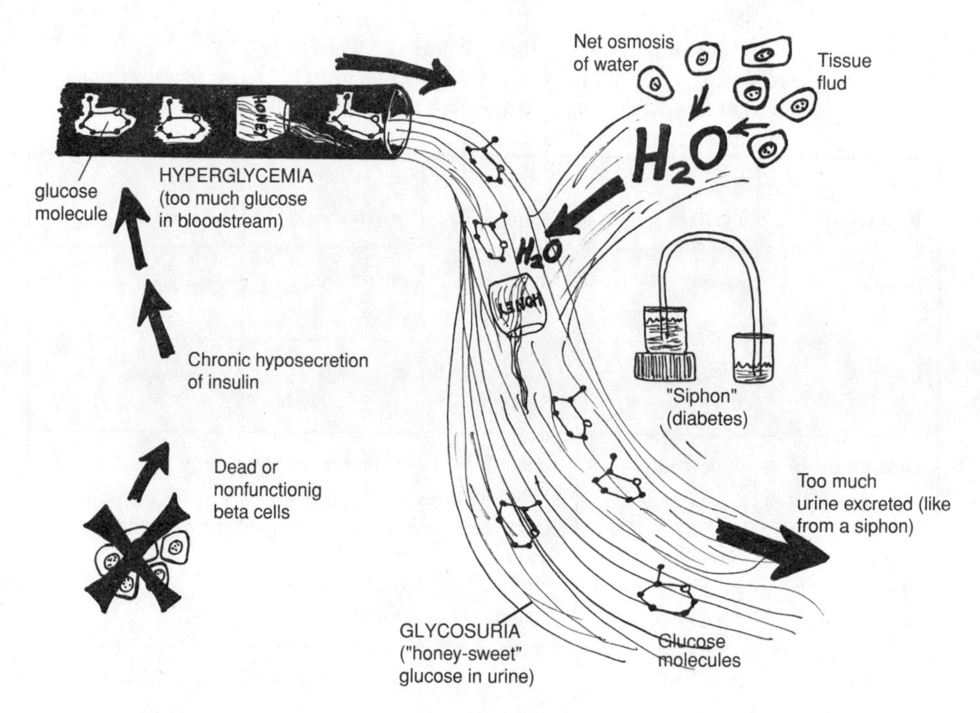

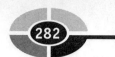

Fig. 10.7 Explaining some signs and symptoms of diabetes mellitus.

"*Why* does the person excrete glucose (which is something "sweet") in his or her urine, Dr. Hippocrates? Is this *normal*?" No, Dear Reader. As we will soon learn (Chapter 13), glucose is *not* normally excreted into our urine. We knew this even in my day, when the physicians of Ancient Greece and Rome quickly dipped their fingertips into the patient's urine. They tasted the "sweetness" of the excreted glucose that was in it. The reason for glucose in the urine is because of the patient's severe *hyperglycemia* (**high**-per-glye-**SEEM**-e-uh). "What does hyperglycemia mean in common English, Dr. H?" [**Word dissection prompt:** Help Hippocrates' Ghost answer this reader's question by dissecting *hyperglycemia* using three slash marks. Label the resulting word parts as prefix, root, and suffix, then see how far you can go in completely translating the term on your own.]

Cutting up this term with slash marks yields:

Prefix	*Root*	*Suffix*
HYPER /	GLYC /	EMIA
"excessive"	**"sweetness"**	**"blood condition of"**

Therefore, hyperglycemia is a "blood condition of excessive sweetness." The basic underlying problem is a chronic hyposecretion of insulin. The hyposecretion ("below normal secretion") of insulin may be related to dead or

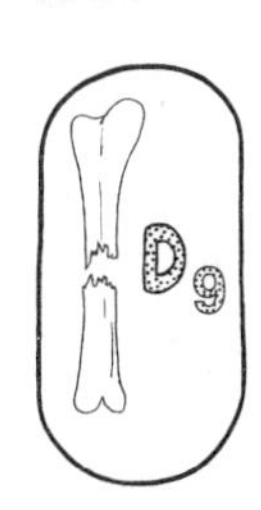

nonfunctioning beta cells in the pancreas. Without adequate insulin to move glucose out of the bloodstream and into the tissue cells, far too much glucose remains in the blood. The blood glucose level just keeps building higher and higher every time the diabetic person eats something with sugar in it! The resulting hyperglycemia causes too much glucose to be filtered into the *kidney tubules* (**TOO**-byools), the "little tubes" (*tubul*) in the kidney. Some of the glucose remains within the kidney tubules and is eventually excreted out of the body in the urine. (This explains the glycosuria.) Because so many glucose molecules are in the kidney tubules, they lower the water concentration in the kidney tubules below that of the surrounding tissue fluid. Consequently, there is a *net osmosis* (**ahs-MOH**-sis) or "condition of thrusting" (*osm*) of water molecules out of the bloodstream and into the kidney tubules. With so much added water from the tissue fluid, an increased amount of watery urine is excreted. (This explains the diuresis.)

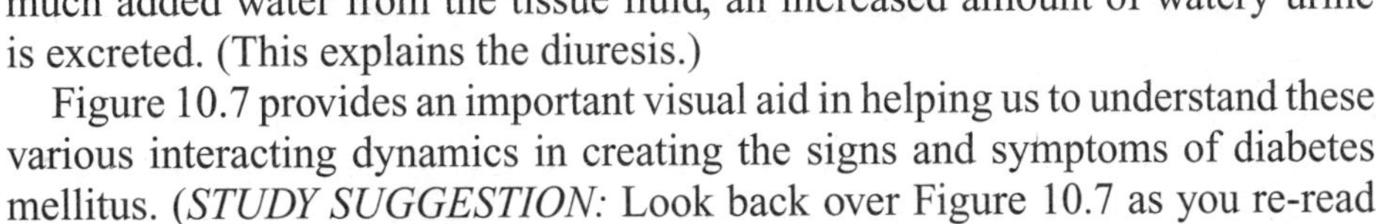

Figure 10.7 provides an important visual aid in helping us to understand these various interacting dynamics in creating the signs and symptoms of diabetes mellitus. (*STUDY SUGGESTION:* Look back over Figure 10.7 as you re-read the preceding paragraph.)

Insulin overdose and diabetic coma

Mrs. Penny S., a lady in her late forties, had been suffering from *insulin-dependent diabetes mellitus* for the past few years. Until that time, she was able to maintain *normoglycemia* (**nor**-moh-gleye-**SEE**-me-uh) without need of external insulin. She did this by limiting the consumption of sugar and other refined carbohydrates in her diet. However, after the recent death of her husband and two children in a tragic car accident, Mrs. S. became severely depressed. She took to consuming thousands of extra calories every day, using eating as an emotional coping mechanism. Unfortunately, this excess *caloric* (kah-**LOR**-ik) consumption put her into a condition of *morbid* (**MOR**-bid) *obesity* (oh-**BEE**-sih-tee). This is a "condition of" (*-ity*) "sick" (*morbid*) "fatness" (*obes*).

This obesity swelled hundreds of thousands of lipid-stuffed *adipocytes* (**AD**-ih-poh-**sights**) or "fat" (*adip*) "cells" (*cytes*) in the patient's body. Her chronic *hypoinsulinism* (**high**-poh-**IN**-sul-in-izm) was thus made far worse. Her pancreatic beta cells simply could not secrete enough additional insulin to handle this increased metabolic requirement for cellular glucose energy. As a result, Mrs. S's formerly insulin-*independent* diabetes mellitus, which was "not" (*in-*) "dependent" upon external insulin therapy, transformed into a severe *insulin-dependent* diabetes mellitus (IDDM).

The patient began a regular daily regimen of insulin self-injection *subQ*—that is, *subcutaneously* (**sub**-kyoo-**TAY**-nee-us-lee). Injections were made into the anterior aspect of the thigh. Because of her inexperience with self-treatment, Mrs. S decided to give herself an intravenous injection to achieve a "quick fix" by rapid administration of the hormone directly into her bloodstream. She accidentally gave herself a tenfold overdose of insulin! So much glucose rushed out of the bloodstream, into the patient's *insulin target cells*, that a dramatic drop in circulating blood glucose concentration resulted.

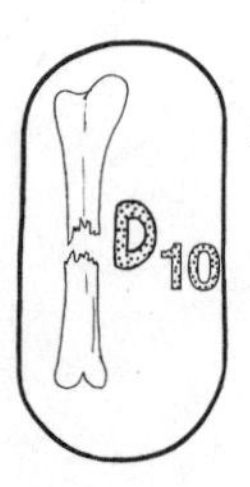

This created severe *hypoglycemia* (**high**-poh-gleye-**SEEM**-e-uh). The patient went into sudden *insulin shock.*

Her symptoms included diaphoresis, *tremor* (**TREM**-or) or "shaking," and *vertigo* (dizziness). There was also a *diplopia* (dih-**PLOH**-pea-uh)—"condition of" (*-ia*) "double vision" (*diplop*). This was soon followed by *delirium* (dih-**LIR**-e-um), which is a "condition of" (*-um*) "crazy raving" (*deliri*). Convulsions, then *diabetic coma* (**KOH**-muh) followed. (A *coma* is an "abnormally deep sleep" [*com*].)

A concerned neighbor found Mrs. S. the next morning, still unconscious. She was lying *prostrate* (**PRAHS**-trayt) on the kitchen floor. Her body was "thrown down" flat, with her face resting on the tiles. Unhappily, the patient had been *comatose* (**KOH**-mah-tohs)—in an "abnormally deep sleep" condition—for far too long. Large intravenous injections of glucose solution in the ER of a local hospital, were unable to revive her.

Probe of case history

(**A**) Subdivide *normoglycemia* by inserting slash marks. Label the resulting word parts (prefix, root, or suffix), then translate this term into its common English equivalent. (**B**) If an insulin injection is made *subcutaneously*, and *cutane* is a root for "skin," then what does the whole term mean in regular English? [Check your short answers with the key near the end of this chapter.]

Quiz

Refer to the text in this chapter if necessary. A good score is at least 8 correct answers out of these 10 questions. The answers are listed in the back of this book.

1. "Refers to" the body's "covering":
   (a) Digest/ive
   (b) Dia/gnost/ic
   (c) Integument/ary
   (d) Glandul/ar

2. You should really see a _____ for treating your acne!
   (a) Oncologist
   (b) Neurosurgeon
   (c) Dermatologist
   (d) Cosmetologician

3. Thin layer that lies upon the connective tissue layer of the true skin:
   (a) Melanoma
   (b) Dermis
   (c) Muscular
   (d) Epidermis

4. Diagnosing a patient with chronic hyperhidrosis suggests that they:
   (a) Suffer from long-lasting extreme hunger
   (b) Experience occasional episodes of coma
   (c) Have to go to the bathroom very frequently!
   (d) Are dealing with a long-range problem of excessive sweating

5. The black-colored cells that darken our skin and hair:
   (a) Melanocytes
   (b) Leukocells
   (c) Erythrocytes
   (d) Fibroblasts

6. *Glandul/ar* facts literally refer to those involving:
   (a) "Big listeners"
   (b) "Tiny secretors"
   (c) "Fiber formation"
   (d) "Little acorns"

7. Exocrine glands are those that:
   (a) Secrete hormones into the bloodstream
   (b) Subdivide continuously into ever-smaller groups of cells
   (c) Secrete useful products into ducts
   (d) Contain two or more different types of basic body tissue

8. The main hormone that decreases blood glucose concentration:
   (a) Insulin
   (b) Glucagon
   (c) Growth hormone
   (d) Melatonin

9. Pituitary gigantism involves a hypersecretion of:
   (a) Cholesterol
   (b) Growth hormone

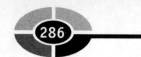

(c) Hemoglobin
(d) Glucose

10. The main body function of hairs is probably:
(a) Memory retention
(b) Antigen-antibody reactions
(c) Hemostasis via clotting
(d) Sensory reception

Memory Pillboxes for Chapter 10

Several key facts were tagged with numbered icons in the page margins of this chapter. Write a short summary of each of these key facts into a numbered cell or compartment within the appropriate type of *Memory Pillbox* that appears below.

Background and History **Pillboxes for Chapter 10:**

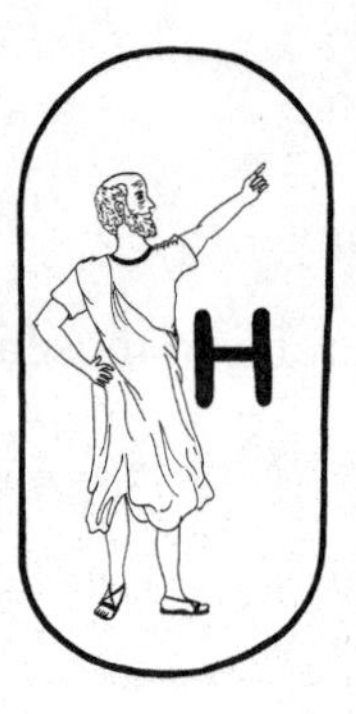

1

***Anatomy* Pillboxes for Chapter 10:**

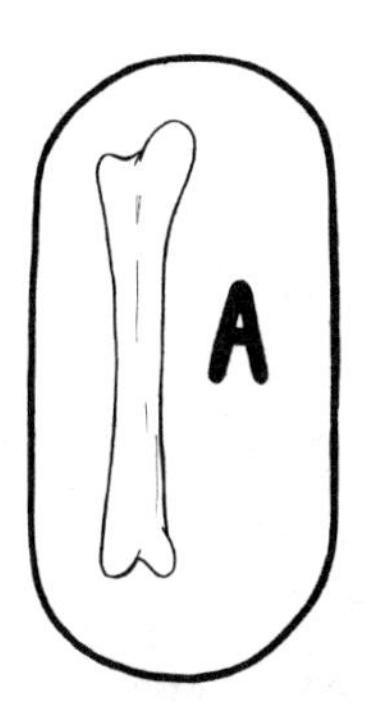

1	
2	3
4	5

6	7

Physiology Pillboxes for Chapter 10:

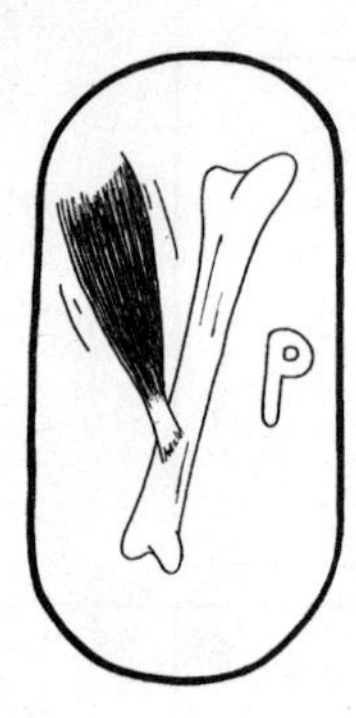

1	2

3	4

5	6

7

***Disease/Injury* Pillboxes for Chapter 10:**

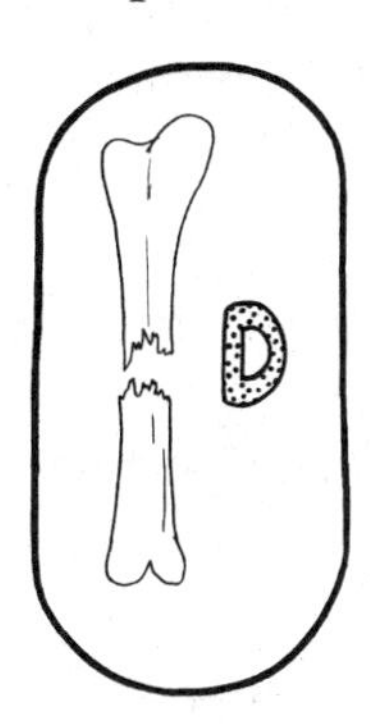

1	2

3	4
5	6
7	8
9	10

Answers for Chapter 10 Summary Tables

FOR SUMMARY TABLE 10.1

1. "referring to covering"
2. "relating to little acorns"
3. "presence of skin"
4. "presence of (something) upon skin"

5. "process of water (moving) from skin"
6. "black tumor"
7. "pertaining to (a condition) without symptoms"
8. "one who specializes in studying the skin"
9. "process of breathing through"
10. "abnormal condition of excessive sweating"

FOR SUMMARY TABLE 10.2

1. "relating to a pine"
2. "presence of a secreting out of"
3. "presence of a secreting into"
4. "neutral substance/ protein (involving) little islands"
5. "pertaining to all flesh"
6. "condition of secreting normally"
7. "condition of deficient secreting"
8. "condition of excess secreting"

Answers to Probe of Case History

(**A**) normo (prefix) /glyc (root) /emia (suffix) = "blood condition of normal sweetness."

(**B**) "Pertaining to" (*-ously*) something "below" (*sub-*) the "skin" (*cutane*).

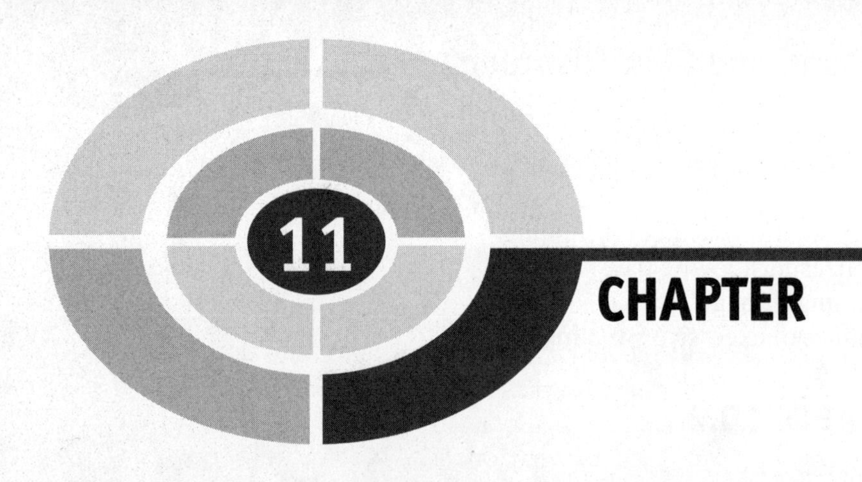

Terms Related to Disorders of the Nervous System and Special Senses

The skin and glands have their own means of communication. The skin has sensory receptors, while the glands have their secretions. But the main flow of body information goes into and out of the brain and spinal cord. And the *special senses*, such as those of hearing and vision, also head that way.

Background and History

When we talk about the *nervous system*, of course, we are talking about an organ system that literally "pertains to" (*-ous*) the "nerves" (*nerv*). A nerve is a collection of *nerve fibers*. These fibers are really just long, thin, fiber-like extensions of the cytoplasm of various *neurons* (**NUR**-ahns), or nerve cells. The fibers of the *sensory neurons*, for example, carry information (like touch, pressure, temperature, or pain) from the sensory receptors (Chapter 10) located in the skin and elsewhere. "And to *where* do they carry this sensory information, Good Hippocrates?" Why, they carry it toward the brain and spinal cord! Hence, we can state this convenient introductory equation:

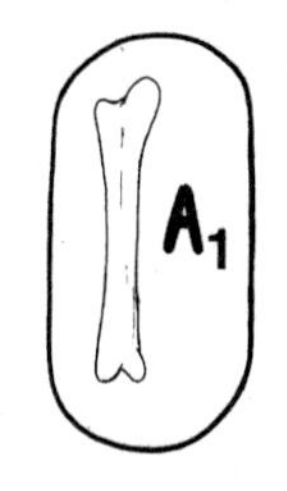

THE NERVOUS SYSTEM = BRAIN + SPINAL CORD + NERVES + SENSORY RECEPTORS

Speaking broadly, the nervous system (along with the endocrine glands) is one of the body's major systems for communication and control of the internal environment. Now, both the brain and spinal cord are centrally located, right in the middle of the body (Figure 11.1). Therefore, together they make up the *Central Nervous System* (CNS).

The nerves and sensory receptors are part of the *Peripheral Nervous System* (PNS). This is because they are located in the body edge or periphery (per-**IF**-er-**ee**), far from the middle. Capsulizing all of the preceding, we have:

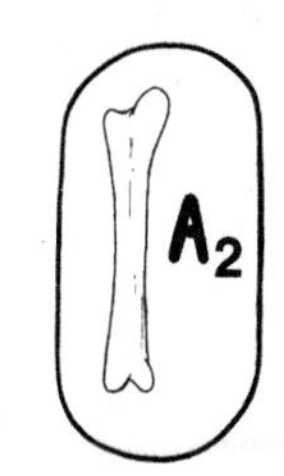

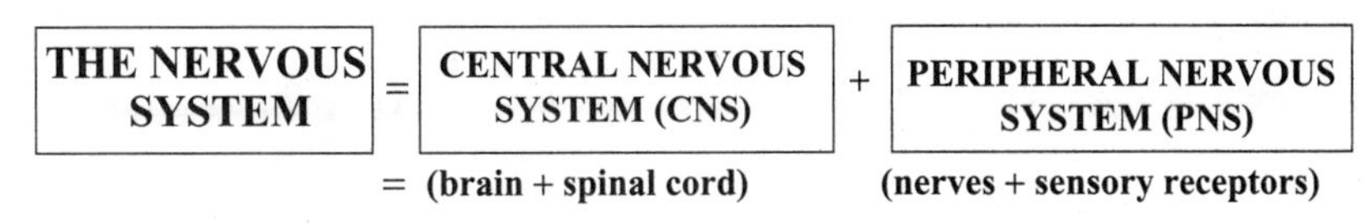

Small humps of nerve activity are called *action potentials* or *nerve impulses*. These are actually traveling waves of excitation. The action potentials (nerve impulses) are the kind of chemical "information" that is carried by nerve fibers.

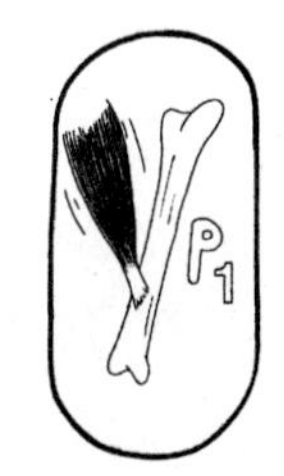

In addition to the sensory info (action potentials) coming *into* the CNS from the peripheral receptors, there is also *motor info* going *out of* the CNS. The motor info (like the motor or engine of your car) makes things "move," such as the skeletal muscles in the body limbs. The motor info stimulates skeletal muscle *effectors* (e-**FEK**-tors) to contract, thereby having some "effect" upon the body.

A *sensory neuron* (Figure 11.1) brings information about a *stimulus* (**STIM**-you-lus) or "goad," such as the fact that you are stepping upon the sharp point of a nail! Conversely, a *motor neuron* and its nerve fiber causes body movements to occur.

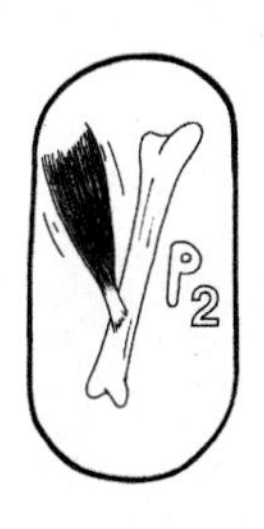

THE BRAIN AND ITS ORGANIC PROBLEMS

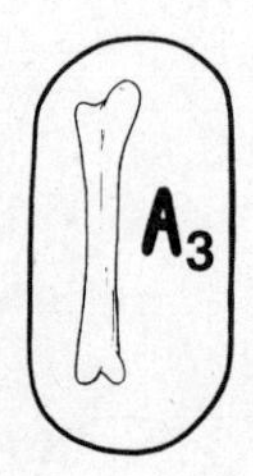

The brain is alternately called the *encephalon* (en-**SEF**-ah-lahn). This is because the brain is the superior portion of the CNS, which is "present" (*-on*) "within" (*en-*) the "head" (*cephal*). Figure 11.2 illustrates the basic anatomy of the encephalon (brain). Most noticeable is the cerebrum (main brain mass). Also note the *cerebellum* (sahr-eh-**BEL**-um) or "little cerebrum" (*cerebell*) that is "present" (*-um*) behind and below it. And even farther below the cerebellum, we see the *brainstem*. The brainstem is the narrow, tapered, stem-like, inferior portion of the brain. Collecting this info yields:

THE BRAIN (ENCEPHALON) = **CEREBRUM** (major brain mass) + **CEREBELLUM** (minor brain mass) + **BRAINSTEM**

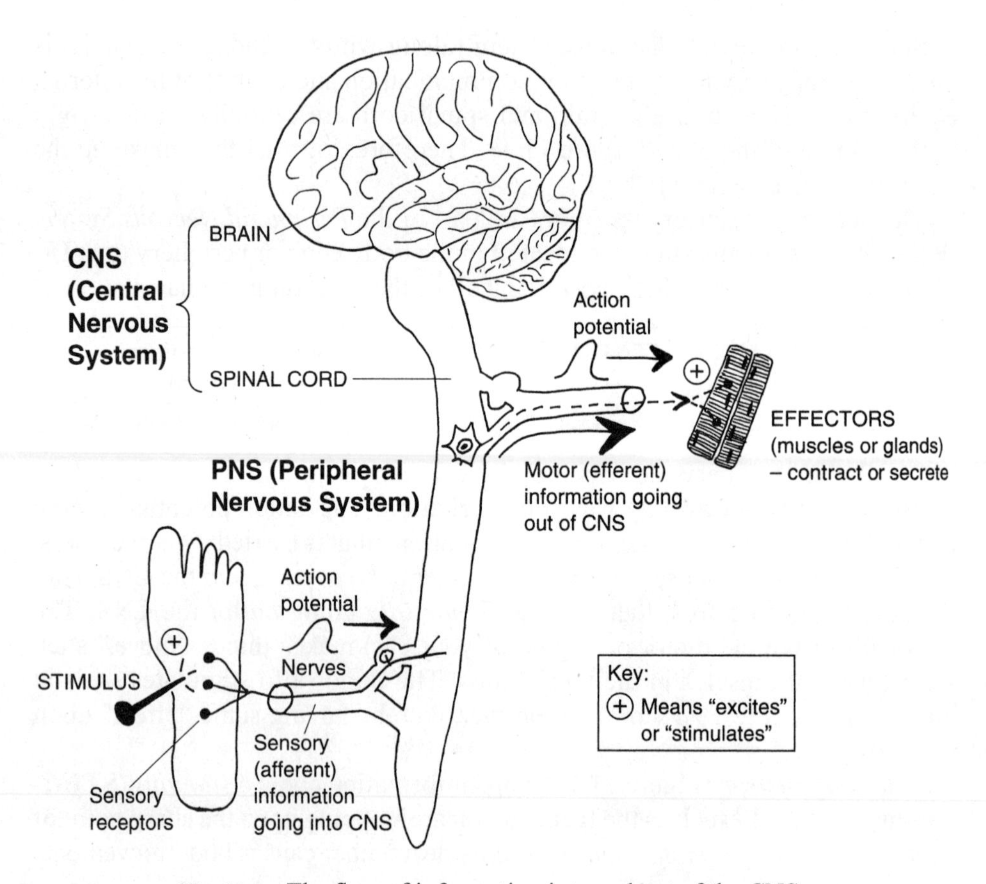

Fig. 11.1 The flow of information into and out of the CNS.

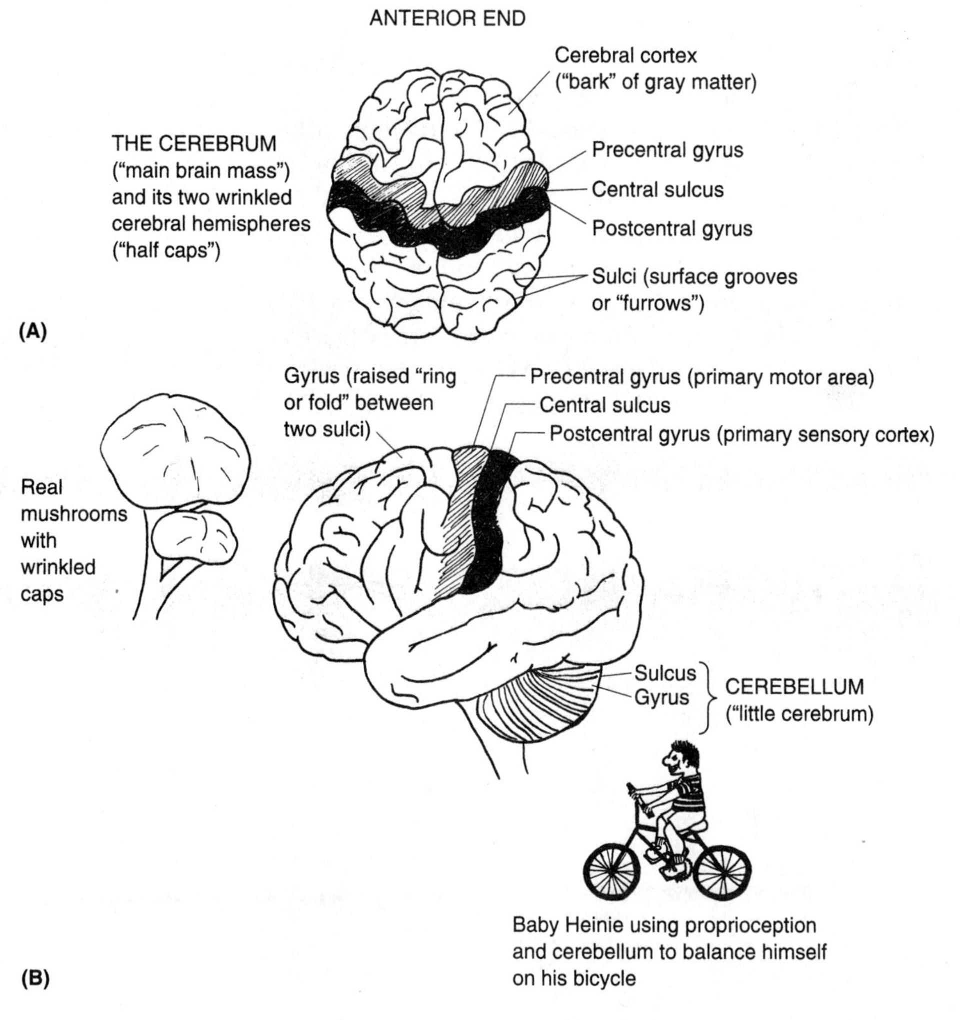

Fig. 11.2 A look at the brain or encephalon.

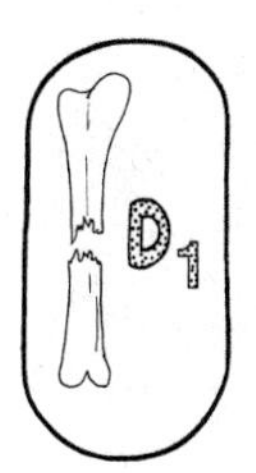

If the entire brain (encephalon) becomes "inflamed," the result is called *encephalitis* (en-**sef**-ul-**EYE**-tis). This problem may be *viral* (**VEYE**-ral)—"referring to a virus"—in origin, and carried by mosquito vectors. (You have probably heard of *viral encephalitis*, for example.)

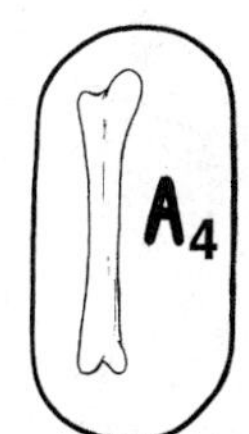

Both the cerebrum and cerebellum are covered by a thin "bark" or *cortex* (**KOR**-teks) of *gray matter*. In the case of the cerebrum, this bark is called the *cerebral* (seh-**REE**-bral) *cortex*. Notice the occurrence of many *gyri* (**JEYE**-rye)—raised, wormlike "rings or folds" (*gyr*). You can also see numerous *sulci* (**SUL**-see)—surface grooves or "furrows" (*sulc*). Taken as a whole, the gyri and sulci create a wrinkled surface of the cortex. This pattern makes the cerebrum and cerebellum resemble two big, spongy mushrooms with wrinkled caps!

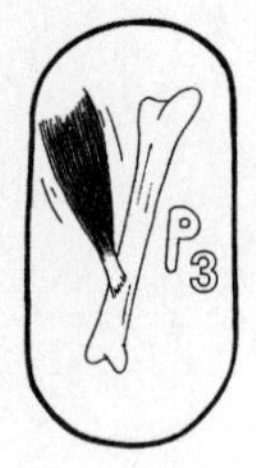

There are several sulci (fissures) and gyri (folds) of cerebral cortex that are especially important. The *central sulcus*, for instance, is a groove that runs down the center of each *cerebral hemisphere* (**HEM**-is-**feer**) or "half sphere." The *precentral* (**pree-SEN**-tral) *gyrus* is located just "before" (*pre-*) the "central" sulcus. It is the body's *primary motor area*. This means that the precentral gyrus orders and controls most voluntary movements. Millions of motor nerve fibers descend from this gyrus, cross the *midline*, and then finally terminate on the *contralateral* (**KAHN**-trah-**lat**-er-al) or "opposite" (*contra-*) "side" (*later*) of the body. (Carefully study Figure 11.3.) It's almost as if

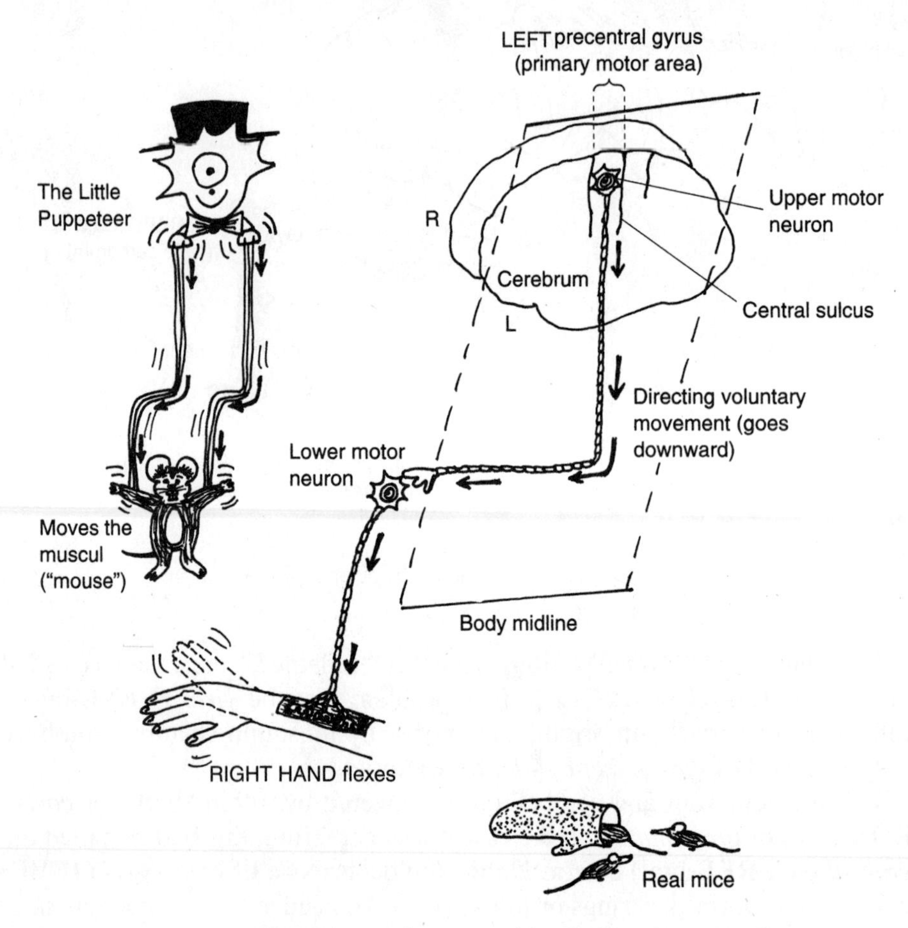

Fig. 11.3 The precentral gyrus and its "hidden puppeteer."

there is a hidden puppeteer in the precentral gyrus who is pulling the strings and moving the "little mice" or skeletal muscles on the opposite side of the body!

Now, assume that you are right-handed (like the vast majority of people). Therefore, the *left* precentral gyrus (*not* the *right* precentral gyrus) is ordering most of the voluntary movement of your right hand! [**Understanding probe:** From what you have just been reading, why doesn't the *right* side of the cerebrum mainly control movements on the *right* side of the body?]

Suppose you suffer a stroke or cerebrovascular accident (CVA, Chapter 8) that interrupts blood flow to the *left* precentral gyrus. The result is a partial or total *paralysis* (puh-**RAL**-uh-sis). This means that there is a "disabling" of some or all voluntary movements on the *right* (contralateral) side of the body. [**Study suggestion:** Imagine making a big black *X* through the motor pathway shown in Figure 11.3. This *X* represents the blocking or interfering effects upon body movement that would result from a stroke that damaged the precentral gyrus.] Summarizing the preceding facts, we write:

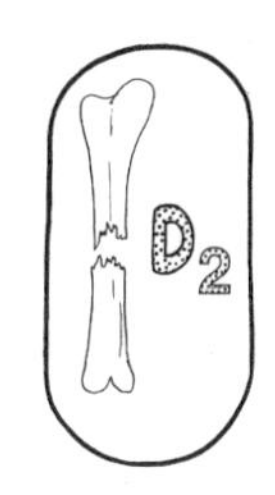

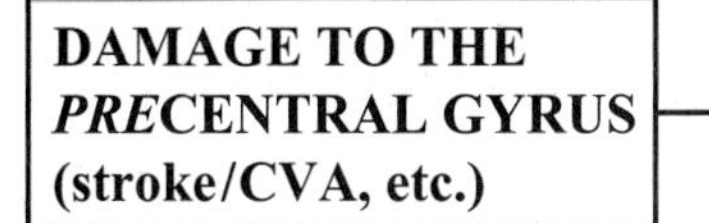
DAMAGE TO THE *PRE*CENTRAL GYRUS (stroke/CVA, etc.) → **PARTIAL OR TOTAL *PARALYSIS* ON THE *OPPOSITE* (*CONTRALATERAL*) SIDE OF THE BODY**

Again, look back at Figure 11.2. Just "after" (*post-*) the "central" sulcus lies the *postcentral* (**pohst-SEN**-tral) *gyrus*. The postcentral gyrus area is the body's *primary or general sensory cortex*. This region of the cerebral cortex receives information about most general body sensations, such as touch, pressure, pain, and temperature. And, like the precentral gyrus, the postcentral gyrus has a largely contralateral (opposite side of the body) hook-up.

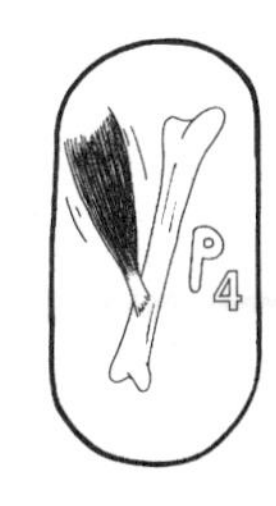

This intriguing situation is visualized for us in Figure 11.4. Using our helpful imaginations, we can almost "see" a cute *sensory homunculus* (hoh-**MUNG**-kyuh-lus)— a "little feeling man or dwarf" (*homuncul*)! This little dwarf is perched just above the postcentral gyrus of the *left* cerebral hemisphere. General body sensations that start, say, from the *right* hand will ascend (go up), cross the midline, and then end in the *left* postcentral gyrus. Hence, if you prick your right hand with a sharp nail, you will mainly experience the pressure and pain sensations within your left postcentral gyrus.

This contralateral hook-up for sensory nerve info (like that for motor nerve info) can be blocked or interrupted by a CVA. [**Study suggestion:** Again, imagine a big black *X*, this one being placed into the sensory pathway shown in Figure 11.4.] Specifically, a stroke or CVA that damages the *left* postcentral gyrus will result in partial or total anesthesia ("loss of feeling," Chapter 2) on

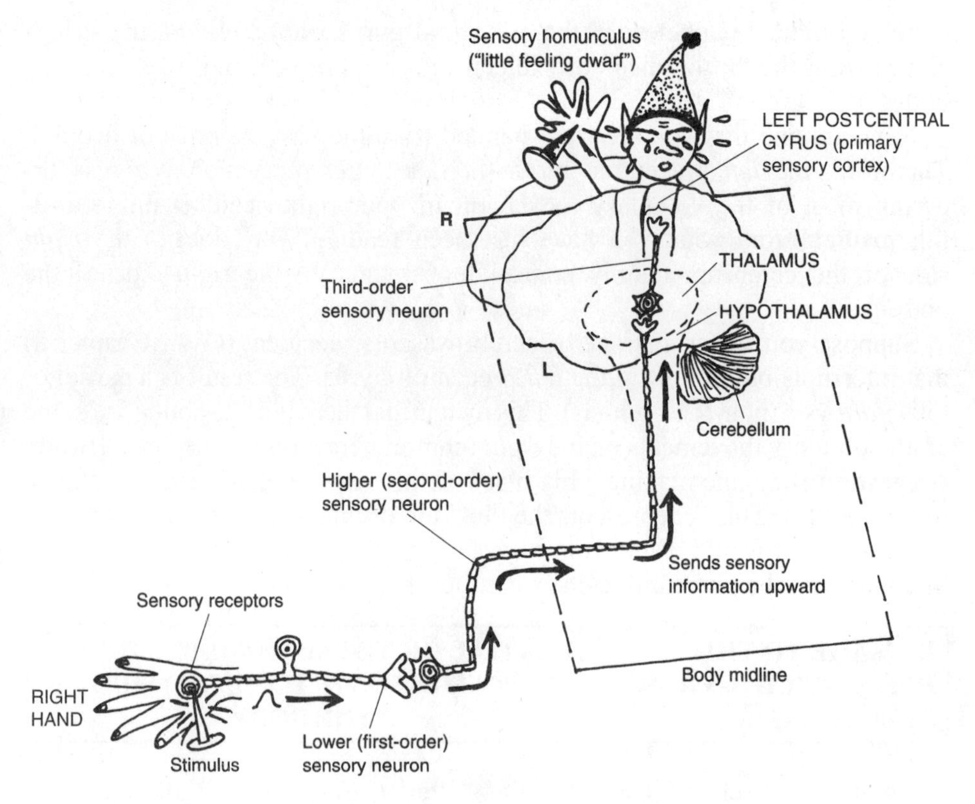

Fig. 11.4 Our "little feeling dwarf" finds a sensory home.

the *right* side of the body. This is because the cerebral cortex destination for the sensory information is destroyed or blocked. Summarizing, we have:

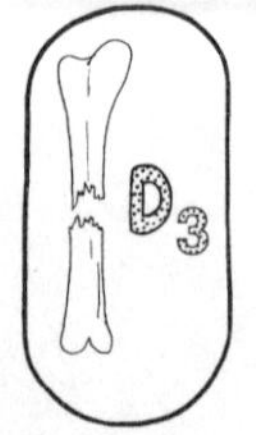

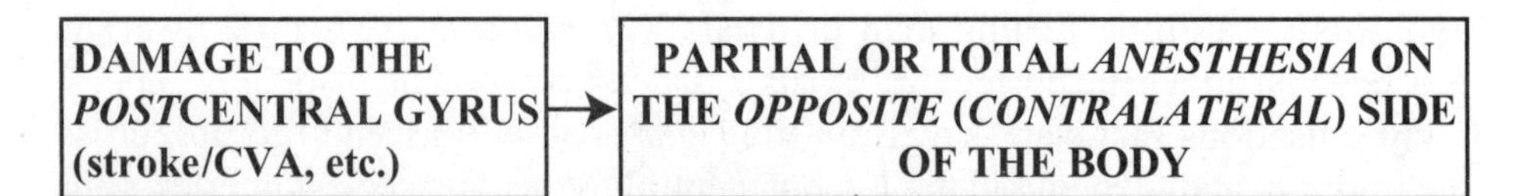

[Further reading prompt: Our fun and different friend, *BIOLOGY DEMYSTIFIED*, provides more background and details about this important subject!]

"This is just *great* stuff, Hippocrates! I'm really starting to *understand* what happened to my Grandma when she had that stroke last year! But we still haven't talked about the *cerebellum* very much, have we?" Yes, let's go back to

Figure 11.2 for just a minute. Here we again see our rather mischievous little sidekick, Baby Heinie, successfully riding his bicycle. The naughty little kid is making use of *proprioception* (**proh**-pree-oh-**SEP**-shun). This is the "process of" (*-tion*) "receiving" (*cept*) information about "one's own" (*propri*) self. By self, we mean the positions of your own self (body and body parts) in space.

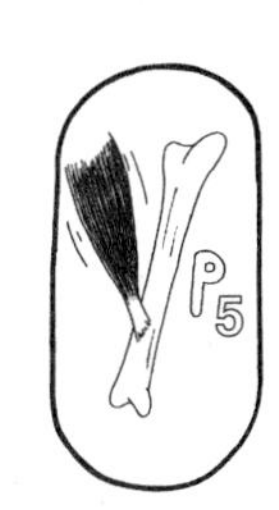

The cerebellum coordinates various automatic *reflexes* and helps maintain Baby Heinie's upright posture and balance on his bicycle, via proprioception. Suppose there is some kind of lesion (damage) to the cerebellum, say from a sharp blow to the base of the skull. This damage might be reflected in *cerebellar* (**sahr**-eh-**BEL**-er) *ataxia* (ah-**TAK**-see-ah)—a "loss of" (*a-*) "order" (*tax*) in balance. The person suffering cerebellar damage may thus walk much like a drunk, weaving and falling down because of the ataxia.

Organic brain disorders

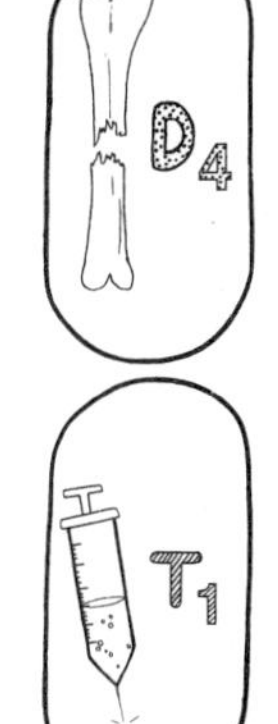

What do encephalitis, paralysis, anesthesia, and cerebellar ataxia, discussed in the previous section, have in common? They are all *organic* brain disorders, also called *organic brain syndromes*. By organic, it is meant that these disorders have some identifiable *structural* (anatomical) or *functional* (physiological) cause. Brain tumors (malignant or benign) are also organic lesions.

Neurology (nur-**AHL**-uh-jee)—"the study of nerves"—is the branch of medicine often consulted for treating organic diseases and injuries of the nervous system. And *neurosurgery* (**nur**-oh-**SURJ**-er-ee) is the branch of medicine that focuses on surgical correction of structural brain problems.

Some additional organic *mental* ("referring to the mind") disorders are: *Alzheimer's* (**ALZ**-high-mers) *disease*, *senile* (**SEE**-nile) *dementia* (deh-**MEN**-chyuh) and *amnesia* (am-**NEE**-zhuh) or "loss" (*a-*) of "memory" (*mnes*). This list of organic brain problems also includes various *seizure disorders*, such as *epilepsy* (**EP**-in-**lep**-see).

SOME NEUROSES AND PSYCHOSES

Mental disorders in general may be subdivided into two broad classes: the *neuroses* versus the *psychoses* (sigh-**KOH**-seez). A *neurosis* (nur-**OH**-sis) is literally an "abnormal condition of" (*-osis*) the "nerves" (*neur*). Thus, a crushed nerve in the arm, for instance, could technically be considered a neurosis. But more commonly, a neurosis is an abnormality in thinking that does not involve a loss of reality. In an *anxiety neurosis*, for instance, the affected person suffers a vague anxiety or fear to the point where it interferes with their normal daily life.

A *psychosis* (sigh-**KOH**-sis) is "an abnormal condition" (*-osis*) of the "mind" (*psych*). But in a practical sense, a psychosis is an abnormality in thinking that is so severe that the personality disintegrates and there is a loss of contact with reality. Hospitalization of the *psychotic* (sigh-**KAHT**-ik) patient, therefore, is often required.

One well known type of psychosis is *schizophrenia* (**skits**-oh-**FREN**-ee-uh). This is a "condition of" (*-ia*) "split" (*schiz*) "mind" (*phren*). What appears to "split" apart is the victim's total personality. He or she behaves in one way on some occasions and the exactly opposite way on other occasions. Another characteristic feature of this psychosis is the occurrence of *autism* (**AW**-tizm)—"a condition of" (*-ism*) "self" (*aut*) obsession. The *schizoid* (**SKITZ**-oid) person is *autistic* (**aw-TIS**-tik) or self-absorbed, to the point of almost completely withdrawing from normal social interactions with others.

A *psychiatrist* (sigh-**KEYE**-uh-trist)—"one who treats" (*-iatrist*) the "mind" (*psych*)—is often consulted for those with various *psychoses* (sigh-**KOH**-seez). A *clinical psychologist* (sigh-**KAHL**-uh-jist)—"one who studies" (*-ologist*) the "mind" (*psych*)—is somewhat different. Psychology (compared to psychiatry) is often more focused upon changing self-destructive and antisocial behaviors, such as various forms of *addiction*.

Summarizing (all of) the preceding information yields the following series of statements:

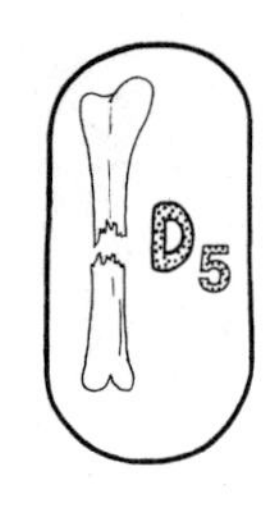

NEUROSES = **Mental disorders that do *not* involve loss of sense of reality**

whereas

PSYCHOSES = **Mental disorders that *do* involve loss of sense of reality**

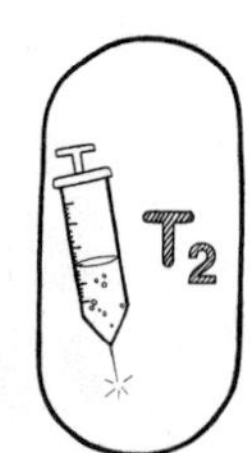

NEUROLOGISTS → **Treat organic nervous orders traceable to specific disorders in *neuroanatomy and/or neurophysiology***

whereas

PSYCHIATRISTS → **Treat mental disorders involving defects in *emotions* and *thinking* (both neuroses and psychoses)**

and

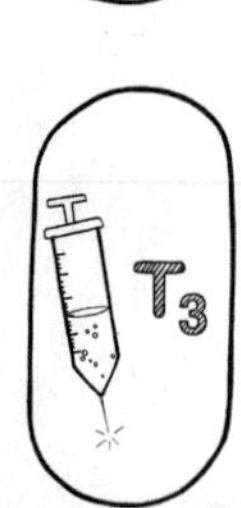

PSYCHOLOGISTS → **Focus upon intervening and correcting various defects in *behavior (such as addictions)*.**

SUMMARY TABLE 11.1

Consult Summary Table 11.1 for a quick review of some important words and word parts.

Summary Table 11.1 Words and Word Parts

Write in the *exact* meaning (literal English translation) for up to 10 key terms selected from the preceding block of text. After you are done, check your word meanings with the correct answers, which are given at the end of this chapter.

Key Terms	Prefixes	Roots	Suffixes	Exact Meanings
nervous	(none)	nerv "nerves"	-ous "pertains to"	1. ________
encephalon	en- "within"	cephal "head"	-on "presence"	2. ________
sulcus	(none)	sulc "furrow"	-us "presence of"	3. ________
cerebellum	(none)	cerebell "little cerebrum"	-um "presence of"	4. ________
precentral	pre-"before"	centr "center"	-al "referring to"	5. ________
postcentral	post-"after"	centr "center"	-al "relating to"	6. ________
contralateral	contra- "opposite"	later "side"	-al "pertaining to"	7. ________
neurosis	(none)	neur "nerves"	-osis "abnormal condition of"	8. ________
psychosis	(none)	psych "mind"	-osis "abnormal condition of"	9. ________
schizophrenia	(none)	schiz "split"; phren "mind"	-ia "condition of"	10. ________

PHILIPPE PINEL UNCHAINS THE INSANE

Throughout the ages, even in the days of Hippocrates, psychotic individuals have sometimes shown *transitory* (**TRANS**-ih-**tor**-ee) *mania.* For a short time, they "go across" (*transit*) into a severely overactive "madness" (*mani*) and frenzy.

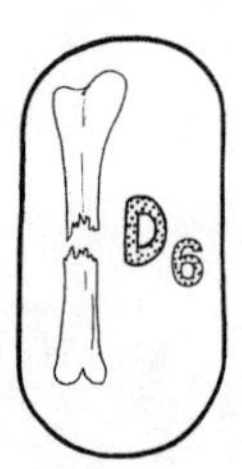

They carry out actions that are potentially dangerous to themselves or others. There are also many cases of *manic depression*, also known as *bipolar* (**buy-POH-**lur) *disorder*. Here the afflicted person alternates between 2 *poles* (opposite mental states). They intermittently show a frenzied and hyperactive mania that alternates with other episodes of deep emotional withdrawal, unresponsiveness, and depression. (NOTE: Since bipolar disorder occurs in varying degrees of severity, the affected individual is not necessarily psychotic.)

Obviously, anyone in the presence of a manic person has a very difficult time trying to help or control them! This was especially true before the advent of tranquilizers (calming drugs) and advanced *antipsychotic* (**an**-tie-sigh-**KAHT**-ik) *drugs*. Manic people were beaten, then strapped into chairs and repeatedly dunked into ice-cold water for *shock treatments*. Even worse, some were burned at the stake as witches! After giving up on trying to reason with them, many doctors and caretakers simply kept these patients in chains, like violent and unpredictable animals!

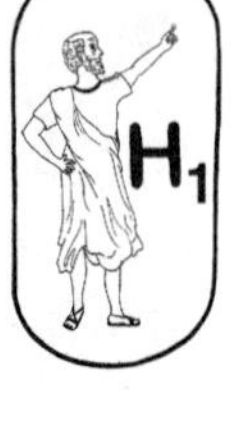

In 1793, however, a very sympathetic French psychiatrist named *Philippe Pinel* finally unchained the insane in two local *asylums* (ah-**SIGH**-lums) or "sanctuaries." (See Figure 11.5, A.) To nearly everyone's surprise, many of these mentally ill people responded favorably to such kindness and compassion and were *rehabilitated* (**re**-hah-**BIL**-ih-**tay**-ted)—"returned to (proper) aptitude"—enough to leave the asylums. But even when the manic had been unchained, before the advent of modern tranquilizers, *straitjackets* were used to temporarily restrain them (Figure 11.5, B). Starting in the mid-twentieth century, oral *antidepressants* (**an**-tie-de-**PRESS**-unts) such as *Prozac* (**PROH**-zak) helped reduce the severity of many patients' manic-depressive states.

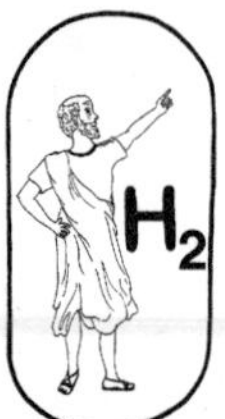

Pinel's pioneering attitude was carried farther by *Jean Charcot* (shar-**KOH**) (1825–1893), a French physician who is often considered the Father of

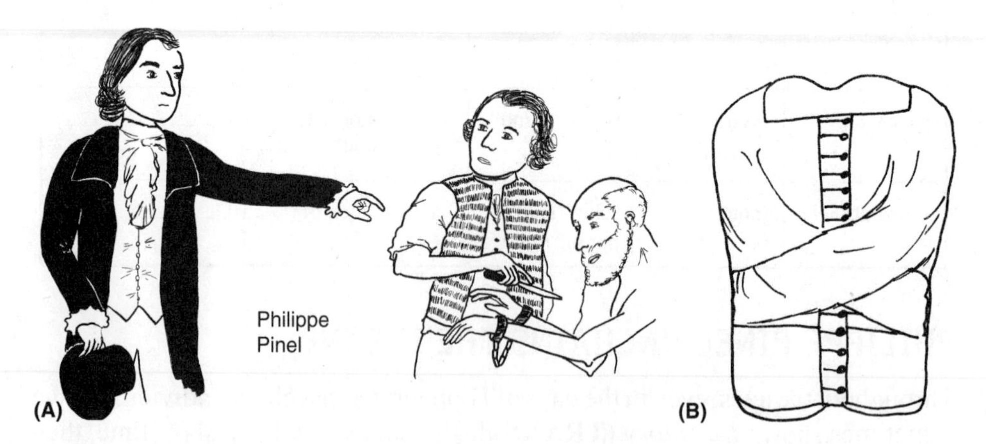

Fig. 11.5 Pinel unchained the insane, but the straitjacket remained. **(A)** Philippe Pinel unchains the insane in mental asylum. **(B)** An old type of straitjacket.

Neurology. His student, *Sigmund Freud* (**FROYD**), developed the psychiatric procedure known as *psychoanalysis* (**sigh**-koh-uh-**NAL**-uh-sis).

SPINAL CORD DISORDERS

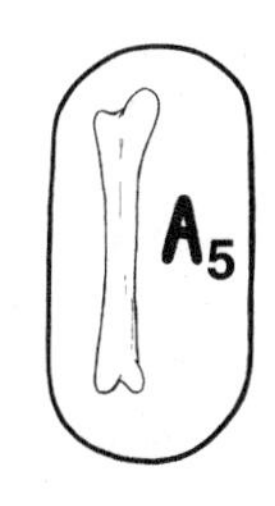

The spinal cord is the long, narrow, cord-like, inferior portion of the CNS. It lies within the *vertebral column* (backbone), below the brainstem. (Review Figure 11.1 if desired.) The spinal cord carries millions of sensory and motor nerve fibers up and down from the brain. Thus, it is critically involved in body sensations and movements. Consider, for instance, the effects of a *spinal transection* (**tran-SEK**-shun). This is a "cut" (*sect*) made all the way "across and through" (*trans-*) the "spinal cord" (*spin*), as in an injury or car accident! Some degree of paralysis and anesthesia is sure to follow!

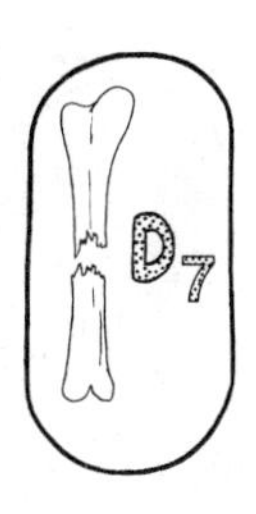

Another heartbreaking damage to the spinal cord is *spina* (**SPY**-nah) *bifida* (**BIH**-fih-dah) *cystica* (**SIS**-tih-kah). This is the "presence of" (-a) a "cleft or split" (*bifid*) "backbone" (*spin*). In spina bifida cystica, there is an open cleft or gap in the posterior wall of the vertebral column. The spinal cord and some of the *meninges* ("membranes" covering the CNS) may thus stick out. (Study Figure 11.6.) The protruding cord and meninges are enclosed within a *cyst*—a fluid-filled sac or "bladder." The cyst (bladder) is filled with *cerebrospinal fluid* (CSF). Spina bifida is generally a *congenital* (kun-**JEN**-ih-tal) skeletal defect—one that comes "with" (*con-*) "birth" (*genit*). The affected newborn is usually paralyzed from the site of the spina bifida on down. Numerous other organ system failures often make the prognosis for the child's continuing survival very poor.

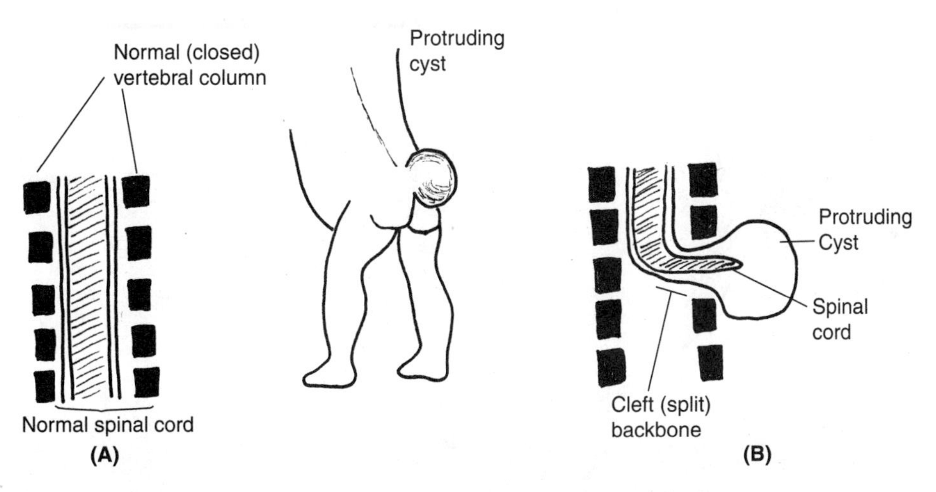

Fig. 11.6 Spina bifida: Cleft spine. **(A)** Vertebral column (backbone) is closed. **(B)** Spina bifida cystica: Backbone has a cleft, with spinal cord protruding inside a cyst.

SOME DISORDERS OF VISION AND HEARING

The bulk of our discussion so far has been about normal neuroanatomy and neurophysiology versus *neuropathology* (**nur**-oh-path-**AHL**-uh-**jee**). This medical term involves "the study of nerve diseases." Our attention has been focused upon the CNS. Let us now consider the so-called "special senses"—in particular, vision and hearing.

Visual dynamics and disorders

There are two main situations to consider when discussing both normal and abnormal vision. These are: (*1*) the anatomy and physiology of the eyeball itself, and (*2*) the anatomy and physiology (A&P) of the *optic* (**AHP**-tik) *nerve* and the visual processing areas of the cerebrum. The A&P of the normal eyeball is displayed in Figure 11.7, while Figure 11.8 suggests the processing of visual information by the brain.

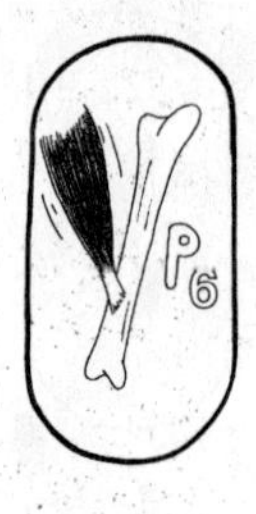

Figure 11.7 shows the beginning of the visual process. Light rays first cross through the *conjunctiva* (kahn-**JUNK**-tih-vuh). This is the thin, transparent membrane that "joins" (*junct*) "together" (*con-*) the lining of the eyelid and the surface of the eyeball. The *cornea* (**KOR**-nee-ah), coming next, is the tough, "horny" (*corne*). This is outer coat of the eyeball itself. The cornea is the transparent anterior portion of the *sclera* (**SLAIR**-uh)—the "hard" (*scler*) white

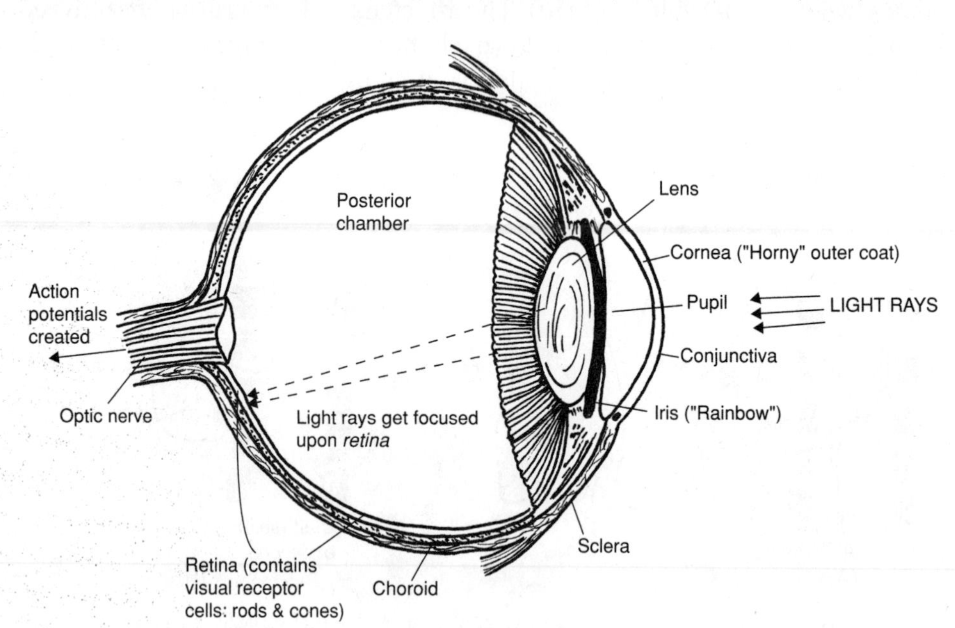

Fig. 11.7 Internal anatomy of the eyeball.

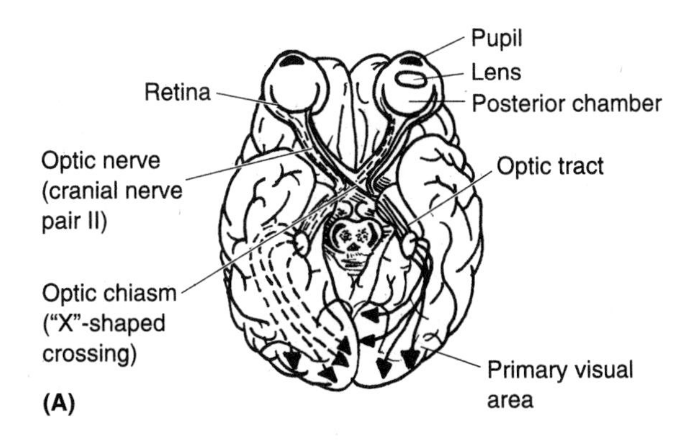

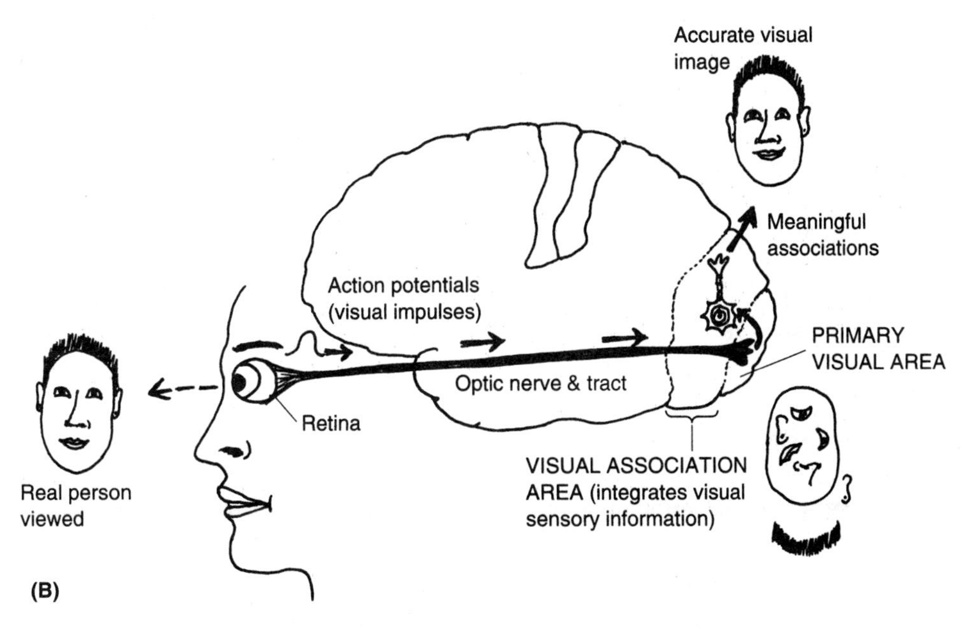

Fig. 11.8 The optic ("seeing") nerves travel to the back of the brain. **(A)** Optic nerves, optic chiasm, and optic tracts shown on base of cerebrum (behind eyeballs). **(B)** Pathway to visual areas of cerebrum.

portion of the eye. Light rays then pass through the *pupil*, a black hole in the middle of the *iris* (**EYE**-ris). The iris is the circular ring that appears in several colors, like a "rainbow" (*ir*).

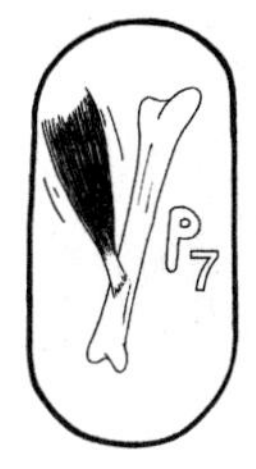

After passing through the pupil, light rays are bent by the *lens* and continue through the *posterior chamber* of the eye. The rays finally come to a focus upon the *retina* (**RET**-ih-nah). The retina is a "network" of *visual receptor cells*—the *rods* and the *cones*—located in the back of the eye. From the retina, action potentials (nerve impulses) are generated, and they leave the eyeball via the optic nerve.

As Figure 11.8 (A) pictures, the optic nerves cross over one another to create the X-shaped *optic chiasm* (**KEYE**-asm) at the base of the brain. From here, the *optic tracts* pass to the *primary visual area*, which is located in the extreme rear end of the cerebrum (Examine Figure 11.8 [B]). At first, the visual images are inverted (upside down) within the primary visual area. But the nearby *visual association area* of the brain integrates the visual information to make an accurate and meaningful "seeing" picture of reality.

Potential visual disorders, therefore, can occur anywhere along this total *visual pathway* we have outlined above. What are some specific clinical disorders often suffered that disturb normal vision? Let's list about half a dozen *ocular* (**AHK**-yoo-lar) or *ophthalmic* (ahf-**THAL**-mik) disorders that literally "refer to" (*-ar* or *-ic*) the "eyes" (*ocul* or *ophthalm*):

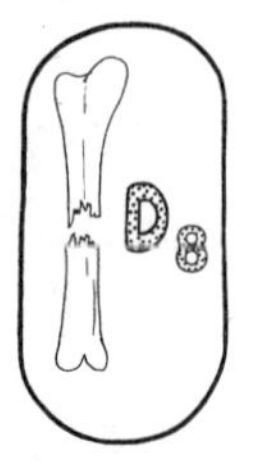

1. *Acute conjunctivitis* (kun-**JUNK**-tih-**VEYE**-tis) or "sudden inflammation of the conjunctiva." This is also known as *pink eye*. The pinkness is due to the deep red *conjunctival* (kun-**JUNK**-tih-val) blood vessels that are *dilated* (**DIE**-lay-ted) or "widened" during the *inflammatory* (in-**FLAM**-ah-tor-ee) *process*. This inflammation is the result of infection with viruses or bacteria, or irritation of the conjunctiva by allergies to pollen or dust. It is the most common eye disease in the Western world.
2. *Blepharitis* (**blef**-ar-**EYE**-tis) or "inflammation of the outer edges of the "eyelids" (*blephar*). Blepharitis is quite common and has symptoms of eye irritation, burning, and pruritus (itching). The eyes look "red-rimmed," and small scales can be seen clinging to the eyelashes. A common etiologic agent is pathogenic staphylococci.
3. *Chronic glaucoma* (glaw-**KOH**-muh) or "long-term" (*chron*) "silver-gray" (*glauc*) eye "tumor" (*-oma*). This is not really a tumor or growth. The silver-gray (*glauc*) part of the name probably refers to the late-stage occurrence of seeing halos around lights. The primary problem occurs when fluid drainage is blocked from the interior of both eyeballs. (The disease is generally bilateral). Usually, the *intra-ocular* (**in**-trah-**AHK**-yoo-lar) or "within the eyeball" *pressure* is about 10 to 25 mmHg. The abnormal fluid buildup within the eyes during glaucoma, however, can push the intra-ocular pressure up out of its normal range and into a dangerous hyper-state. The slender optic nerve becomes progressively damaged by such excessive pressure. This eventually causes *optic nerve atrophy* (shrinkage). The atrophy progresses over a span of months or years, causing a slight loss of *peripheral vision*. This is vision of objects on the "edge" or side of a person's total *field of vision*. Eventually, complete blindness may result.

4. *Cataract* (**KAT**-ah-rakt) literally means a "dashing-down or steep waterfall" that creates a cloudy mist of spray. In human eyes, this weird metaphor is employed to describe a progressive *opacity* (oh-**PASS**-uh-tee) or "condition of" (*-ity*) "darkness" (*opac*) of the lens. In healthy people, the lens is described as the *crystalline* (**KRIS**-tah-lin) *lens*. This is because it is clear and transparent like a diamond or other "crystal." Such clarity lets light rays easily pass through the lens and then come to a focus, a visual image upon the retina in back of the eye. However, in some people (usually older people), an *ophthalmoscope* (**ahf-THAL**-muh-skohp) or "instrument used to examine the eye" can reveal something very interesting. A cataract or "cloudy waterfall"–like image may be seen within the *dilated* (**DIE**-lay-ted) pupil. In other words, a cataract is an abnormally cloudy lens (View Figure 11.9). Cataracts may partially result from many years of lens exposure to ultraviolet (UV) radiation in sunlight. These rays may progressively

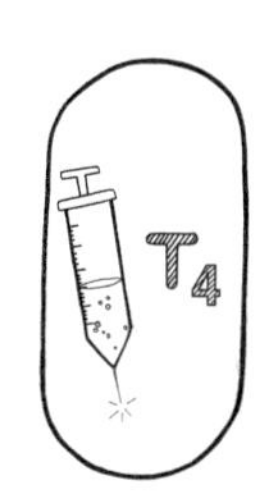

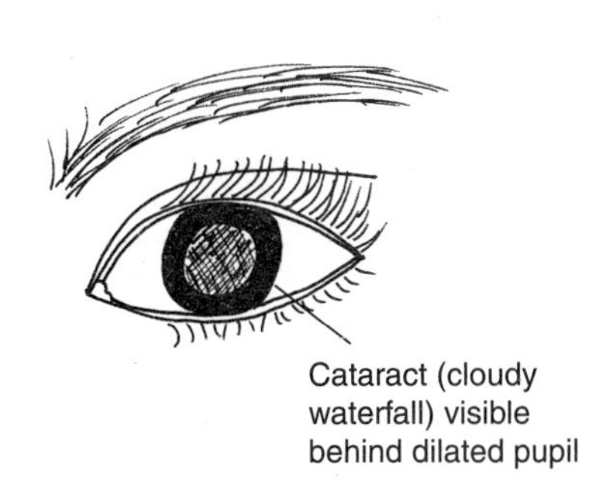

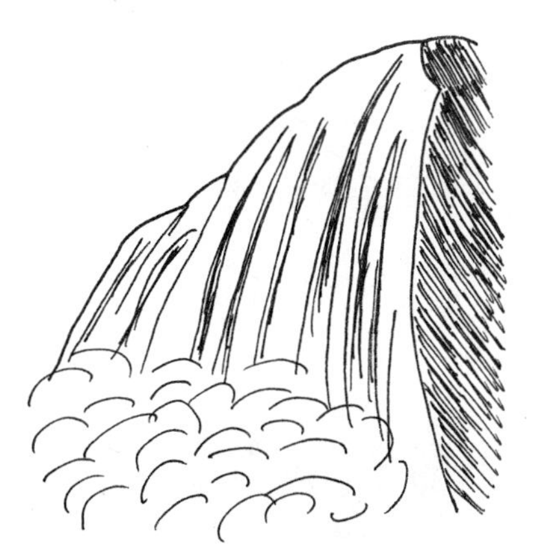

Fig. 11.9 A cataract seen behind the pupil.

cross-link the proteins within the crystalline lens, thereby turning the lens opaque (dark) and cloudy. If not removed, cataracts can result in blindness. [**Health hint:** Wear sunglasses with UV protection!]

5. Finally, there may be errors in *refraction* (re-**FRAK**-shun). Refraction is the "process of breaking or bending" rays of light entering the eye. Two very common types of *refractive* (re-**FRAK**-tiv) errors are *myopia* (**my-OH**-pea-uh) and *hyperopia* (**high**-per-**OH**-pea-uh). Myopia is "a condition" (*-ia*) of "nearsightedness" (*myop*). The *myopic* (my-**AHP**-ik) person is said to be nearsighted because the eyeball is too *long*. Therefore, light rays from distant objects come to a focus *in front* of the retina, rather than directly on it. (Study Figure 11.10, A.) Hyperopia is a "condition of" (*-ia*) light rays focusing "beyond" (*hyper-*) the retina of the "eye" (*op*). The *hyperopic* (**high**-per-**OH**-pik) or "farsighted" individual has an eyeball that is too *short*. As a result, light rays come to a focus *in back of* the retina rather than directly on it. (Study Figure 11.10, B.)

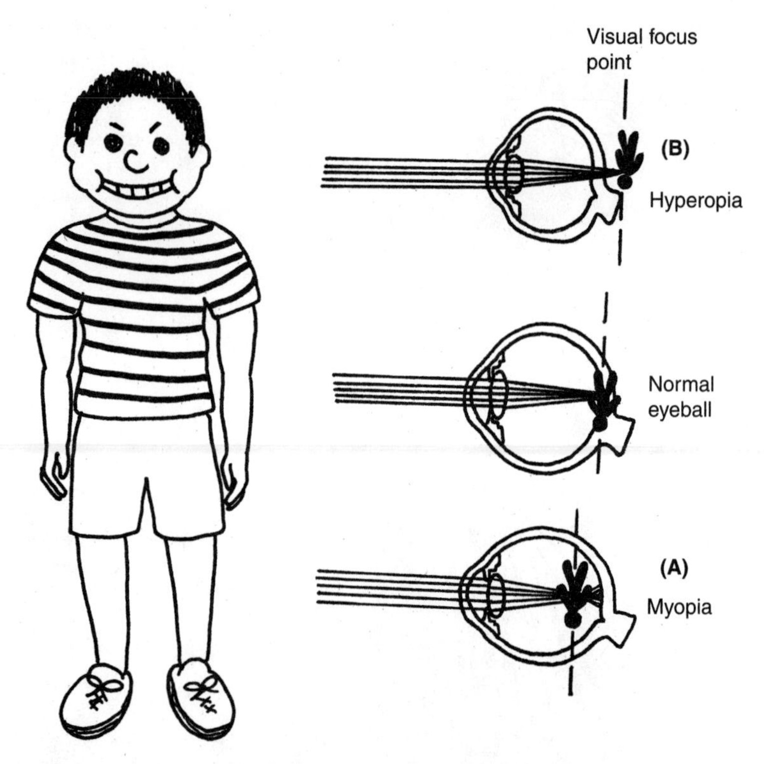

Fig. 11.10 Errors in seeing Baby Heinie: Myopia versus hyperopia. **(A)** Myopia ("nearsightedness"): Eyeball too *long*; inverted image comes to focus *in front of* retina. **(B)** Hyperopia ("farsightedness"): Eyeball too *short*; inverted image comes to focus *beyond (in back of)* retina.

Summarizing, we have:

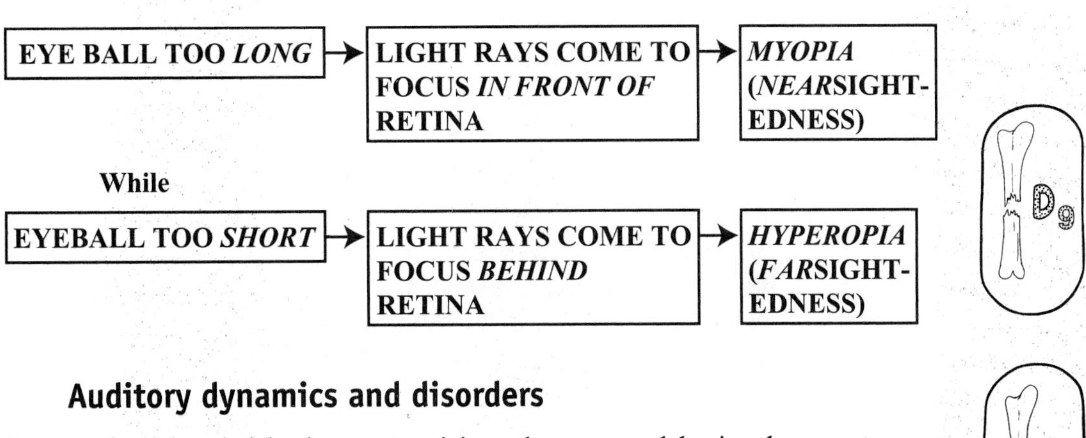

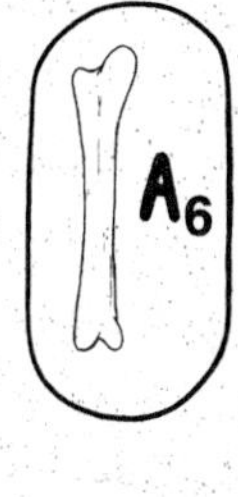

Auditory dynamics and disorders

Just as the eyes and brain create vision, the ears and brain also create *audition* (aw-**DIH**-shun). This is the "process of" (*-ion*) "hearing" (*audit*). Figure 11.11 provides a brief overview of the normal *auditory* (**AW**-dih-**tor**-ee) *sequence*. Sound waves pass through the *auricle* (**OR**-ih-kul, "little ear") on

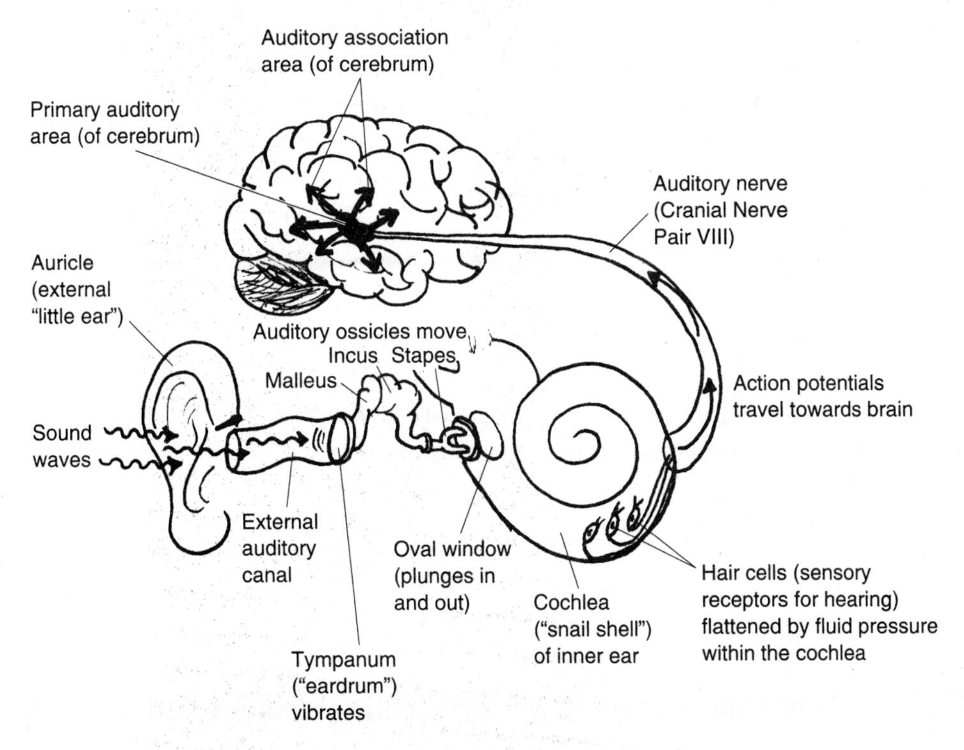

Fig. 11.11 The auditory nerve and hearing.

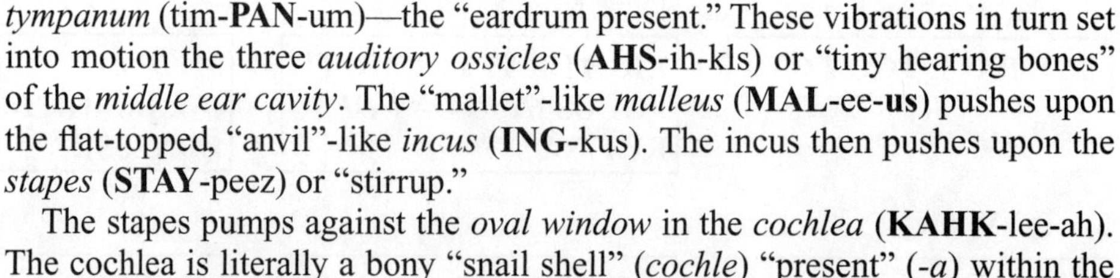

the side of the head. They enter the *external auditory canal* and vibrate the *tympanum* (tim-**PAN**-um)—the "eardrum present." These vibrations in turn set into motion the three *auditory ossicles* (**AHS**-ih-kls) or "tiny hearing bones" of the *middle ear cavity*. The "mallet"-like *malleus* (**MAL**-ee-**us**) pushes upon the flat-topped, "anvil"-like *incus* (**ING**-kus). The incus then pushes upon the *stapes* (**STAY**-peez) or "stirrup."

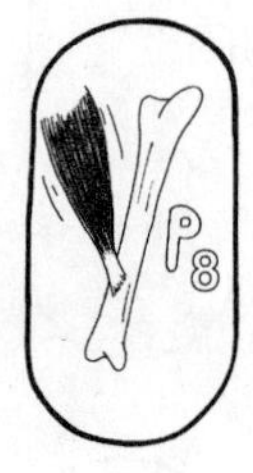

The stapes pumps against the *oval window* in the *cochlea* (**KAHK**-lee-ah). The cochlea is literally a bony "snail shell" (*cochle*) "present" (*-a*) within the *inner ear*. Its tiny *auditory receptors*, the *hair cells*, are bent by the pressure of the inner ear fluid, as the result of the pumping of the stapes. Action potentials (nerve impulses) are then created. They travel to the *primary auditory area* of the brain via the *auditory* (hearing) *nerve*. This is where the brain first "hears" sounds. But it takes the *auditory association area* of the cerebrum to put these sounds into the meaningful patterns we interpret as language—such as the sounds creating or own name!

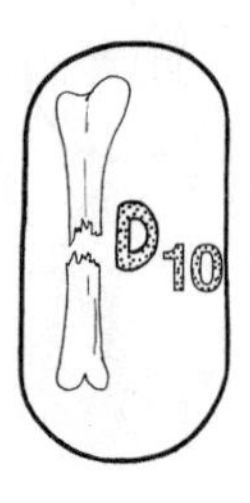

A very common auditory problem is *acute otitis* (oh-**TIE**-tis) *media* (**MEE**-dee-uh). This is a "sudden" (*acute)* "inflammation of" (*-itis*) the "middle" (*medi*) "ear" (*ot*) cavity. Consider what can happen following an upper respiratory infection, such as acute coryza. A variety of pathogenic bacteria can travel into the middle ear cavity from the nose (especially if you blow it too hard!). Streptococci, staphylococci, and other types of pathogenic cocci lodge in the mucous—"pertaining to" (*-ous*) "slime" (*muc*)—membrane that lines the middle ear cavity.

The inflammatory process creates a tissue edema (swelling). The buildup of fluid bulges out the *tympanic* (tim-**PAN**-ik)—"referring to" (*-ic*) "eardrum" (*tympan*)—*membrane.* This bulging irritates local sensory nerves. The result is *otalgia* (**oh**-**TAL**-juh)—that is, "ear" (*ot*) "pain" (*-algia*). Other typical symptoms include a feeling of fullness in the ear. This can contribute to *anacusia* (**an**-ah-**KYOO**-see-ah), "a condition" (*-ia*) "without" (*ana-*) "hearing" (*cus*). This may be accompanied by fever, chills, and a *suppuration* (**sup**-yuh-**RAY**-shun). Suppuration is literally a "process of" (*-tion*) "forming pus" (*suppur*). The pus is then discharged through the external ear (auricle).

SUMMARY TABLE 11.2

Consult Summary Table 11.2 for a quick review of some important words and word parts. (Please see Table on next page.)

Medical Case History: Cerebrovascular Accident and Aphasia

Mr. Tom J., 54, suffered a stroke (CVA) after lifting heavy weights in the gym. The damaging effect of the resulting ischemia (blood supply deficiency) largely

Summary Table 11.2 Words and Word Parts

Write in the *exact* meaning (literal English translation) for up to 10 key terms selected from the preceding block of text. After you are done, check your word meanings with the correct answers, which are given at the end of this chapter.

Key Terms	Prefixes	Roots	Suffixes	Exact Meanings
antipsychotic	anti- "against"	psychot "(a disturbed) mind"	-ic "relating to"	1.________
bifida	(none)	bifid "cleft or split"	-a "presence of"	2.________
congenital	con- "with"	genit "birth"	-al "referring to"	3.________
neuropathology	(none)	neur "nerve"; path "diseases"	-ology "study of"	4. ________
iris	(none)	ir "rainbow"	-is "present"	5. ________
optic	(none)	opt "eye"	-ic "pertaining to"	6.________
blepharitis	(none)	blephar "eyelids"	-itis "inflammation of"	7. ________
ophthalmoscope	(none)	ophthalm "eyes"	-scope "instrument used to examine"	8. ________
myopia	(none)	myop "nearsightedness"	-ia "condition of"	9. ________
auditory	(none)	audit "hearing"	-ory "pertaining to"	10. ________

depended upon what *local part* of Mr. J's brain was actually being deprived of oxygen.

A computed axial tomography scan (or CAT scan; Chapter 5) was done. It showed that *Broca's* (**BROH**-kahs) *area*, also called the *motor speech area*, was severely affected. This cerebral region was named after *Pierre Paul Broca* (**BROH**-kah), a French surgeon who lived from 1824 to 1880. Dr. Broca was

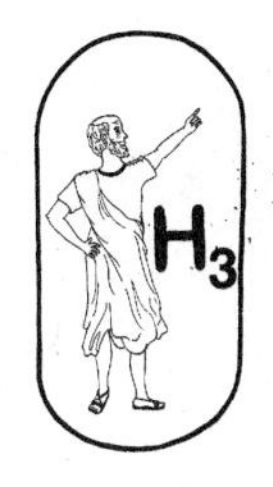

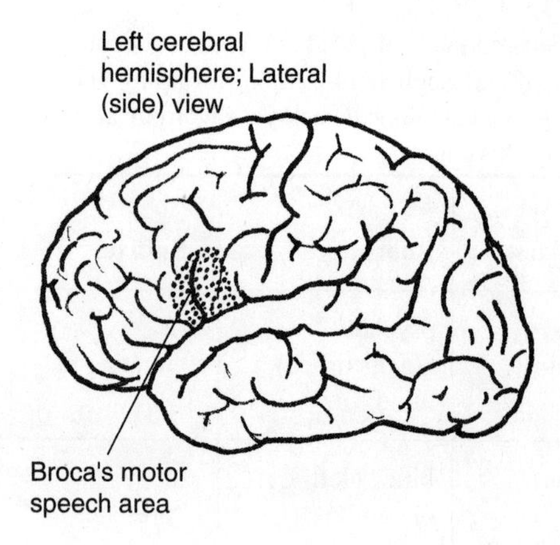

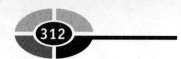

Fig. 11.12 Broca's motor speech area of the brain.

the first to localize the motor speech area: it is near the base of the precentral gyrus, usually in the *dominant* cerebral hemisphere (Figure 11.12). This region is mainly responsible for forming and using words in speaking, reading, and writing. Broca's motor speech area also plays an important role in controlling movements of the tongue, lips, and vocal cords.

Because Mr. J. was right-handed, his dominant cerebral hemisphere was the one on the *left*. [**Memory probe:** Why would a right-handed person have their *left* cerebral hemisphere as the dominant one? What is the anatomical explanation that we made earlier in this chapter?] Therefore, Mr. J's Broca's area was located around the base of his left precentral gyrus. It was quickly obvious that Broca's area had been damaged by the CVA because of the sudden occurrence of *aphasia* (uh-**FAY**-zee-ah). This medical term indicates the "condition of" (*-ia*) a "lack" (*a-*) of "speech" (*phas*). *Total aphasia* was suffered by Mr. J. In this condition, the stricken person is able to *hear* words. However, the person just can't process, understand, or express their *own* words in response! (Talk about complete frustration!)

Probe of case history

(**A**) Assume that the *aphasic* (ah-**FAY**-zik) patient was suffering from a *neuroma* (nur-**OH**-muh) that was damaging Broca's area. Dissect *neuroma* by inserting slash marks. Label the resulting word parts as prefix, root, or suffix. Write the common English translation. (**B**) *Plegia* (**PLEE**-jee-uh) means "a condition of stroke or paralysis." Using the prefix in *hemisphere*, build a single term that means "a condition of paralysis of half (the body)." [Check your short answers with the key near the end of this chapter.]

Quiz

Refer to the text in this chapter if necessary. A good score is at least 8 correct answers out of these 10 questions. The answers are listed in the back of this book.

1. The nervous system equals the:
   (a) Brain + Peripheral Nervous System
   (b) CNS + spinal cord
   (c) Brain + spinal cord + nerves + sensory receptors
   (d) Cranial neurons minus the motor nerve fibers
2. The technical term for the brain is:
   (a) Brainokete
   (b) Neuroma
   (c) Cerebellum
   (d) Encephalon
3. "Refers to the opposite side" of the body:
   (a) Contralateral
   (b) Medial
   (c) Superior
   (d) Lateral
4. Surface grooves or "furrows" in the cerebral cortex:
   (a) Gyri
   (b) Hallucinations
   (c) Sulci
   (d) Optic nerves
5. *Homunculus* is properly dissected as:
   (a) Homuncul/us
   (b) Ho/munc/ulus
   (c) Homunc/ul/us
   (d) Homunculu/s
6. "The study of nerves":
   (a) Psych/ology
   (b) Path/ology
   (c) Psych/iatry
   (d) Neur/ology
7. *Schizophrenia* translates as:
   (a) "Presence of a sick brain"
   (b) "Removal of the main brain mass"

(c) "Inflammation of the sciatic nerve"
(d) "Condition of split mind"

8. *Psychoses* are mental disorders that always involve:
(a) Extensive need for neurosurgery
(b) No loss of the sense of reality
(c) Ruptures of the tympanic membrane
(d) Lack of a sense of who one really is

9. A stop-smoking clinic would most likely be run by what type of mental health professional?
(a) Psychiatrist
(b) Psychologist
(c) Phrenologist
(d) Physiologist

10. Psychiatrist who is famous for unchaining the insane:
(a) Philippe Pinel
(b) Aldous Huxley
(c) Sigmund Freud
(d) Albert Schweitzer

Memory Pillboxes for Chapter 11

Several key facts were tagged with numbered icons in the page margins of this chapter. Write a short summary of each of these key facts into a numbered cell or compartment within the appropriate type of *Memory Pillbox* that appears below.

Background and History **Pillboxes for Chapter 11:**

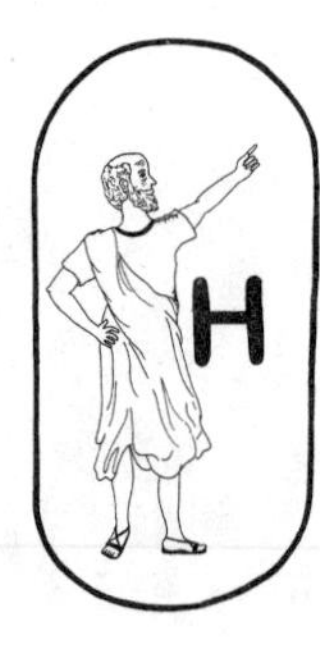

1

2	3

***Anatomy* Pillboxes for Chapter 11:**

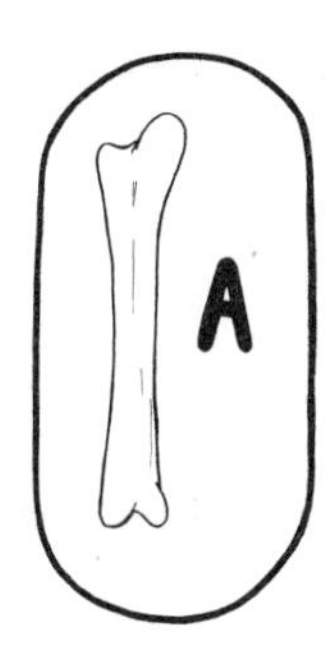

1	2

3	4

5	6

***Physiology* Pillboxes for Chapter 11:**

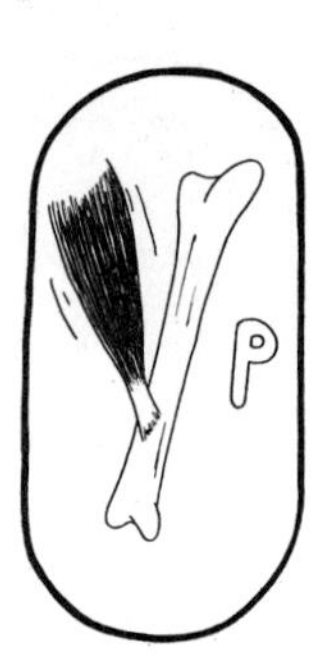

1	2

3	4

5	6

7	8

***Disease/Injury* Pillboxes for Chapter 11:**

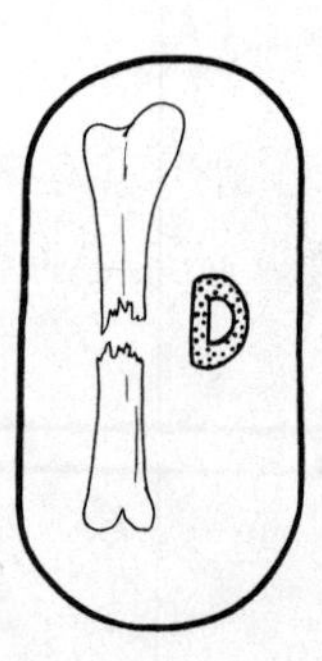

1	2

3	4

5	6

7	8

9	10

Treatment/Therapy **Pillboxes for Chapter 11:**

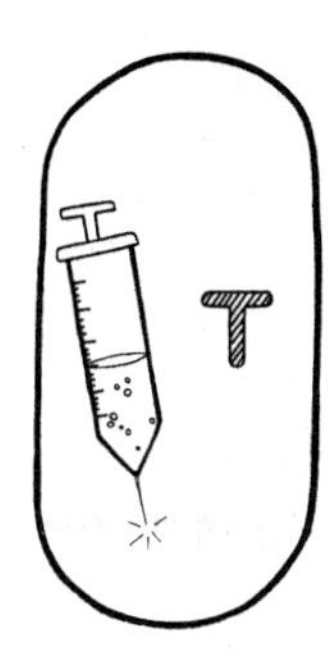

1	2

3	4

Answers for Chapter 11 Summary Tables

FOR SUMMARY TABLE 11.1

1. "pertains to nerves"
2. "presence of (something) within the head"
3. "presence of a furrow"
4. "presence of a little cerebrum"
5. "referring to (something) before the center"
6. "relating to (something) after the center"
7. "pertaining to the opposite side"
8. "abnormal condition of nerves"
9. "abnormal condition of mind"
10. "condition of split mind"

FOR SUMMARY TABLE 11.2

1. "relating to (something) against (a disturbed) mind"
2. "presence of a cleft or split"
3. "referring to (something) with birth"
4. "study of nerve diseases"
5. "rainbow present"
6. "pertaining to the eye"
7. "inflammation of the eyelids"
8. "instrument used to examine the eyes"
9. "condition of nearsightedness"
10. "pertaining to hearing"

Answers to Probe of Case History

(**A**) neur (root) /oma (suffix) = "a tumor of nerves" (**B**) *Hemiplegia* (**hem**-ih-**PLEE**-jee-ah).

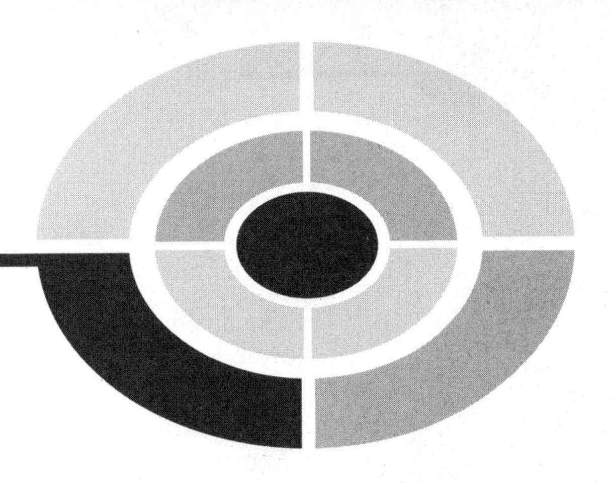

Test: Part 5

DO NOT REFER TO THE TEXT WHEN TAKING THIS TEST. A good score is at least 18 out of 25 questions correct. The answers are in the back of the book. It's best to have a friend check your score the first time so you won't memorize the answers if you want to take the test again.

1. Organ system literally consisting of "little acorns":
   (a) Circulatory
   (b) Digestive
   (c) Glandular
   (d) Genitourinary
   (e) Nervous
2. "One who specializes in study of the skin":
   (a) Dermatology
   (b) Endocrinologist
   (c) Dermatological
   (d) Integumentectomy
   (e) Dermatologist
3. Asymptomatic is properly dissected as:
   (a) A/symp/to/matic

(b) Asy/mpto/ma/tic
(c) A/symptomat/ic
(d) Asym/pt/o/ma/tic
(e) Asymptomati/c

4. The exact opposite in meaning to endocrine is:
(a) Holocrine
(b) Sebaceous
(c) Integument
(d) Exocrine
(e) Hemoglobin

5. "Black tumor" of the skin:
(a) Carcinoma
(b) Leukocytosis
(c) Sporozoite
(d) Mycoma
(e) Melanoma

6. A hypersecretion of hormone X implies that hormone X:
(a) Is being released in excessive or above-normal amounts
(b) Has multiple body effects
(c) Is quickly inactivated and destroyed upon contact with the bloodstream
(d) Is being secreted in deficient or below normal amounts
(e) Really isn't being secreted at *all!*

7. The ______ glands secrete "grease" into the hair follicle:
(a) Anterior pituitary
(b) Sweat
(c) Pancreatic acinar
(d) Islet
(e) Sebaceous

8. Baldness, or "fox mange," is technically called:
(a) Glaucoma
(b) Alopecia
(c) Allowicious
(d) Decubitus ulcer
(e) Papillitis

9. A teenager may be embarrassed because he has too many ______, or "pimples," on his face.
(a) Comedoes

(b) Papules
(c) Hydrocarbons
(d) Villi
(e) Carbohydrates

10. You may give your favorite uncle an antiperspirant for his birthday present, because:
(a) He suffers from diapedesis
(b) His sweat pores are clogged
(c) He has a problem with diaphoresis (hyperhidrosis)
(d) Thermoregulation is failing!
(e) Those big birthday cakes are just getting too darn expensive!

11. The _/_ gland is named for its resemblance to a pinecone.
(a) Pituit/ary
(b) Pine/al
(c) Thyr/oid
(d) Pancre/at
(e) Nephr/on

12. Secrete insulin into the bloodstream:
(a) Alpha cells
(b) Pancreatic acinar cells
(c) Gluca-goners!
(d) Beta cells
(e) Islets of Alfredo

13. Disease resulting from chronic hyposecretion of insulin:
(a) Hypoglycemia
(b) Insulin shock
(c) Diabetes mellitus
(d) Acromegaly
(e) Diabetes insipidus

14. The most inferior portion of the Central Nervous System:
(a) Brainstem
(b) Cerebellum
(c) Spinal cord
(d) Cerebral cortex
(e) Frontal lobe

15. The primary motor area:
(a) Central sulcus
(b) Broca's area

(c) Medulla oblongata
(d) Cornea
(e) Precentral gyrus

16. A good professional to seek out for help with schizophrenia:
(a) Neurosurgeon
(b) Physiatrist
(c) Neurologist
(d) Pharmacologist
(e) Psychiatrist

17. A spinal cord transection refers to:
(a) A cut made all the way across and through the cord
(b) An operation to remove a spinal tumor
(c) Surgical repair of the cerebellum
(d) Proprioception alone
(e) An operation involving slicing through the cerebral cortex

18. A mixed gland:
(a) Thyroid
(b) Pineal
(c) Trachea
(d) Pancreas
(e) Sebaceous

19. Someone with blepharitis would be suffering from inflammation associated with what particular body structure?
(a) Tear gland
(b) Lens of the eye
(c) Eyelid
(d) Optic nerve
(e) Auricle

20. A network of rods and cones on the back of the eyeball:
(a) Retina
(b) Optic chiasm
(c) Cornea
(d) Iris
(e) Pupil

21. Cousin George's eyeball is abnormally short! Therefore, he probably suffers from:
(a) Hyperopia
(b) Retinal detachment

(c) Myopia
(d) Iriditis
(e) Conjunctival fusion

22. The __/__ is a "snail shell present" within the inner ear.
(a) Cochle/ar
(b) Stape/s
(c) Cochle/a
(d) Mito/chondrion
(e) Nas/al

23. In the word, *intraocular,* the root is:
(a) Intra
(b) In
(c) Ular
(d) Ocular
(e) Ocul

24. *Ophthalmoscopic* (**ahf**-thal-mah-**SKAHP**-ik) literally translates as:
(a) "Relating to an instrument used to examine the ear"
(b) "Presence of a device employed for food foraging"
(c) "Pertaining to a scope that scoops up blackheads"
(d) "Referring to an instrument used to examine the eye"
(e) "The process of removing the eyeball using a special scope"

25. *Otitis media* represents:
(a) A defect in visual refraction
(b) Special types of bacteria infecting the middle ear cavity
(c) Conditions of near-blindness due to aging lenses
(d) Cataractous eyeballs, but without glaucoma
(e) A process of hardening of the three auditory ossicles

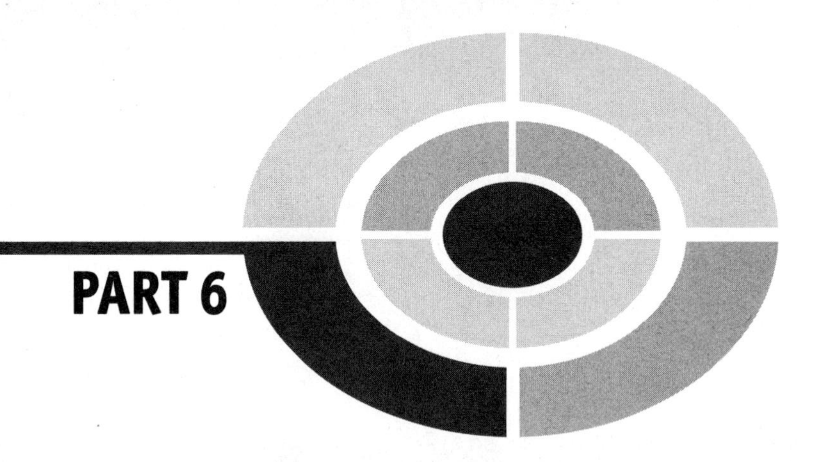

PART 6

Welcome to Life in the Land "Down Under"!

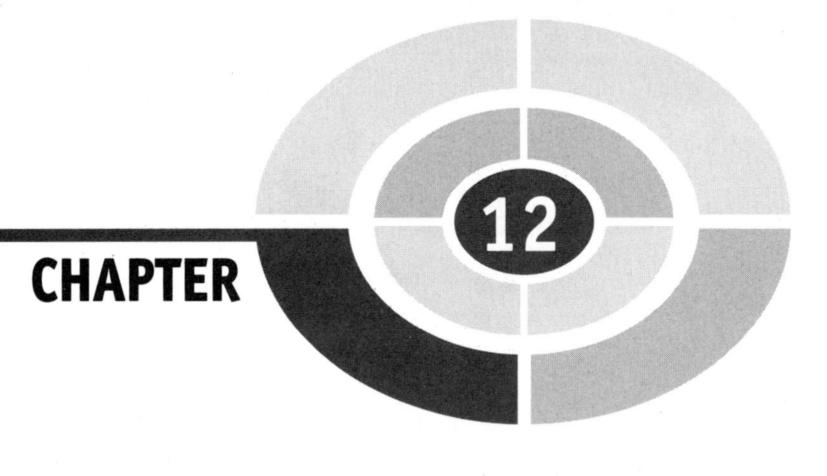

Terms Related to Disorders of the Digestive Tract

This final unit of our study takes us to the Land "Down Under"! No, we don't mean Australia! We are referring to the *digestive* (**die-JES**-tiv) *system* (here in Chapter 12) and the *genitourinary* (**jen**-ih-toh-**UR**-ih-**nair**-ee) *system* (Chapter 13).

Background and History

The digestive system is also called the *digestive tube* or *tract*. This tube extends from the mouth (oral cavity) all the way down to the *anus* (**AY**-nus). (View Figure 12.1.) The anus is literally the small, muscular "ring" (*an*) "present" (*-us*) at the terminal end of the digestive tube/tract.

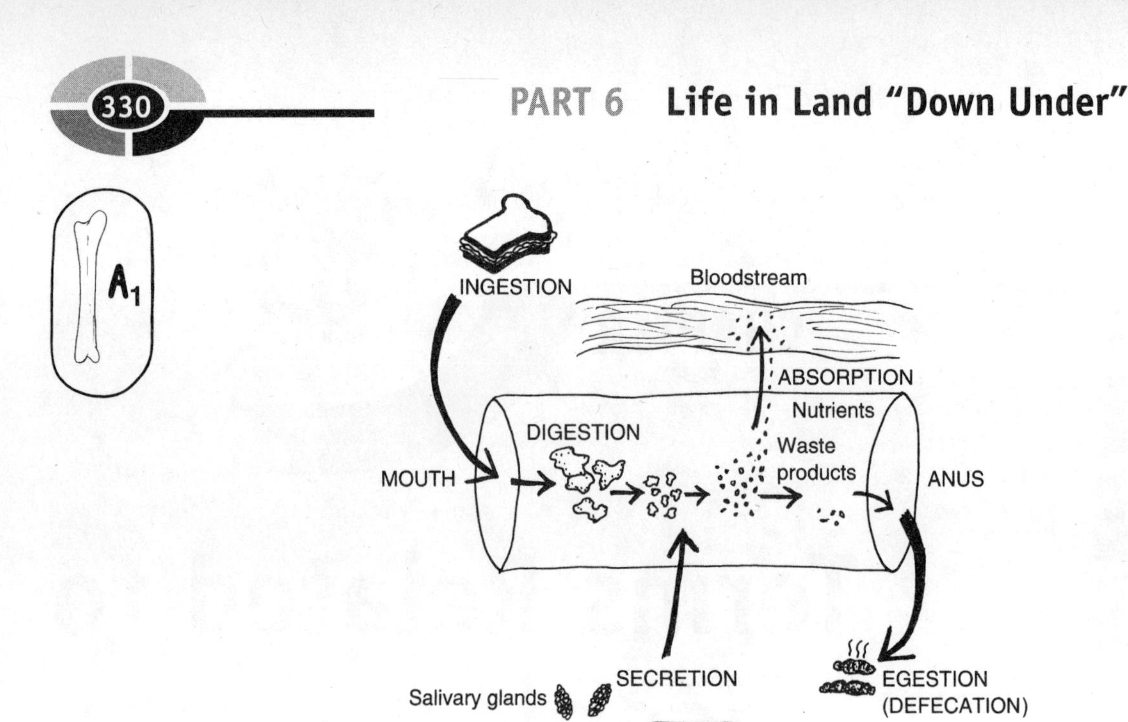

Fig. 12.1 The digestive tube and its general functions.

THE FIVE MAJOR FUNCTIONS OF THE DIGESTIVE TRACT

The word, *digest* (die-**JEST**), comes from the Latin for "separate, carry apart, or dissolve." *Digestive* therefore "pertains to" (*-ive*) "carrying apart." It should be no surprise that one of the major functions of this tube is *digestion* (die-**JES**-chun). This word literally means the "process of" (*-ion*) "carrying or breaking apart" (*digest*) food. Digestion begins very soon after *ingestion* (**in-JES**-chun), which "carries (food) in" (*ingest*). The process of digestion begins in the mouth, where the food is chewed and mixed with "spit" or *saliva* (sah-**LIE**-vah). An *ingested* (**in-JES**-ted) ham sandwich, for instance, quickly becomes a food *bolus* (**BOH**-lus). This soft "ball" (*bol*) is digested into small fragments of nutrients (such as glucose and other simple carbohydrates). These tiny nutrient particles then undergo *absorption*. Absorption is the movement of material from the lumen (light space) of the digestive tube into the bloodstream. By the process of absorption, then, ingested glucose molecules that used to be part of the bread in a ham sandwich eventually move out of the digestive tract and become *blood glucose* molecules.

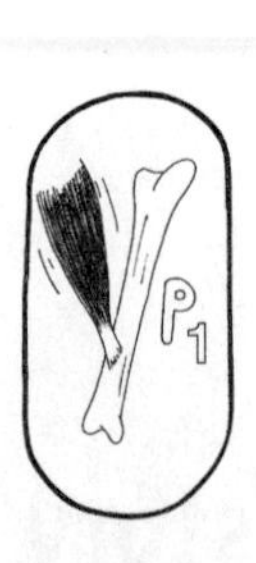

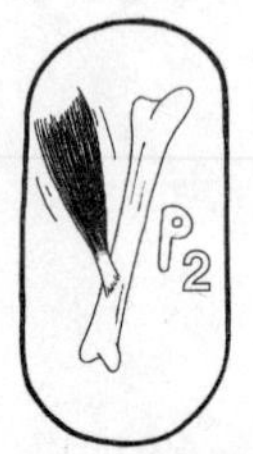

Besides ingestion, digestion, and absorption, a fourth major function associated with the digestive tract is *secretion*. Figure 12.1 shows that there are several *accessory* (**ak-SESS**-or-ee) *digestive organs* that add *secretions* to the digestive tube lumen. These include the *salivary* (**SAH**-lih-**vair**-ee) *glands*, *liver, pancreas*, and *cholecyst* (**KOH**-leh-**sist**) or "gall" (*chole*) "bladder" (*cyst*). It is the salivary glands, of course, that secrete the sticky saliva into the oral cavity.

Finally, the last major function of the digestive tube is called *egestion* (**ee-JES**-chun) or *defecation* (**deh**-feh-**KAY**-shun). Egestion is the "process of" (*-ion*) "carrying" (*gest*) waste matter "out" (*e-*) of the anus. Its synonym, *defecation,* is the "process of" (*-tion*) releasing *feces* (**FEE**-sees) "from" (*de-*) the anus.

Summarizing the above info yields:

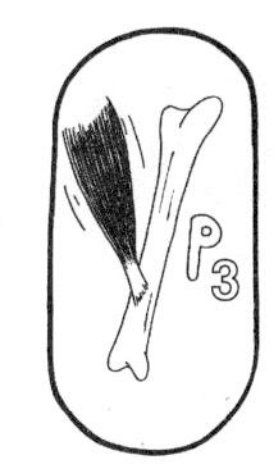

GENERAL DIGESTIVE TRACT FUNCTIONS = **Ingestion + Digestion + Absorption + Secretion + Egestion (defecation)**

MAJOR ORGANS OF THE DIGESTIVE TRACT

Figure 12.2 displays the major organs of the human digestive tract. Observe that after the oral cavity lies the pharynx (throat). [**Memory probe:** What other major organ system besides the digestive system includes the pharynx? Do you remember its name? (Hint: Look back at Chapter 9.)]

After the pharynx lies the *esophagus* (eh-**SAHF**-uh-**gus**) or "gullet." The esophagus (gullet) is the muscle-walled tube that leads down into the stomach. The liver, cholecyst (gallbladder), and pancreas, along with the stomach, all empty their contents into the *duodenum* (dew-**AH-**den-um). The duodenum is the first or proximal portion of the *small intestine.* A close-up view of the duodenum and its friendly neighbors is provided by Figure 12.3. This figure illustrates a curious fact (known to Hippocrates and many early Greek anatomists): the word, *duodenum*, means "presence of" (*-um*) "twelve" (*duoden*). This odd name comes from the ancient method of measuring the length of various body structures by adding together fingerbreadths (finger wideness). The duodenum, therefore, is approximately twelve fingerbreadths long!

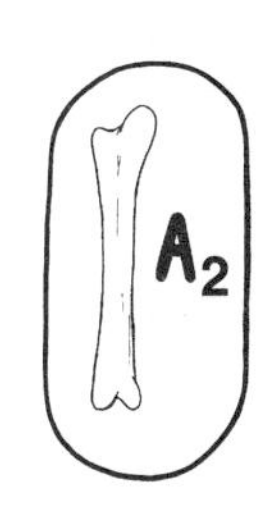

As is evident from Figure 12.3, the duodenum is the common destination for *pancreatic juice* from the pancreatic duct (Chapter 10), as well as for *bile* from the liver. Bile is stored and intermittently released by the cholecyst (gall or bile bladder). The bile travels into the duodenum through the *common bile duct.* Bile is a brownish-green detergent substance (much like dish soap). It acts to *emulsify* (ih-**MUL**-sih-feye)—"milk out" (*emulsif*)—big globs of ingested fat into a foam of tiny fat bubbles.

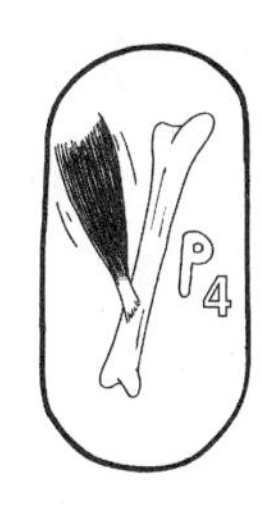

Continuing on our journey down the digestive tube, after the duodenum comes the last two sections of the small intestine. These are, in order, the *jejunum* (jeh-**JOO**-num) and the *ileum* (**IL**-ee-um). "Oh, Noble Ghost of Hippocrates,

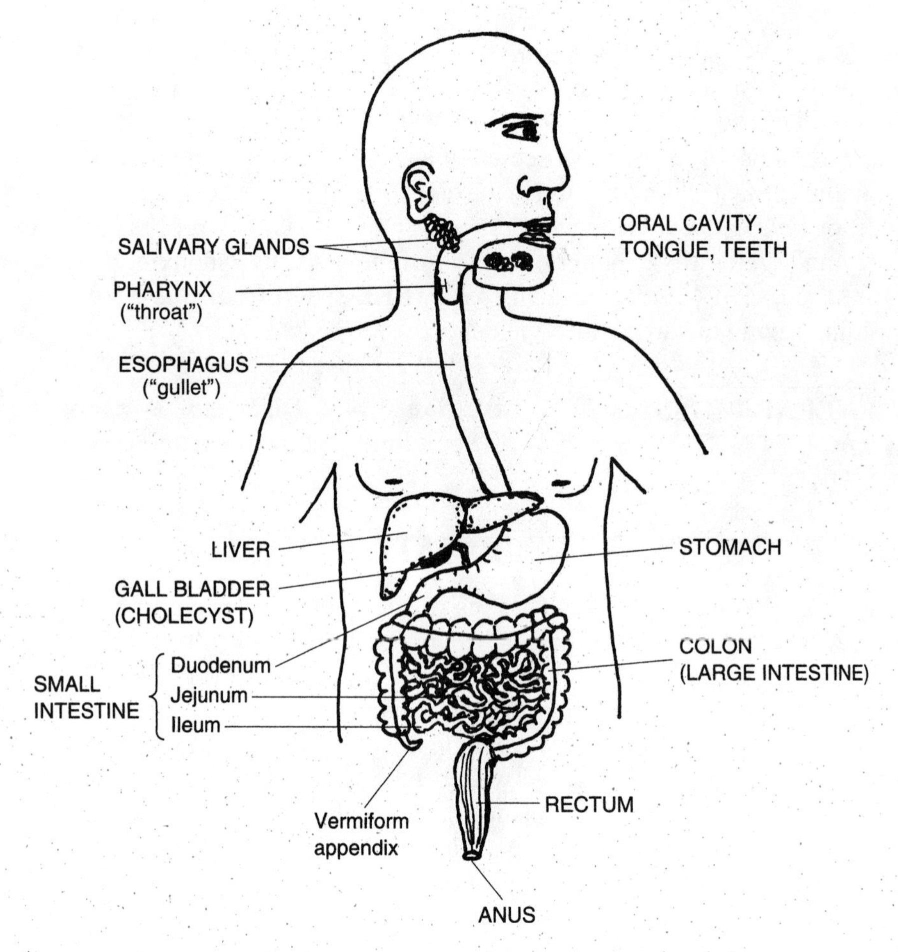

Fig. 12.2 Major organs of the human digestive tract.

how did these two sections of the small intestine get their names?" Well, Dear Reader, in ancient times our Greek and Roman anatomists described the jejunum as "something" (*-um*) "empty" (*jejun*) when they dissected it. Further, they localized the end of the small intestine as being within the "flank" (*ile*)—hence its name.

Following the small intestine is the much wider *large intestine* (Figure 12.4), alternately called the *colon* (**KOH**-lun). The colon begins with the *cecum* (**SEE**-kum). This is a rounded, "blind" (*cec*), dead-ended pouch. The *vermiform* (**VERM**-ih-form) *appendix* is a slender, "wormlike" (*vermiform*) "attachment" (*appendix*). Figure 12.4 shows that it is hooked onto the base of the cecum.

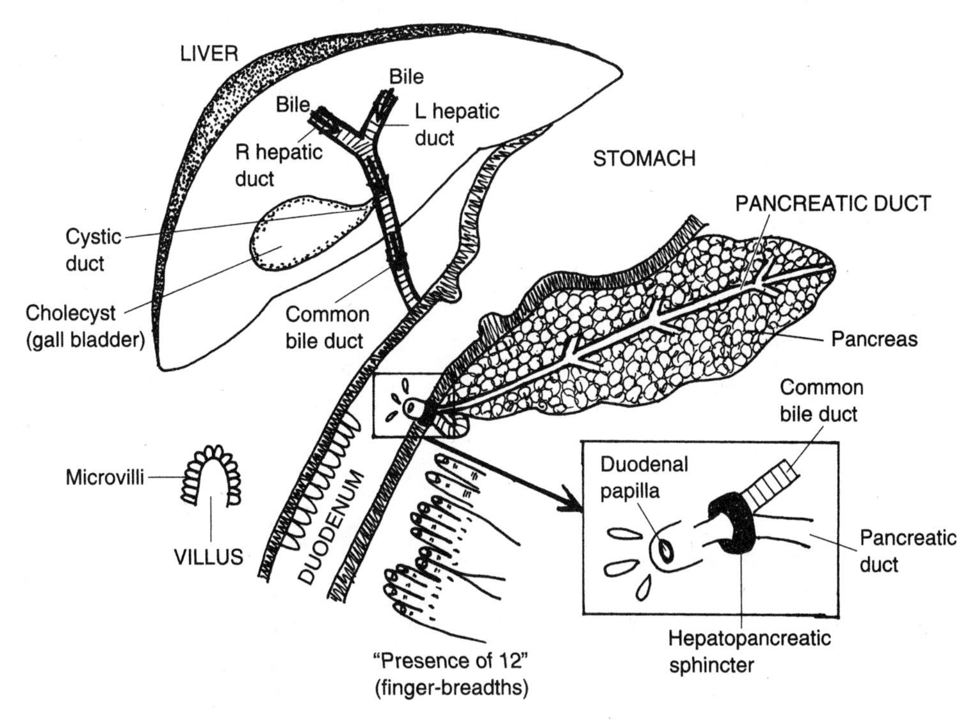

Fig. 12.3 The duodenum and its friendly neighbors.

Composed of lymphatic connective tissue, the vermiform appendix also contains lymphocytes and plasma cells (Chapter 5). Therefore, it plays a minor role in the body's immunity or self-defense.

Rising "upward" from the cecum is the *ascending colon*. It then "turns" (*vers*) and moves "across" (*trans-*) the body as the *transverse colon*. Going "downward" from this point is the *descending colon*. This snakes over into the "S-resembling" *sigmoid* (**SIG**-moyd) *colon*. Note (Figure 12.4) the presence of several *sphincter* (**SFINGK**-ter) muscles. A sphincter is literally a "band" or "squeezer." A sphincter is a circular band of muscle that forms a ring around a body opening. When the sphincter muscle contracts, it constricts (narrows) a body opening, often completely closing it off. Observe in Figure 12.4, for example, the *internal* and *external anal sphincters*. These sphincters are located within the *rectum* (**REK**-tum)—a "straight" (*rect*), muscular tube that empties feces into the anus. When the external anal sphincter contracts, it completely "squeezes" shut the opening into the anus. This allows us to select the appropriate time and place for carrying out defecation (egestion)!

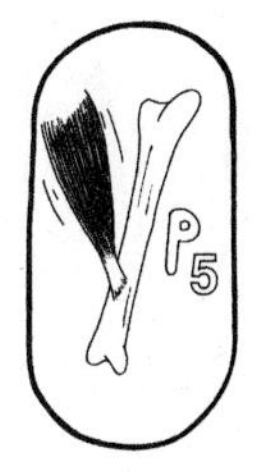

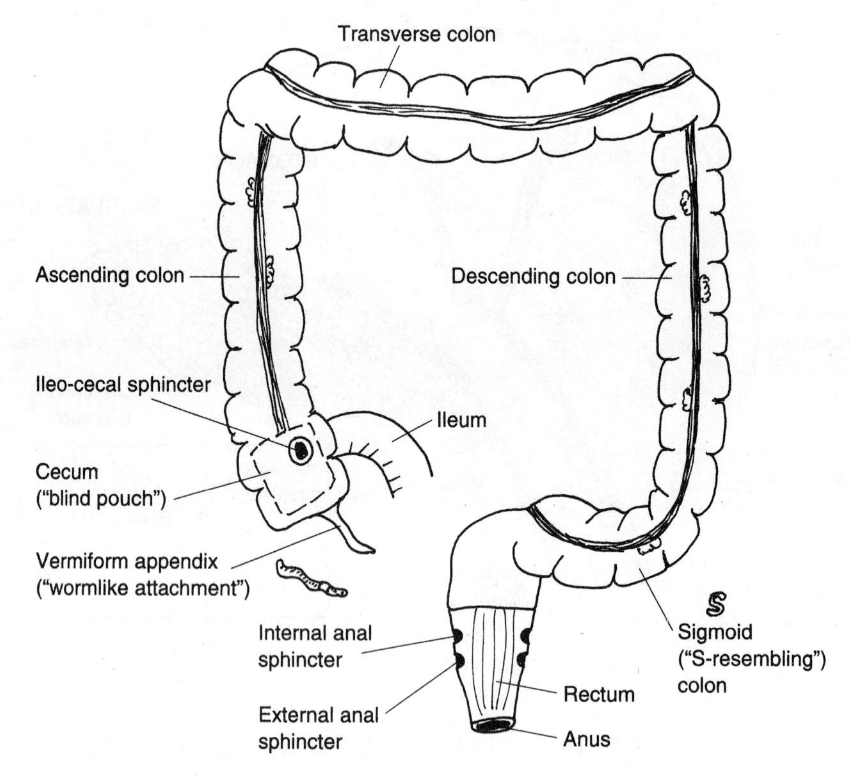

Fig. 12.4 The human colon (large intestine).

SUMMARY OF DIGESTIVE TRACT ANATOMY

Now that we have briefly introduced all of the major digestive organs, let us put them all together into a convenient summary equation:

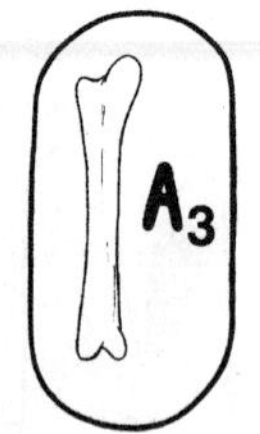

DIGESTIVE TRACT = **ORAL CAVITY + PHARYNX + ESOPHAGUS + STOMACH + SMALL INTESTINE + LARGE INTESTINE (COLON)**

A DETAILED LOOK AT THE STOMACH

When we are dealing with the *medical* terminology of the digestive tract, we are essentially dealing with its *disorders*. In theory, then, medical terms of the digestive tract could describe problems with *any* of the five major *functions* (digestive *physiology*) or any of the six major *structures* (digestive *anatomy*) that we have listed in our equations.

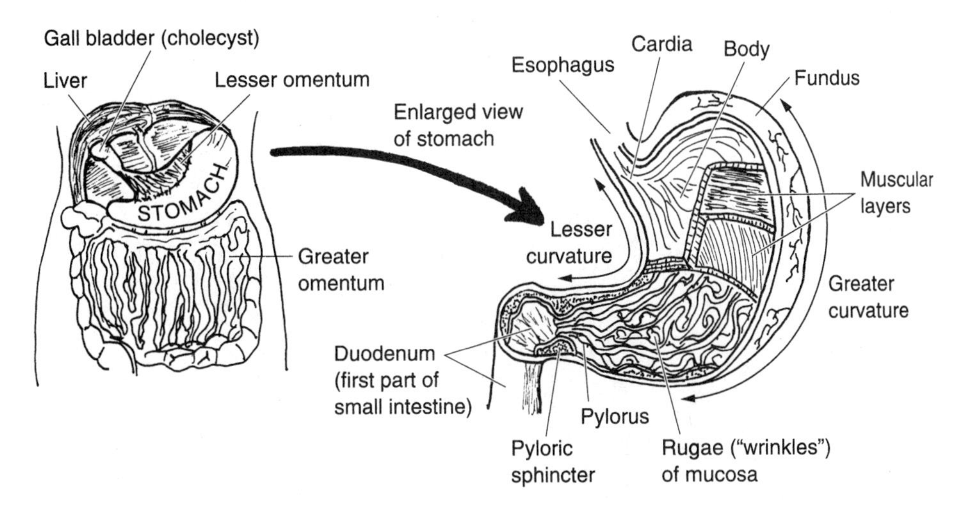

Fig. 12.5 The anatomy of the stomach.

When you think of *gastrointestinal* (**GAS**-troh-in-**TES**-tih-nul) or *GI* upsets, however, what is the *first* thing that comes to mind? As the term, *gastrointestinal*, suggests, don't we usually think about upsets of our "stomach" (*gastr*) or our "intestines" (*intest*)? Therefore, (GI) upsets by definition involve disorders of only the stomach and intestines. Nevertheless, these disorders are so common that the *whole* digestive tube is sometimes *incorrectly* labeled as the GI tract!

Figure 12.5 provides us with a detailed view of both the internal and external anatomy of the stomach. Observe that the *cardia* (**KAR**-dee-ah) is the superior portion of the stomach and connects directly to the esophagus above it. The *body* is the major central portion. The stomach also has a *fundus* (**FUN**-dus). In general, a fundus is "a bottom or base" (*fund*) of some organ that is "present" (*-us*) farthest from its opening. In the case of the stomach, the fundus is a rounded region toward the top and side, rather than the bottom. But it is the area farthest from the opening of the stomach into the duodenum. Finally, the *pylorus* (pie-**LOR**-us) is the "gatekeeper" (*pylor*) area "present" (*-us*) as a small pouch just before the duodenum of the small intestine.

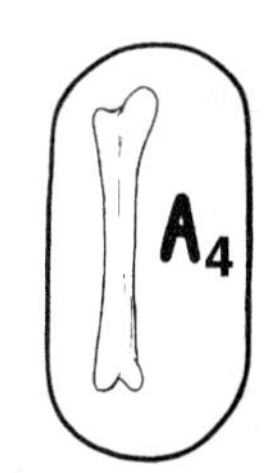

Dr. Beaumont gets a "window" in the stomach

"What exactly goes on within these regions of the stomach, Hippocrates?" Well, back in my day (ancient Greece and Rome), we physicians speculated that the stomach was something like an oven. It baked and broke down ingested food by its own internal heat! But all of this speculation ended after that fateful day of June 6, 1822, at wilderness *Fort Mackinac* (**MAK**-ih-**naw**), on tiny Mackinac

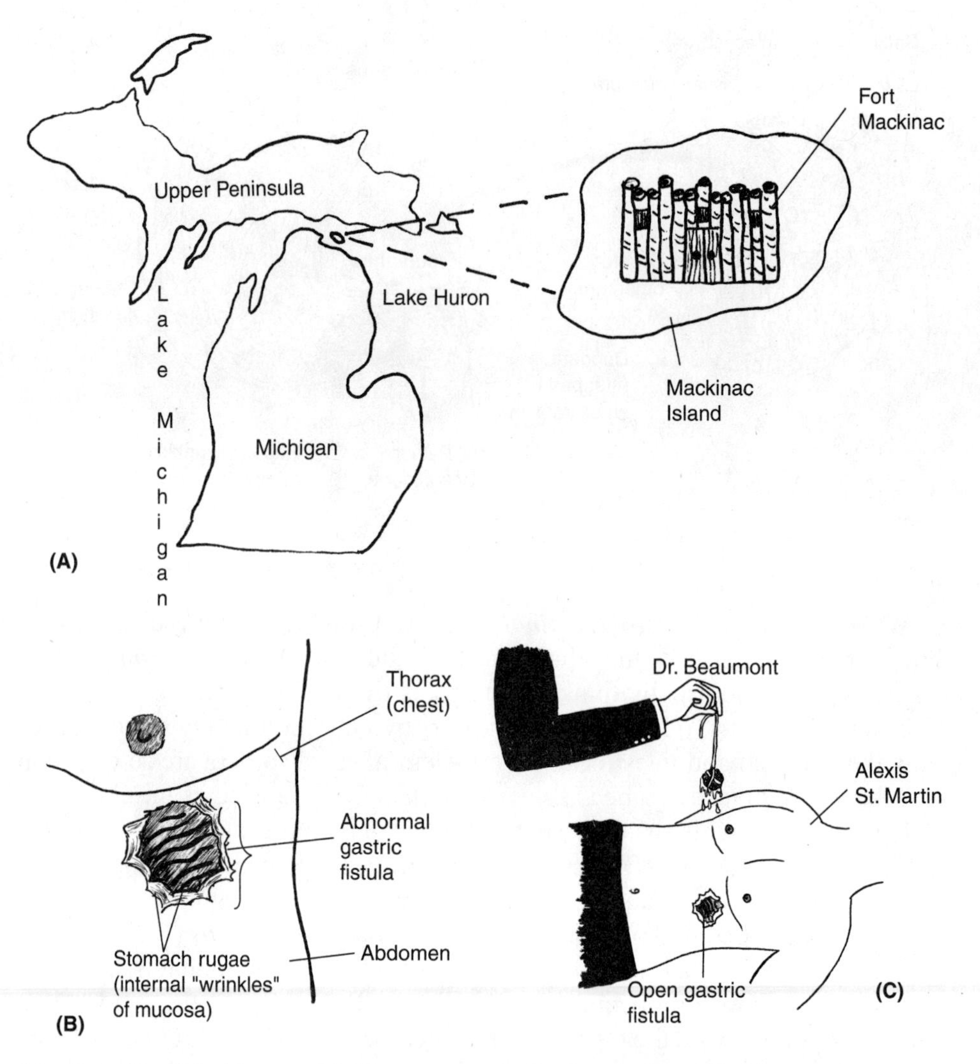

Fig. 12.6 Fort Mackinac and its famous gastric fistula. **(A)** Fort Mackinac and Mackinac Island. **(B)** Close-up view of Alexis St.Martin's artifical gastric fistula, showing the interior rugae. **(C)** Dr. Beaumont inserting meat into the fistula, observing gastric juice effect upon digestion.

Island between Lake Superior and Lake Huron. (See Figure 12.6, A.) It was here that a 19-year-old French *voyageur* (**vwah**-yah-**ZHUR**) or canoe "traveler" named Alexis St. Martin accidentally dropped his musket onto the ground. The musket shot him in his upper left abdomen (trunk midsection) and lower thorax (chest) with a powerful blast at close range! As a result, a large hole was blasted into St. Martin's left side, through which several broken ribs, a burnt lobe of the lung, and part of the stomach hung out!

The voyageur's life was saved by *Dr. William Beaumont*, the fort doctor. After many months of rehabilitation, St. Martin was still weak, and a large *fistula* (**FIS**-tyoo-lah)—"pipe"-like abnormal passage—remained in the side of his stomach. (Consult Figure 12.6, B.) The technical name for this abnormal opening is a *gastric* (**GAS**-tric)—"pertaining to" (*-ic*) "stomach" (*gastr*)—*fistula*. The fistula was about 2.5 inches in circumference—large enough for Dr. Beaumont to insert his entire forefinger deep into the cavity of the stomach. When not covered with a dressing, swallowed food and liquid would continually pour out of the fistula!

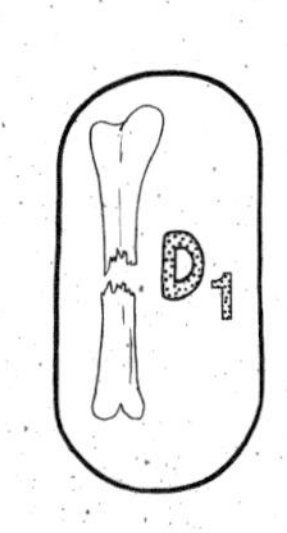

This fistula extended through all the layers of the stomach wall. Thus the *rugae* (**ROO**-guy) or raised "wrinkles" in the *mucosa* (mew-**KOH**-sah) could clearly be seen by Dr. Beaumont. (Review Figure 12.5, if desired.) The mucosa is the innermost mucous membrane lining the entire digestive tract.

Now, Dr. Beaumont suspected that the mucous ("slimy") secretions of the stomach mucosa were something different from the actual *gastric juice*. But since no one had ever done digestive experiments on the stomach of a living person, the truth was not known for sure. Seeing St. Martin's gastric fistula as a permanent "window on the living stomach," Dr. Beaumont had him live for many years in his home, where he served as his paid experimental subject. Dr. Beaumont would tie silk threads around various kinds of meat, then lower them into St. Martin's stomach through the large fistula in his side (Figure 12.6, C).

"What is some of the exact stuff that Dr. Beaumont lowered into St. Martin's gastric fistula, Hippocrates?" Well, being Hippocrates' Ghost, I was there, watching, all the time! So I know that Dr. Beaumont put in raw salted beef, raw salted pork, boiled corn beef, stale bread, and heads of raw cabbage into the hole! Why, at one time the Doc even pushed twelve raw oysters into the fistula! Is it any wonder that poor St. Martin eventually got sick of this treatment and left?

But Dr. Beaumont was a sharp and studious experimenter, carefully timing how long it took to digest this great variety of foodstuffs. He even extracted small samples of gastric juice with a tube and described it as being *acidic*. Beaumont eventually wrote a famous book, *Experiments and Observations on the Gastric Juice and Physiology of Digestion*, which was published in 1833. This established him as the first *gastric physiologist*.

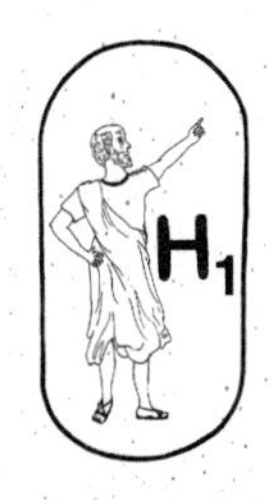

Because he was forced to work under primitive conditions in the wilderness, and no sophisticated chemical analysis was available in the early 1800s, Dr. William Beaumont paved the way for a thorough understanding of the gastric juice. We know now that the main component of the gastric juice is *hydrochloric* (**HIGH**-droh-**klor**-ik) *acid*, or HCl. Another major chemical is *pepsin* (**PEP**-sin), an enzyme that helps break down proteins in ingested food. Hydrochloric

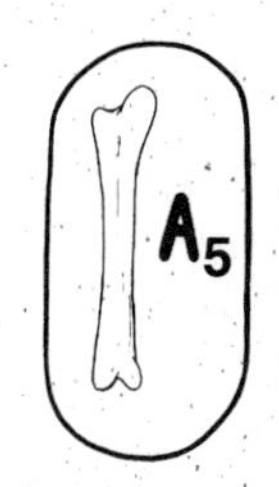

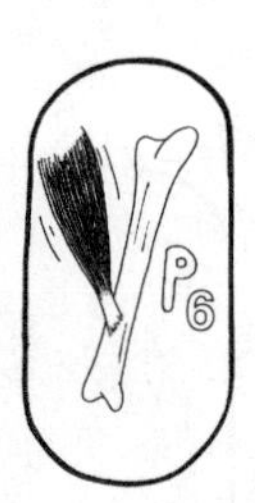

acid (HCl) is a very strong acid, donating or giving off many highly reactive H+ (hydrogen) ions. These H+ ions basically dissolve and break down practically anything they encounter! Thus, the gastric juice, with its heavy concentration of HCl and pepsin, quickly digests a food bolus entering the stomach. It changes the bolus into what Dr. Beaumont called the *chyme* (**KIGHM**), a thick, soupy, shapeless mass of partially digested food. Since chyme is almost a liquid, it is basically a "juice" (*chym*) that leaves the stomach through its "gatekeeper," the *pyloric* (pie-**LOR**-ik) *sphincter*. [**Review suggestion:** Go back and observe this sphincter in Figure 12.5. Since the entire pylorus is called the gatekeeper, then the pyloric sphincter serves as the muscular door that closes this "gate" into the small intestine!]

DIGESTIVE UPSETS AS DISTURBANCES IN BODY ACID-BASE BALANCE

We have spent considerable time on the stomach and its gastric juice, because it is the source of the most powerful acid in our body, HCl. Now, you might remember that we talked about the general problem of acidosis back in Chapter 9 with regard to the respiratory system. [**Review of word translation:** Insert a single slash mark into *acidosis*. Label the resulting root and suffix. Write out this term's common English translation. If you need help, take a quick trip back to Chapter 9.]

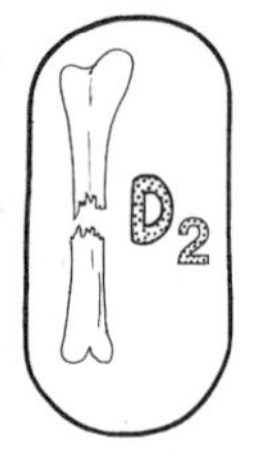

Acidosis is literally an "abnormal condition of" (*-osis*) too much body "acid." The specific type of acidosis talked about in Chapter 9 was *respiratory acidosis*, an abnormal condition of too much body acid resulting from respiratory ("breathing again") problems. A typical cause of respiratory acidosis, you may recall, is hypoventilation. This deficient breathing allowed too much carbon dioxide to build up within the erythrocytes, thereby creating too much body acid (H+ ions).

Such acidosis (like alkalosis) reflects an upset in the normal body acid-base balance. In the digestive tract, body acid-base balance is generally maintained via the *intestinal neutralization* (**new**-tral-ih-**ZAY**-shun) *equation*:

$$NaHCO_3 + HCl \rightarrow NaCl + H_2CO_3$$

$NaHCO_3$	+ HCl	→ $NaCl$	+ H_2CO_3
(sodium bicarbonate: a strong base [alkali] secreted in the pancreatic juice)	**(hydrochloric acid: a strong acid secreted in the gastric juice)**	**(sodium chloride: a common) salt)**	**(carbonic acid: a weak acid)**

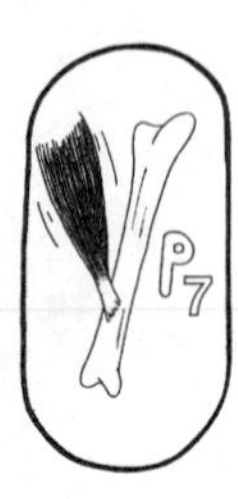

The above reaction normally goes on every single day within the duodenum. The strong base or alkali called $NaHCO_3$ or *sodium bicarbonate*

(buy-**KAR**-buh-**nut**) is secreted into the duodenum as part of the pancreatic juice. Now, every time that the pyloric sphincter relaxes and opens, a slug of acidic chyme enters the duodenum from the stomach. The HCl in the chyme reacts with the sodium bicarbonate ($NaHCO_3$ base) in the small intestine. The products of this reaction are *NaCl—sodium chloride* (**KLOR**-eyed) salt—plus *H_2CO_3—carbonic* (kar-**BAH**-nik) *acid*.

"But doesn't this reaction just substitute *one* acid (HCl) for *another* acid (H_2CO_3), Hippocrates?" Yes, that is correct. "Okay, then why is the whole process called the intestinal *neutralization* equation? It all goes on within the duodenum of the small intestine, but you really aren't completely *neutralizing* (**NEW**-trah-**lie**-zing) the hydrochloric acid, are you?" Good thinking! Neutralization is simply the "process of" (*-tion*) making something "neutral"—that is, neither acidic nor basic. Thus, while the contents of the small intestine are not completely neutralized by the neutralization equation, they have come a lot closer! The reason is that carbonic acid is a *weak* acid and thus donates very few H+ ions. The strong HCl from the stomach is transformed into weak H_2CO_3 within the intestine. This process helps protect the mucosa (inner membrane lining) of the small intestine. from the dangerously *corrosive* (kuh-**ROH**-siv) or "gnawing away" effects of too many H+ ions. The result of this entire process is a rough acid-base balance within the duodenum and the rest of the small intestine (Figure 12.7).

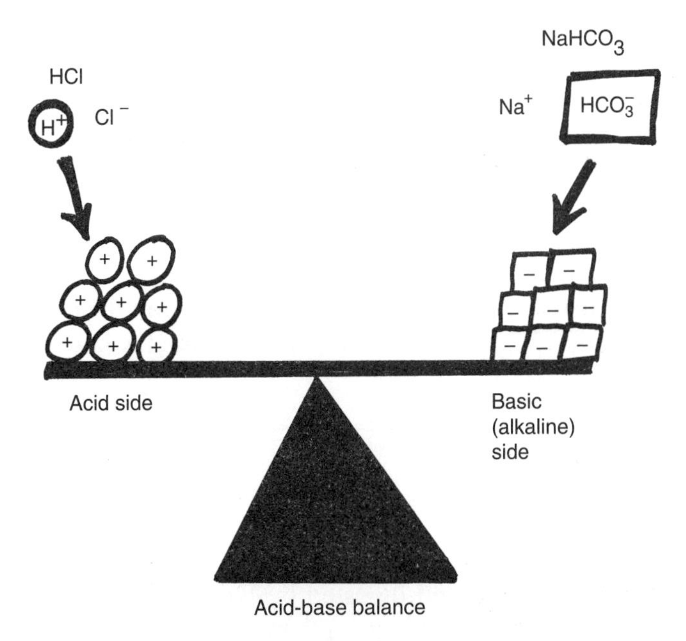

Fig. 12.7 Approximate acid-base balance is preserved within the small intestine.

Severe diarrhea and metabolic acidosis

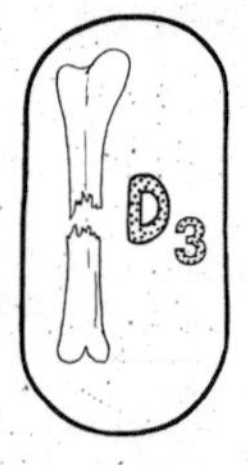

Whenever the intestinal neutralization equation becomes unbalanced, morbidity often results. Consider, for instance, a severe bout of *diarrhea* (**die**-uh-**REE**-ah). This is an excessive amount of liquid stool "flowing" (*-rrhea*) out "through" (*dia-*) the anus. Many times, diarrhea is only a symptom of some more general GI problem. One frequent cause is *gastroenteritis* (**gas**-troh-en-ter-**EYE**-tis). Gastroenteritis is an "inflammation of" (*-itis*) the *mucosal* (myew-**KOH**-sal) lining of both the "stomach" (*gastr*) and "intestines" (*enter*). We often hear it nicknamed the "stomach flu" or "intestinal flu." But what is specifically meant is usually gastroenteritis accompanied by such bothersome symptoms as painful *abdominal* (ab-**DAHM**-ih-nal) cramping and diarrhea. There are any number of possible causes for such a "flu," such as infection of the lower GI tract with pathogenic bacteria or viruses.

When prolonged diarrhea occurs, the contents of the intestines (rather than the stomach) are primarily lost. Such contents chiefly include sodium bicarbonate ($NaHCO_3$) base, lots of water, and lots of *electrolytes* (e-**LEK**-troh-**lights**). Common electrolytes include sodium chloride (NaCl) and other compounds that are "broken down" (*lyt*) by passing an "electrical" (*electr*) current through solutions containing them.

With so much base or alkali ($NaHCO_3$) lost from the intestines, there is very little left to *buffer* or "sop up" the huge number of H+ ions being released by the HCl entering from the stomach. Hence, *metabolic acidosis* may occur. This is an abnormal condition of too much body acid (or not enough base) due to metabolic causes. An important metabolic cause in this case, of course, is the severe diarrhea accompanying gastroenteritis. Along with losing a lot of base, dehydration from water loss may also be present, along with an *electrolyte imbalance*. Summarizing the above information yields what we will call the *diarrhea syndrome*:

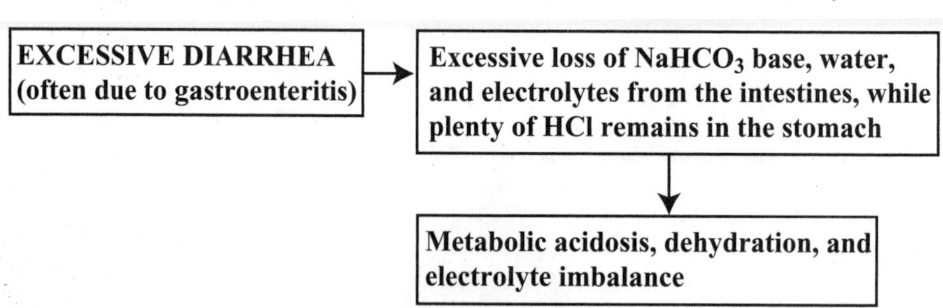

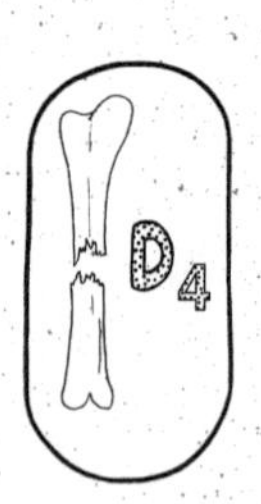

Now, the walls of the duodenum, unlike those of the stomach, are not protected from being dissolved and digested by the H+ ions from HCl. This is because the stomach mucosa secretes a 1-mm-thick layer of highly *alkaline* (**AL**-kah-**lin**) mucus that buffers (sops up) most H+ ions before they do too much damage. But the poor duodenum, unfortunately, lacks this protective mucous film. When too much unbuffered acid and its H+ ions are left behind in the duodenum, therefore, a *duodenal* (dew-**AH**-deh-nal) *ulcer* (**UL**-sir) may result. An *ulcer* is literally a "sore," an area of necrotic (dead) tissue that may also become a deep *ulcer crater*. Summarizing, we have:

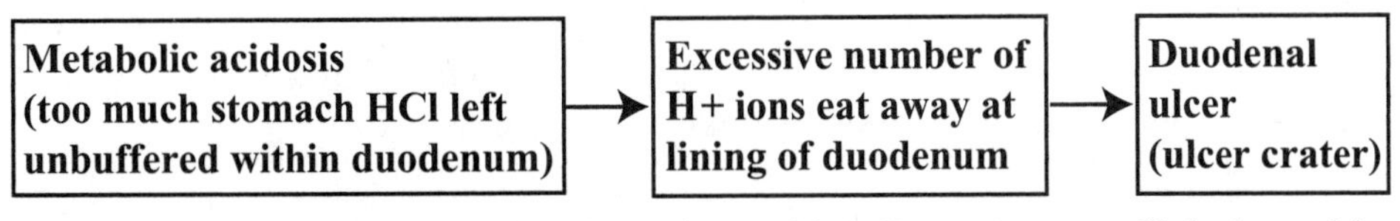

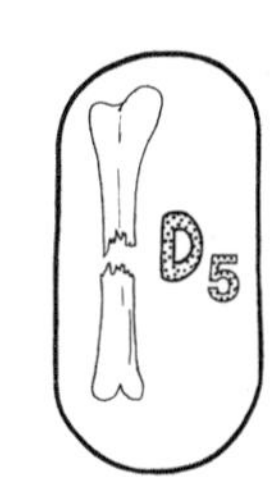

[**Study suggestion:** Look back at Figure 12.5. Draw in a small dark oval in the wall of the duodenum, just below the pyloric sphincter. Now, give the oval area its correct medical name.]

Severe vomiting and metabolic alkalosis

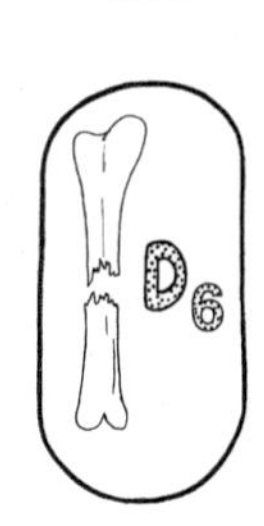

Metabolic *acidosis* is one destructive complication of acid-base imbalance. An exactly opposite complication is called *metabolic alkalosis*. Metabolic alkalosis is an excessive amount of body base or alkali (or a deficiency of body acid) resulting from metabolic causes. One common metabolic cause is excessive *vomiting*, also called *emesis* (**EM**-eh-**sis**). Looking back at the intestinal neutralization equation: if we vomit, large quantities of gastric juice are lost from the stomach. This gastric juice, of course, is rich in HCl. The vomit also contains lots of water and electrolytes from the stomach. But the sodium bicarbonate (base) levels in the duodenum are left mostly unaffected. This situation creates what we can call the *vomiting syndrome*:

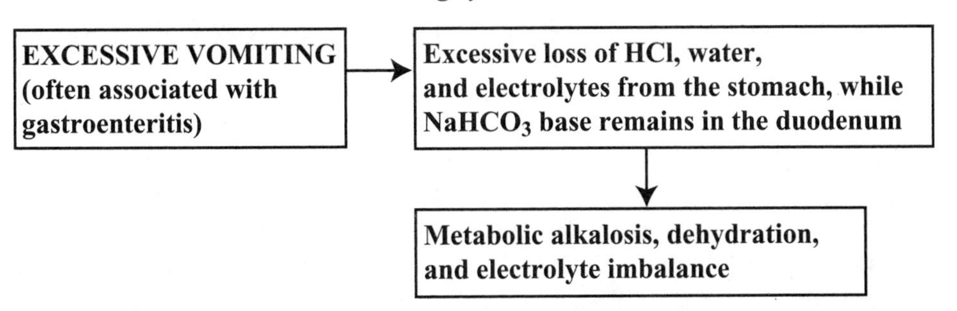

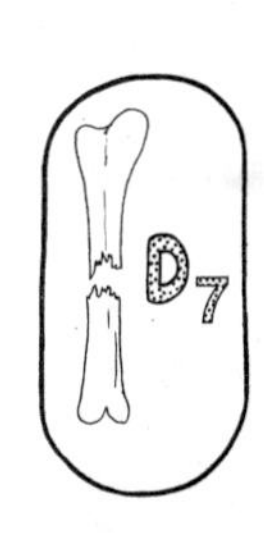

The esophagus, like the duodenum, has no protection against the potent corrosive actions of gastric acid. When the individual repeatedly vomits, HCl is ejected from the mouth, but an acid residue is left upon the *esophageal* (e-**sahf**-uh-**JEEL**) *mucosa*. The possible morbid result is *reflux* (**REE**-fluks) *esophagitis* (eh-**sahf**-uh-**JEYE**-tis). Reflux is literally a "flowing" (*flux*) "backwards" (*re-*). So reflux of the stomach contents during vomiting means that the acid-rich gastric juice goes up out of the cardia region of the stomach, and into

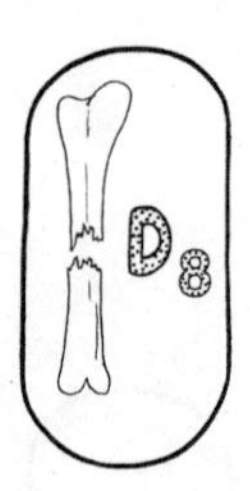

the esophagus. This results in a painful "inflammation of" (*-itis*) the "gullet" (*esoph*). *Pyrosis* (peer-**OH**-sis)—"an abnormal condition of" (*-osis*) "burning" sensations (*pyr*)—is a frequent symptom. The pyrosis is nicknamed "heartburn" because of the anatomic location of the lower esophagus behind the heart. Eventually, severe *esophageal ulcers* can occur. [**Study suggestion:** Go back once more to Figure 12.5 and draw a small dark circle in the wall of the lower esophagus, just above the cardia of the stomach. You now have an ulcer at both ends—one just above the stomach, and one just below it.]

SUMMARY TABLE 12.1

Some important words and word parts appear in Summary Table 12.1. (See next page.)

Medical Case History: An Attack of Acute Appendicitis

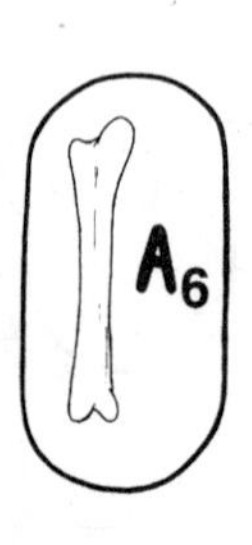

Paul S., age 24, suddenly began to suffer severe pain in the *epigastrium* (**eh**-pih-**GAS**-tree-um). This area is also called the *epigastric* (**eh**-pih-**GAS**-trik) *region.* The name reflects the fact that it is the *abdominopelvic* (ab-**dahm**-ih-noh-**PEL**-vik) *region* that is "present" (*-um*) immediately over and "upon" (*epi-*) the "stomach" (*gastr*). This is one of nine different *abdominopelvic regions* that are marked off upon the body surface, as a rectangular grid matrix (like a rectangular pillbox). (Examine Figure 12.8.) The nine abdominopelvic regions help medical workers localize body structures and symptoms within the "trunk midsection" (*abdomin*) and "bowl" (*pelvic*) area between the two hip bones.

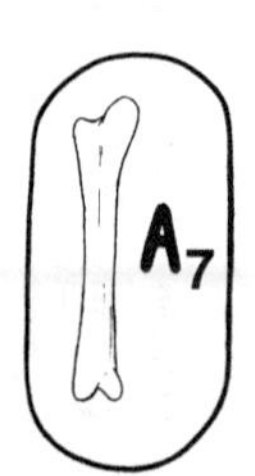

The severe epigastric pain was accompanied by repeated bouts of emesis (vomiting), along with general malaise and moderate hyperthermia. After Paul was taken to the hospital by his father, the emergency physician carefully palpated the abdominal region. She noted that the patient's pain was progressively shifting toward the *right lower quadrant* (**KWAHD**-runt). This is one of "four" (*quadr*) rectangular areas marked off upon the abdominal surface. They are created by an imaginary cross drawn through the patient's *umbilicus* (um-**BIL**-ih-kus)—the central "pit" (*umbilic*) or *navel* (**NAY**-vul). (View Figure 12.9.)

The patient grimaced in pain as the doctor deeply palpated his right lower quadrant. She felt a hard, round lump within his *appendiceal* (**ap**-en-**DISH**-ul) or "pertaining to" (*-eal*) "attachment" (*appendic*) area. More specifically, it was localized in the *right iliac* (**ILL**-ee-ak) abdominopelvic region. The dramatic *appendicular* (**ap**-en-**DIK**-yuh-lar) stretching and dilation was attributed to a large *fecalith* (**FEE**-kah-lith)—hard "stone" (*lith*) of "feces." The fecalith (fecal stone) had become *impacted* (im-**PAK**-ted) or "struck against" the inner wall of the cecum. (Study Figure 12.10, A.)

Summary Table 12.1 Words and Word Parts

Write in the *exact* meaning (literal English translation) for up to 10 key terms selected from the preceding block of text. After you are done, check your word meanings with the correct answers, which are given at the end of this chapter.

Key Terms	Prefixes	Roots	Suffixes	Exact Meanings
digestive	(none)	digest "carrying apart"	-ive "pertains to"	1. ________
ingestion	in- "into"	gest "carrying"	-ion "process of"	2. ________
egestion	e- "out"	gest "carrying"	-ion "process of"	3. ________
defecation	de- "from"	fec "feces"	-tion "process of"	4. ________
duodenum	(none)	duoden "twelve"	-um "presence of"	5. ________
cecum	(none)	cec "blind"	-um "presence of"	6. ________
vermiform	(none)	vermi "worm"	-form "like"	7. ________
gastrointestinal	(none)	gastr "stomach"; intestin "intestin"	-al "referring to"	8. ________
pylorus	(none)	pylor "gatekeeper"	-us "present"	9. ________
esophagitis	(none)	esophag "gullet"	-itis "inflammation of"	10. ________

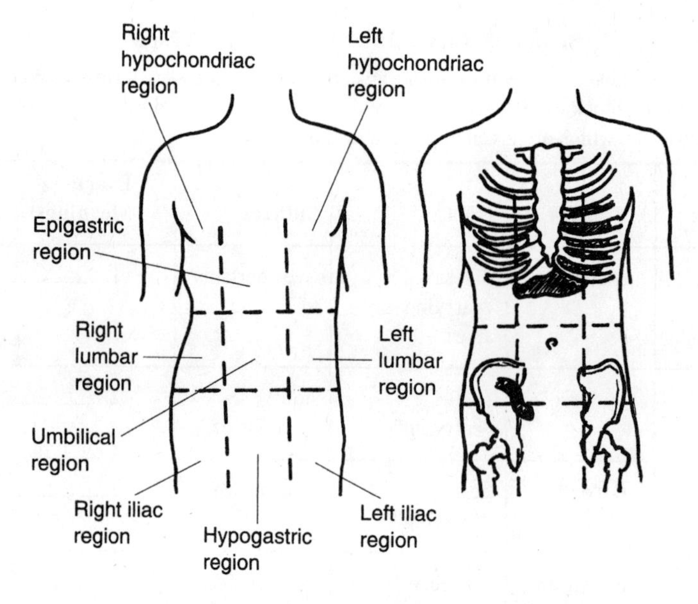

Fig. 12.8 The nine abdominopelvic regions.

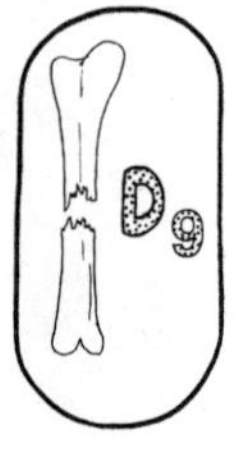

A quick blood sample was drawn. A marked *leukocytosis* (**loo**-koh-sigh-**TOH**-sis), or "abnormal condition of" (*-osis*) too many "white" (*leuk*) blood "cells" (*cyt*), was detected. This strongly suggested the presence of an acute *inflammatory* (in-**FLAH**-mah-tor-ee) *process*. Therefore, a diagnosis of *acute appendicitis* (ah-**pen**-dih-**SIGH**-tis)—"sudden inflammation of the appendix"—was made.

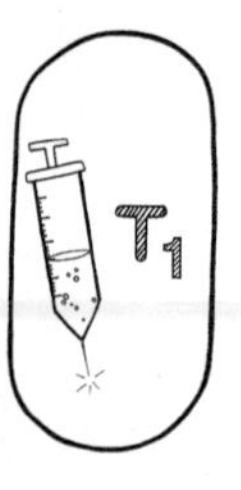

The patient was scheduled for an *emergency appendectomy* (**ap**-en-**DEK**-toh-me). This is literally a "removal of" (*-ectomy*) the "appendix" (*append*). A

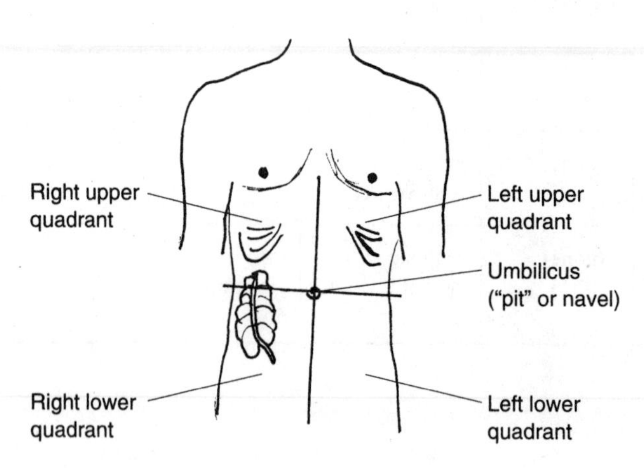

Fig. 12.9 The four abdominopelvic quadrants.

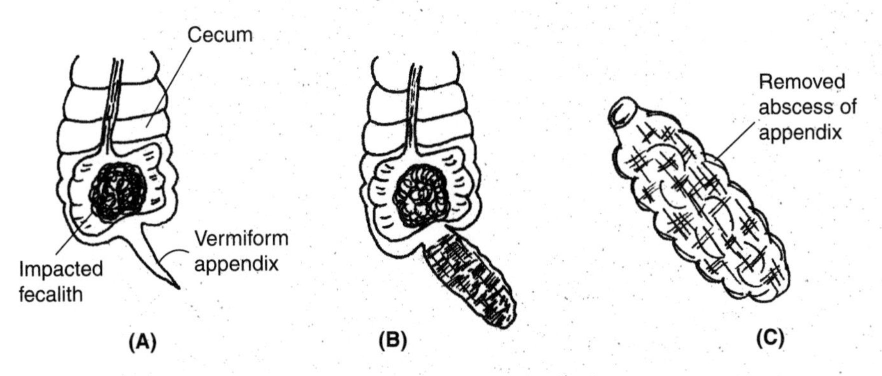

Fig. 12.10 Steps in producing a ganrenous appendix that ruptures. **(A)** Large fecalith becomes impacted above vermiform appendix. **(B)** *Acute appendicitis:* Inflamed and edematous vermiform appendix. **(C)** removed appendix, seen to be gangrenous, with pus-filled abscess.

laparoscope (**LAP**-ah-roh-**skohp**)—"an instrument used to examine" (*-scope*) the interior of the "abdomen or trunk midsection" (*lapar*)—was inserted through a small flank incision. As suspected, the vermiform appendix was severely inflamed and *edematous* (eh-**DEM**-ah-tous, swollen) with fluid pus (Figure 12.10, B). A large fecalith was blocking the lumen to the vermiform appendix and had created a severe tissue ischemia resulting in necrosis. The etiologic agent was the bacterium *Escherichia* (**esh**-er-**EYK**-ee-ah) *coli* (**KOH**-lye), a bacillus that is very common within the GI tract. But because the fecolith put huge numbers of *E. coli* bacilli into constant contact with the vermiform appendix, the immune response of the lymphatic tissue in that area was simply overwhelmed. Tissue death (necrosis) was followed by *secondary gangrene* (**GANG**-green), a "gnawing sore" (*gangren*) that is "present" (*e*).

After the appendix had been removed, close examination showed there was a large *abscess* (**AB**-sess). An abscess is a local collection of pus that, if ruptured, produces a "going away" (leaking out) of the pus and its contained bacteria. The *gangrenous* (**GANG**-greh-nus) appendix of Paul S., fortunately, did not suffer *perforation* (**per**-for-**AY**-shun)—a "process of" (*-tion*) "piercing through" (*perfor*). Otherwise, the contents of the ruptured inflamed appendix, including the feces, pus, and bacteria, would have been released into the normally sterile *abdominopelvic* cavity (Figure 12.10, C). This release could have resulted in a dangerous *peritonitis* (**pair**-ih-toh-**NEYE**-tis), an inflammation of the membrane lining the cavity.

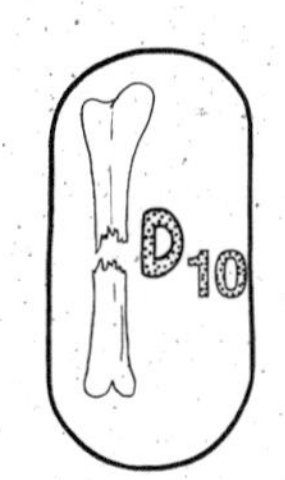

SUMMARY TABLE 12.2

Some important words and word parts appear in Summary Table 12.2.

Summary Table 12.2 Words and Word Parts

Write in the *exact* meaning (literal English translation) for up to 10 key terms selected from the preceding block of text. After you are done, check your word meanings with the correct answers, which are given at the end of this chapter.

Key Terms	Prefixes	Roots	Suffixes	Exact Meanings
epigastric	epi- "upon"	gastr "stomach"	-ic "relating to"	1. ________
abdominopelvic	(none)	abdomin "trunk midsection"; pelv "bowl"	-ic "pertaining to"	2. ________
umbilicus	(none)	umbilic "pit"	-us "presence of"	3. ________
appendiceal	(none)	appendic "attachment"	-eal "pertaining to"	4. ________
fecalith	(none)	fec "feces"	-lith "stone"	5. ________
appendicitis	(none)	appendic "attachment"	-itis "inflammation of"	6. ________
laparoscope	(none)	lapar "abdomen"	-scope "instrument used to examine"	7. ________
appendectomy	(none)	append "appendix"	-ectomy "removal of"	8. ________
gangrenous	(none)	gangren "gnawing sore"	-ous "referring to"	9. ________
perforation	(none)	perfor "piercing through"	-tion "process of"	10. ________

Probe of case history

(**A**) One of the reasons for the patient's appendicitis was a fecalith. What if the patient's problem had been described as a *fecaloma* (fee-kal-OH-mah) instead? Analyze *fecaloma* by inserting two slash marks into it. Label these as root and suffix. What is the literal English translation for this term? (**B**) A laparoscope was used to examine the interior of the abdomen. Build a single term that means "the process of examining the abdomen." [Check your short answers with the key near the end of this chapter.]

Quiz

Refer to the text in this chapter if necessary. A good score is at least 8 correct answers out of these 10 questions. The answers are listed at the back of this book.

1. The word, *digest*, derives from the Latin for:
   (a) "Gnawing hunger"
   (b) "Pretty blueberries"
   (c) "Separate or dissolve"
   (d) "Blow into"

2. An accessory digestive organ that secretes into the oral cavity:
   (a) Salivary gland
   (b) Pancreas
   (c) Tonsil
   (d) Thyroid

3. The *cholecyst* is the technical term for the:
   (a) Liver
   (b) Stomach
   (c) Pylorus
   (d) Gallbladder

4. A synonym (similar word) for *defecation* is:
   (a) Egestion
   (b) Mastication
   (c) Digestion
   (d) Ingestion

5. The unusual root in *duodenum* means:
   (a) "First part"
   (b) "Dynamic duo"

(c) "Twelve"
(d) "Small intestine"

6. If we describe Baby Heinie as *vermiform*, we are describing him as:
(a) Cute
(b) Wormlike
(c) Rascally
(d) Resembling a louse, cockroach, or some other vermin

7. The portion of the digestive tract lying above the stomach equals:
(a) Oral cavity + Larynx + Pharynx
(b) Pharynx + Oral cavity + Cecum
(c) Esophagus + Pharynx + Oral cavity
(d) Larynx + Esophagus + Pharynx

8. Dr. William Beaumont is fondly remembered as being the Father of:
(a) Alexis St. Martin
(b) Tiny Tim
(c) Colonoscopy
(d) Gastric physiology

9. When vomiting occurs without accompanying diarrhea, too much of the ___ component is lost from the intestinal neutralization equation.
(a) HCl
(b) $NaCl$
(c) $NaHCO_3$
(d) H_2CO_3

10. *Gastroenteritis* is properly analyzed as:
(a) Gas/tro/enteritis
(b) Gastr/oen/teri/tis
(c) Gastr/o/enter/itis
(d) Gast/roe/enteritis

Memory Pillboxes for Chapter 12

Several key facts were tagged with numbered icons in the page margins of this chapter. Write a short summary of each of these key facts into a numbered cell or compartment within the appropriate type of *Memory Pillbox* that appears below:

Background and History **Pillboxes for Chapter 12:**

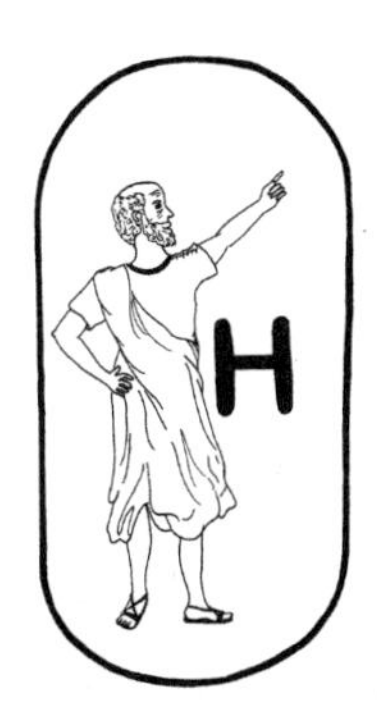

1

Anatomy **Pillboxes for Chapter 12:**

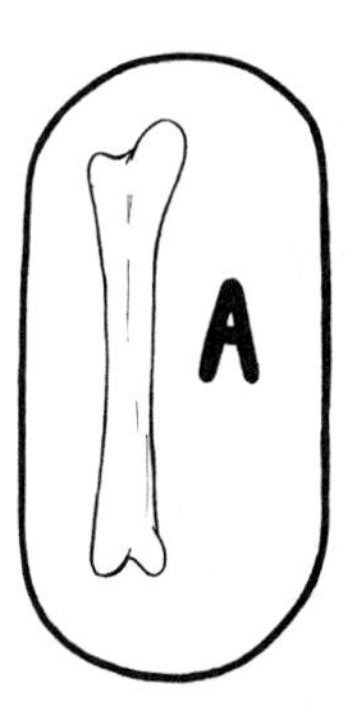

1	2

3	4
5	6
7	

***Physiology* Pillboxes for Chapter 12:**

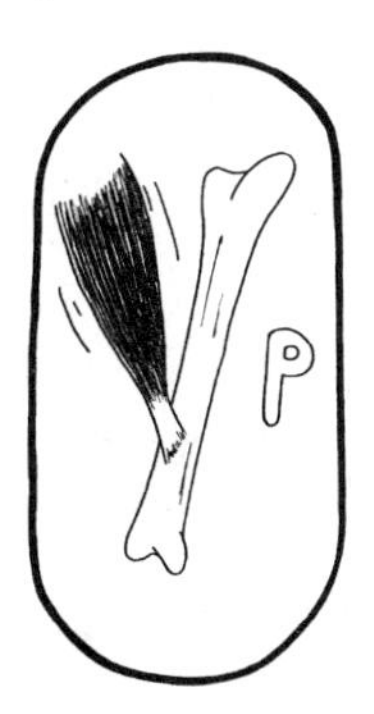

1

2	3

4	5

6	7

***Disease/Injury* Pillboxes for Chapter 12:**

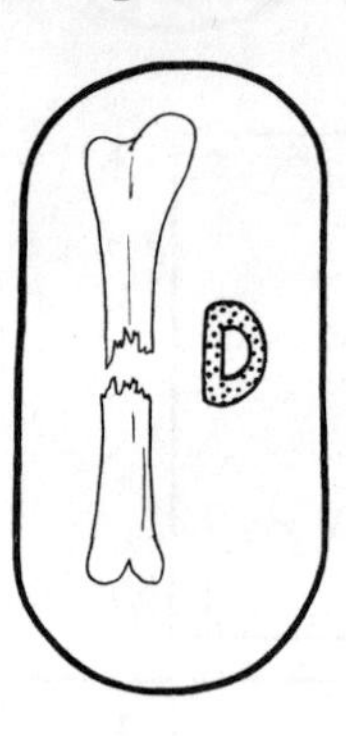

1	2

3	4
5	6
7	8
9	10

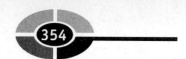

Treatment/Therapy **Pillboxes for Chapter 12:**

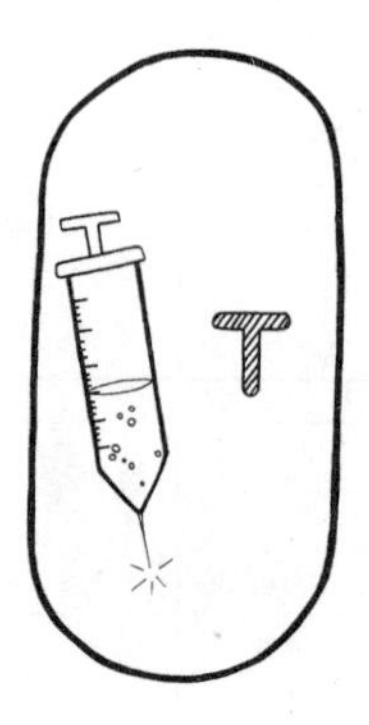

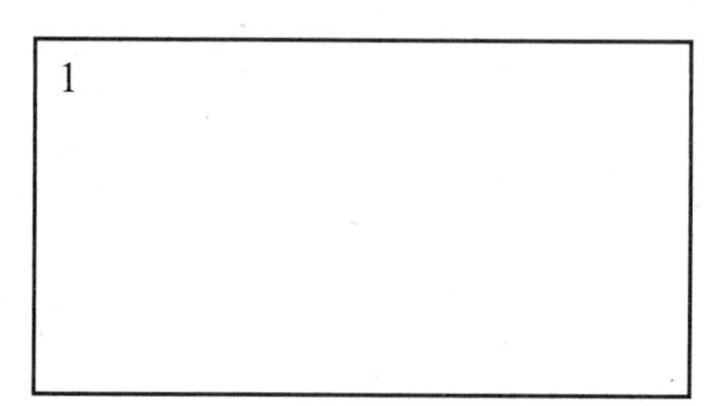

Answers for Chapter 12 Summary Tables

FOR SUMMARY TABLE 12.1

1. "pertains to carrying apart"
2. "process of carrying into"
3. "process of carrying out"
4. "process of (taking) feces away from"
5. "presence of twelve"
6. "presence of (something) blind"
7. "wormlike"
8. "referring to the stomach and intestines"
9. "gatekeeper present"
10. "inflammation of an the gullet"

FOR SUMMARY TABLE 12.2

1. "relating to (something) upon the stomach"
2. "pertaining to the trunk midsection and bowl"
3. "presence of a pit"
4. "pertaining to an attachment"
5. "feces of stone"
6. "inflammation of an attachment"
7. "an instrument used to examine the abdomen"
8. "removal of the appendix"
9. "referring to a gnawing sore"
10. "the process of piercing (something) through"

Answers to Probe of Case History

(**A**) fecal (root) /oma (suffix) = "a tumor of feces." (**B**) laparoscopy (**lap**-ar-**AHS**-koh-pea).

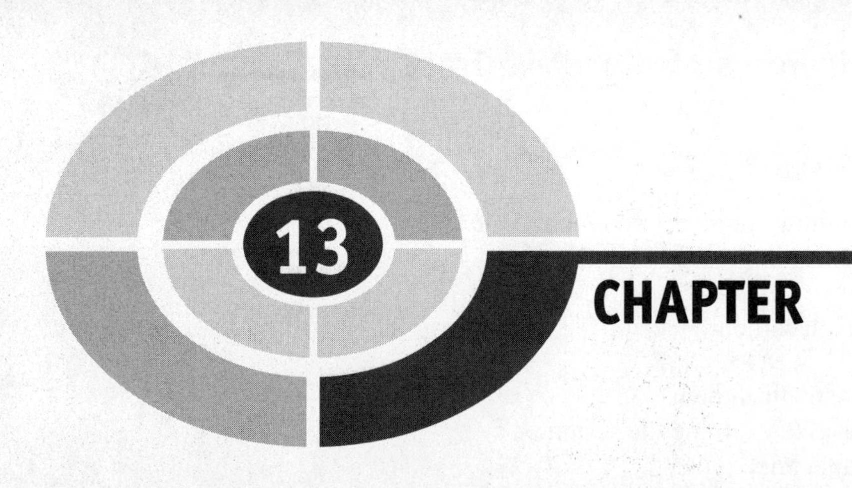

Terms Related to Pregnancy and Urogenital Disorders

In this, our final chapter, we shall seek to *end* this book much as we *began* our life; that is, with the *genitourinary* (**JEN**-ih-toh-**yur**-ih-**nair**-ee) or *urogenital* (**you**-roh-**JEN**-ih-tal) *system*. And in finishing with this system, we will also discuss a few terms relating to pregnancy and birth.

Background and History

If we analyze these two alternate organ system names by inserting slash marks, we get the following results:

R	CV	R	S		R	CV	R	S
GENIT	O	URIN	ARY	=	UR	O	GENIT	AL
"begetting or producing"		*"urine"*	*"pertaining to"*		*"urine"*		*"begetting or producing"*	*"pertaining to"*

And their identical translation is:
"Pertaining to urine and begetting or producing (new human beings)"

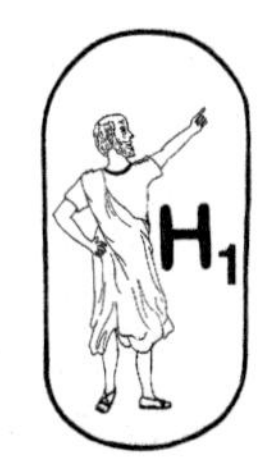

OUR URINARY SYSTEM: THE CRITICAL KIDNEY CONNECTION

The first part of the above translation has to do with the *urinary* (**YUR**-ih-**nair**-ee) *system*, which just "pertains to" (*-ary*) the "urine" (*urin*). Therefore, it is here that we shall begin!

We must look to both *renal* (**REE**-nal) *anatomy* and *renal physiology*, for these give the main story "relating to" (*-al*) the structure and function of the "kidneys" (*ren*). The kidneys, of course, are the major organs of urine excretion. The right and left kidneys are a pair of reddish-brown, bean-shaped organs located quite deep in the back, flanking either side of the vertebral column (backbone). Figure 13.1 provides an overview of gross and microscopic renal anatomy. The kidney is surrounded by the *renal capsule*, a thin whitish membrane of fibrous connective tissue. For purposes of study, the kidney itself is conveniently subdivided into three major areas or zones.

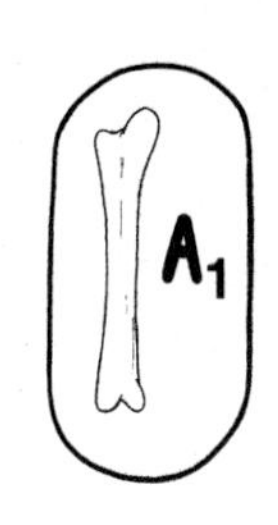

The outer zone is the *renal cortex*. [**Memory probe:** Back in Chapter 11, in discussing the nervous system, what specific organ was mentioned that also had a cortex? What does *cortex* mean in English?] The area "present" (*-a*) in the "middle" (*medull*) of the "kidney" (*ren*) is called the *renal medulla* (meh-**DEW**-lah). Finally, the deepest zone is named the *renal pelvis* (**PEL**-vis) or "kidney bowl." The renal pelvis is the broad, bowl-like *sac* (**SAK**) that receives the urine dripping down from the renal cortex and renal medulla. Summarizing:

THE THREE MAJOR ZONES OF THE KIDNEY	=	RENAL CORTEX	+	RENAL MEDULLA	+	RENAL PELVIS
		(Outer "bark")		***(Broad "middle")***		***(Inner "bowl")***

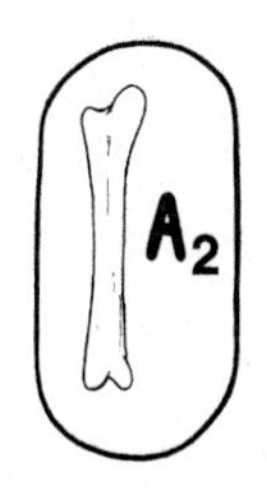

Observe in Figure 13.1 that the renal medulla (middle zone) contains many *renal pyramids*. Shaped much like the flat-topped pyramids of the ancient Aztecs, these renal pyramids have a somewhat striped appearance. This striped look is a result of the presence of microscopic *collecting ducts*. The straight collecting ducts are connected to the more kinked and coiled *renal tubules*

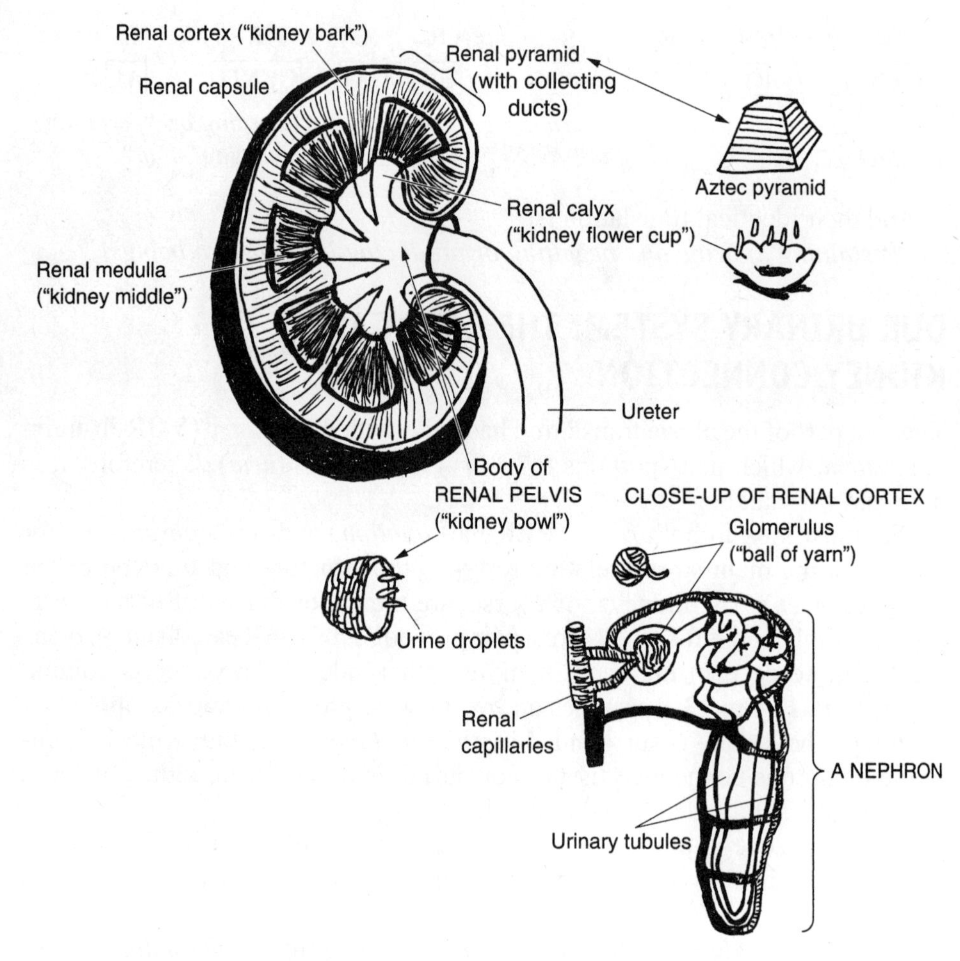

Fig. 13.1 An overview of gross and macroscopic renal anatomy.

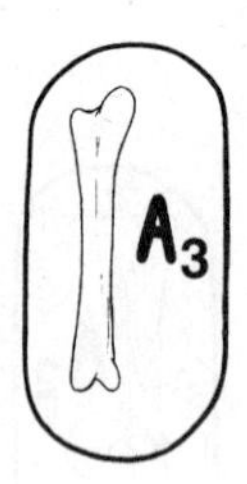

(**TWO**-byools). The renal tubules, in turn, are part of the *nephrons* (**NEF**-rahns). Nephrons are the structural and functional units of urine formation. There are millions of nephrons "present" (*-on*) within each "kidney" (*nephr*). Each nephron begins with a *glomerulus* (gluh-**MAYR**-you-**lus**) or little red "ball of yarn" (*glomerul*). In reality, each glomerulus is a ball-shaped collection of minute *renal capillaries*. Most of each nephron (including the glomerulus) lies within the renal cortex. However, the lower renal tubules, as well as the collecting ducts, travel through the renal medulla.

Urine formation

Figure 13.2 displays the basic mechanism of urine formation that starts with the glomerulus. The relatively high BP (blood pressure) within the glomerulus

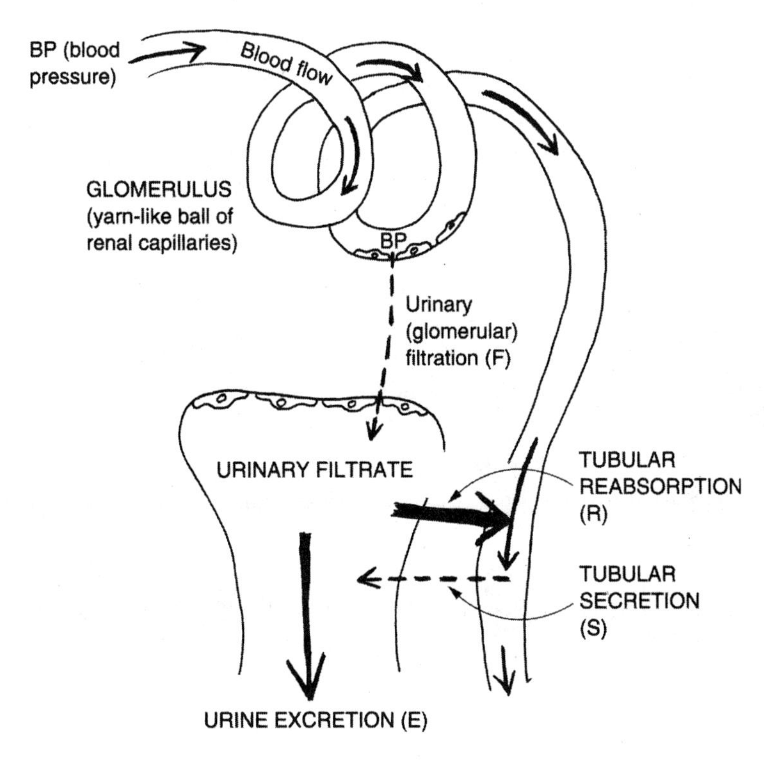

Fig. 13.2 The basic processes in urine formation and excretion.

creates a powerful pushing force. This pushing force results in *urinary* (**YUR**-ih-**nair**-ee) or *glomerular* (gluh-**MAHR**-you-**lar**) *filtration*, abbreviated as F. The fluid that is filtered out of the bloodstream in the glomerulus passes through the very thin walls of the hollow renal tubules, which run nearby. The product is called the *urinary filtrate* (**FIL**-trayt)—"one that" (*-ate*) is "filtered" (*filtr*).

A huge volume of urinary filtrate—about 180 liters in an average-sized adult—is produced every day. Obviously, since there are only about 5 to 6 liters of total blood volume, *most* (about 99%) of the urinary filtrate has to be *taken back* into the *bloodstream*. [**Visualization suggestion:** Pretend that you are eating with friends in a restaurant, and you suddenly get the urge to *urinate* (**YUR**-ih-**nayt**). Writing a short note on a napkin, you excuse yourself and go to the restroom. Now, what do you predict will happen if you urinate all of the fluid present in your urinary (glomerular) filtrate at that time? Would you even *be able* to come back to the table? Why could we speculate that the note you wrote was your *final will and testament*?]

The way we take back 99% of the urinary filtrate is by the process of *tubular reabsorption* (**ree**-ab-**SORP**-shun). Tubular reabsorption is the "absorption" of particular chemicals from the urinary filtrate back into the bloodstream "again" (*re-*). It is called *re*absorption because *absorption* (Chapter 12) is the way in which chemicals entered the bloodstream from the lumen of the digestive tube in the first place. Consider, for example, the glucose molecule. Remember from Chapter 12 that glucose molecules are absorbed into the bloodstream after thorough digestion of a ham sandwich. Eventually, these glucose molecules leave the bloodstream, enter the urinary filtrate, and are actively *reabsorbed* (**ree**-ab-**SORBED**) back into the bloodstream again. It is almost as if a "Magic Chemical Hand" dips down into the urinary filtrate. The hand uses ATP energy (Chapter 6) to actively scoop up all of the glucose molecules. The Hand dumps *all* of the glucose molecules back into the bloodstream *before* they have a chance to go down the steep waterfall (be excreted from the body in the urine). Figure 13.3 depicts this Magic Chemical Hand, which bears the symbolic mark of R, for *tubular reabsorption*.

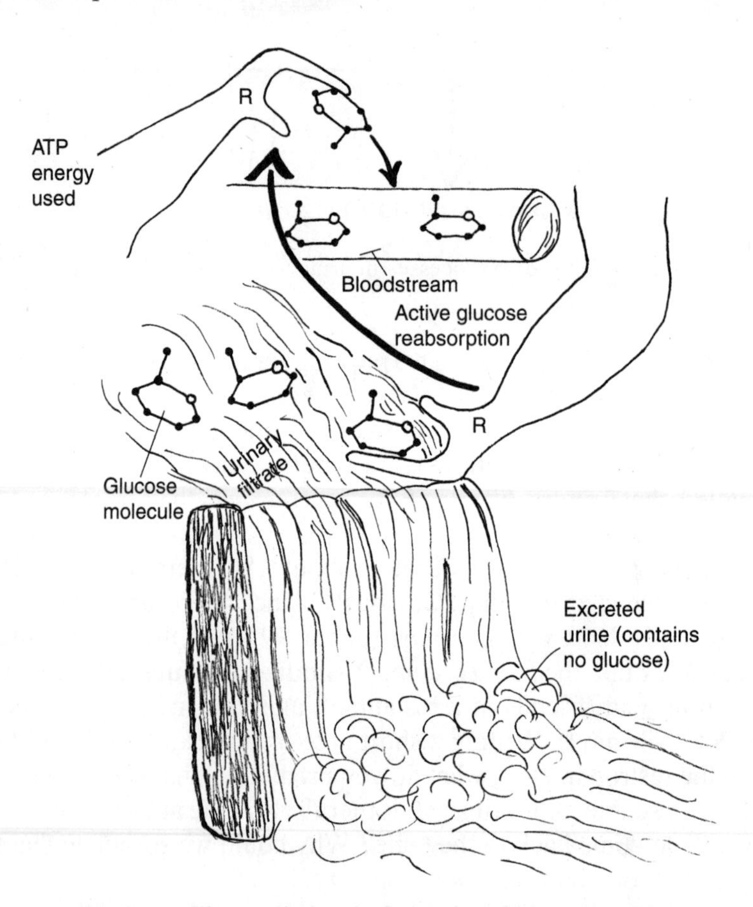

Fig. 13.3 The magic hand of glucose reabsorption (R).

Of course, most of the urinary filtrate is water, so a huge number of H_2O molecules (along with various other particles, like Na+ and Cl– ions) are also reabsorbed back into the bloodstream.

Another imaginary hand is also in operation. This is the "Magic *Mini*-Hand" of *tubular secretion* (S). Tubular secretion is the process of actively secreting "tiny" (*mini*-) amounts of certain substances out across the walls of the blood vessels and into the kidney tubules. It is a way of helping the body excrete small quantities of particles that may be present in excessive amounts (such as H+ ions), as well as large antibiotic drug molecules (such as *penicillin*) that are simply too large to be filtered. Figure 13.4 provides a metaphor of the Magic

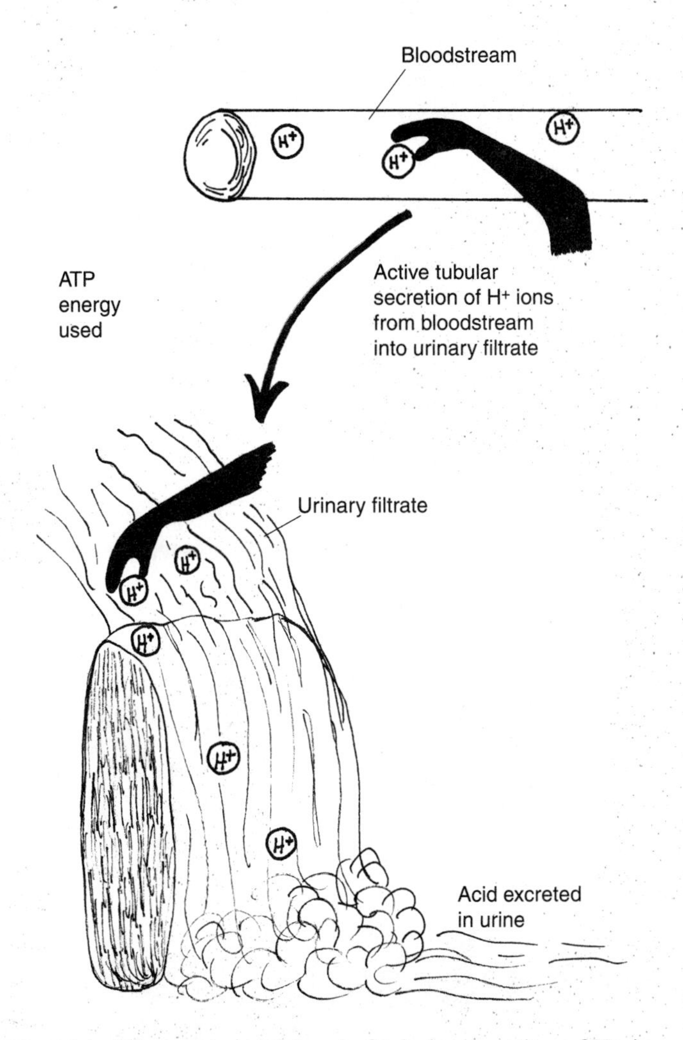

Fig. 13.4 The magic mini-hand of tubular secretion of H+ ions.

Mini-Hand in operation. You can see that it is actively scooping individual H+ ions out of the bloodstream, then dumping them into the urinary filtrate. Eventually, the H^+ ions go down the imaginary waterfall (get excreted from the body within the urine). Even though only a few milliliters of fluid are normally secreted out of the bloodstream each day, this is still important in helping prevent acidosis and other metabolic imbalances.

After the three renal processes of glomerular (urinary) filtration (F), tubular reabsorption (R), and tubular secretion (S) have occurred, the overall result is *urine excretion* (E). Summarizing the preceding block of information yields the *urinary excretion equation*:

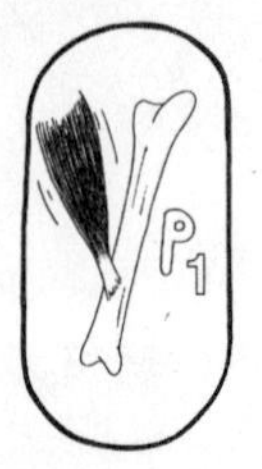

E	=	F	−	R	+	S
1 L/day of urine excreted		**180 L/day**		**179 L/day**		**a few mL/day**
		(filtered)		**(reabsorbed)**		**(secreted)**

The urinary pathway

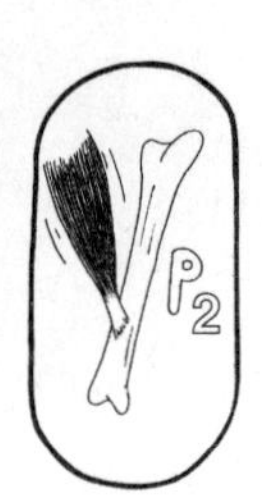

After the urine is formed within the two kidneys' millions of nephrons, it enters the *urinary pathway*. The urinary pathway starts with the urine constantly dripping through the renal pyramids of the renal medulla and then

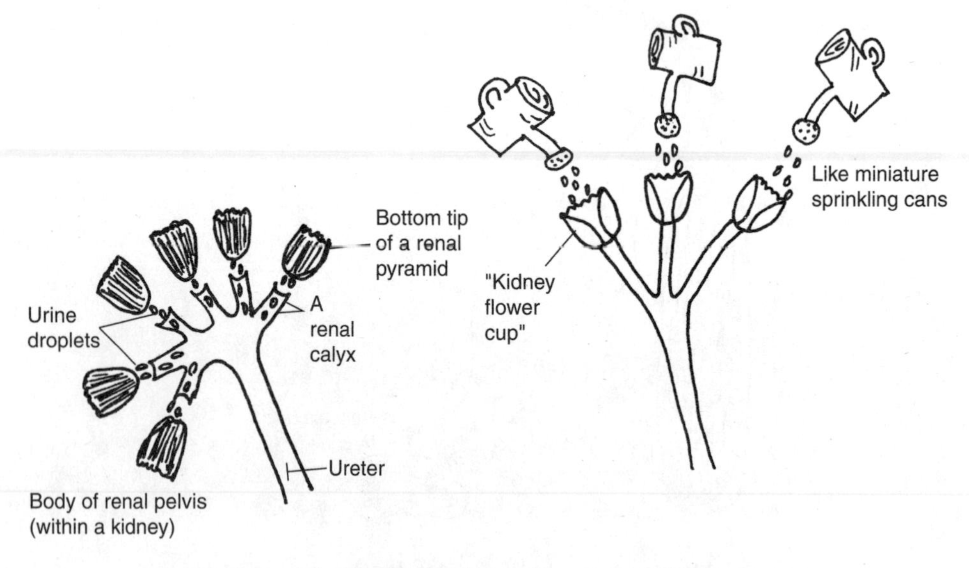

Fig. 13.5 The renal calyces as a bouquet of flower cups.

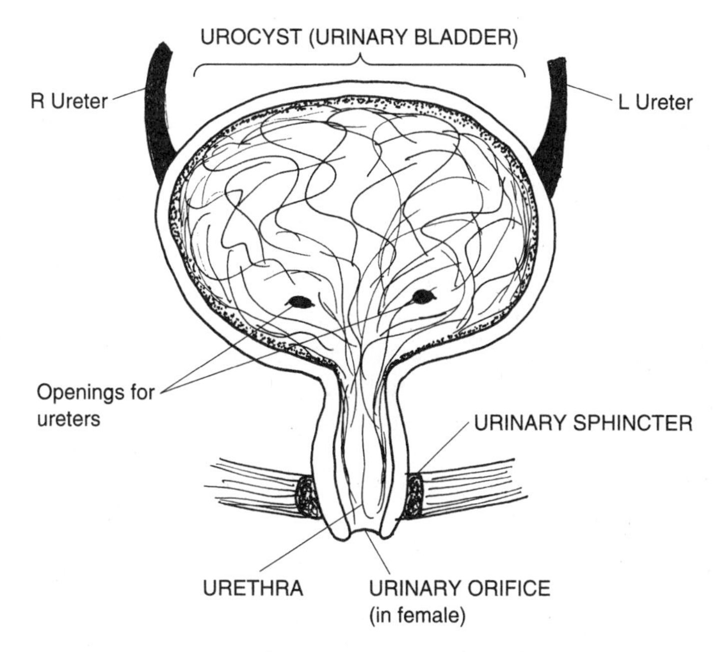

Fig. 13.6 The urinary pathway.

down into the *renal calyces* (**KAY**-lih-**sees**). These are literally the "kidney flower cups." Shown in less detail back in Figure 13.1, but in more detail in Figure 13.5, the renal calyces are the expanded, hollow, flower cup–like extensions of the renal pelvis. Like water from the spouts of miniature sprinkling cans, drops of urine constantly fall through tiny holes in the tip of each renal pyramid. The urine is received by the indented "flower cup" of each *renal calyx* (**KAY**-licks). Perhaps we might visualize the whole group of renal calyces as a striking bouquet of flower cups with wide, hollow stems. These stems eventually merge to create the *body* (central portion) of the bowl-like renal pelvis.

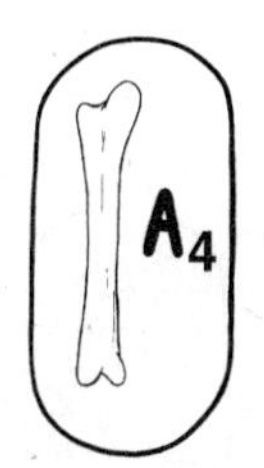

The urine immediately pools within the body of the renal pelvis, then leaves each kidney through a *ureter* (**YUR**-eh-**ter**). The ureter is a muscle-walled tube that constricts and milks urine out of the renal pelvis. Both the right and left ureters travel down into the waiting *urocyst* (**YUR**-oh-**sist**) or "urinary" (*ur*) "bladder" (*cyst*) (View Figure 13.6).

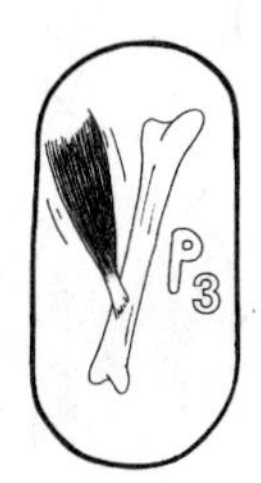

The urocyst (urinary bladder) is a hollow, muscle-walled pouch that temporarily stores the urine produced by both kidneys. Below the urocyst lies the *urethra* (you-**REETH**-rah)—the tube that a person uses to "make water" (*urethr*) by urinating. When the *urinary sphincter* around the urethra voluntarily relaxes, the stored urine passes out of the urocyst. It flows through the urethra, and then exits from the body via the *urinary orifice* (**OR**-ih-**fis**). This is a tiny, "mouth" (*or*) -like opening for excreting the urine.

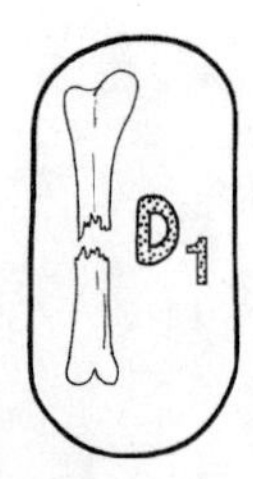

Some urinary disorders

There are two different (but often closely related) basic types of urinary disorders: (*1*) physiological disorders of urine formation or excretion; and (*2*) anatomical disorders of the urinary pathway. Perhaps the most common urinary disorder is *diuresis*. [**Memory probe:** Do you remember the meaning of this term? It was mentioned in Chapter 10 as one of the major symptoms of diabetes mellitus. Speculate, then read on!]

Diuresis, you may recall, is a "process of" (*-esis*) too much "urine" (*ur*) passing out "through" (*di-*) the body. A close synonym of diuresis is *polyuria* (**pahl**-ee-**YUR**-ee-ah). Polyuria is literally "a condition of" (*-ia*) "much" (*poly-*) "urine" (*ur*). We might think of polyuria (diuresis) as a urinary filtration (F) or a tubular reabsorption (R) problem. A basic outline of an *excessive* urinary filtration problem is as follows:

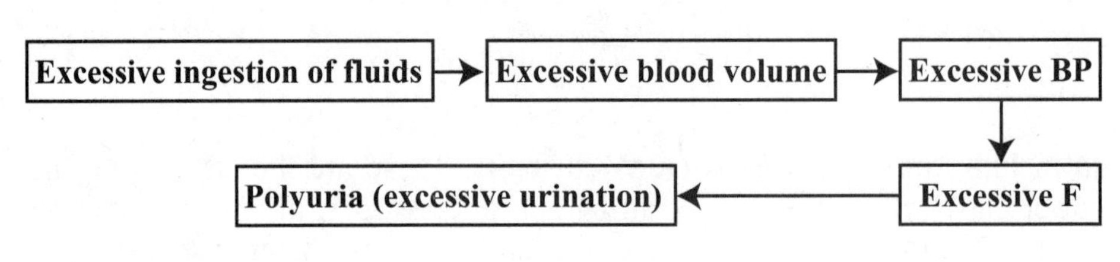

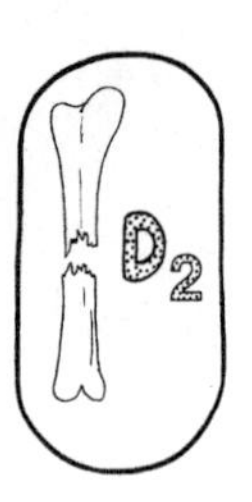

[**Memory probe:** Chapter 8, which discussed the circulatory (cardiovascular) system, included technical terms for "condition of deficient blood volume," which is _______/_______/_______, and "condition of excessive (blood) pressure," which is _______/_______/_______. Try to fill in the word parts of these subdivided medical terms.]

It is normal for an excessive intake of fluid to trigger polyuria, since so much added body water results in a temporary *hypervolemia* (**high**-per-voh-**LEE**-me-ah). Hypervolemia, of course, is a "condition of excessive (blood) volume." This hypervolemia, in turn, creates a temporary hypertension. The high blood volume exerts a greater pushing force upon the vessel walls. In normal, healthy kidneys, however, there is a very efficient *renal compensation* or "process of making up" for these temporary physiological disorders. There is simply a greater amount of urinary filtration (F) of fluid out of the bloodstream and into the kidney tubules. The excess fluid is excreted in the urine, creating diuresis (polyuria). As a result, normovolemia and normotension are soon re-attained.

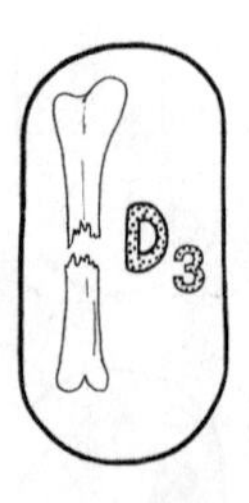

Another type of cause for polyuria, though, involves great deficiencies in tubular reabsorption (R) of water. Many types of *renal diseases* interfere with the

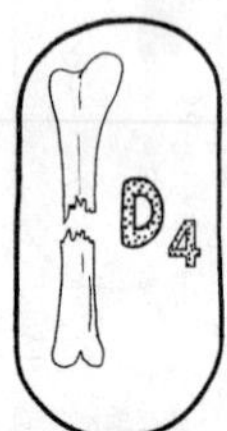

ability of the kidney tubules to reabsorb water from the urinary filtrate, thereby leaving it to be excreted as a huge volume of urine. A special example of this problem is *diabetes insipidus* (in-**SIP**-ih-**dus**). Diabetes (as in diabetes *mellitus*) means an excessive "passing through" (*diabet*) of urine. And *insipidus* indicates the "presence of" (*–us*) something "tasteless" (*insipid*). A person with diabetes insipidus, therefore, passes a huge volume of extremely dilute and watery—hence "tasteless"—urine.

The basic problem here is a familiar one—hormone *hyposecretion*—which we discussed back in Chapter 10. The tubular reabsorption of H_2O from the urinary filtrate is greatly increased by *antidiuretic* (**an**-tee-**die**-yuh-**RET**-ik) *hormone* (ADH). This hormone is described as *antidiuretic* because it acts "against" (*anti-*) "diuresis" (*diuret*). It enlarges the pores in the walls of the collecting ducts, thereby allowing many more H_2O molecules to be reabsorbed back into the bloodstream. This great increase in reabsorption thus helps to prevent the occurrence of diuresis (polyuria). Figure 13.7 (A) provides a symbolic metaphor of a giant body water faucet to help you understand the basic process of reabsorption. With diabetes insipidus, however, a significant

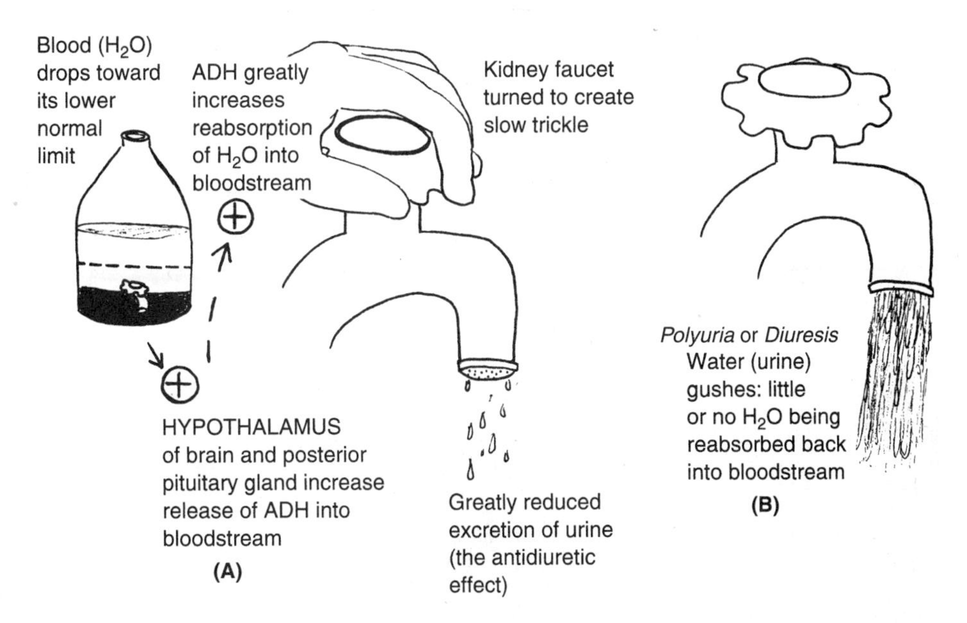

Fig. 13.7 Two giant body water faucets: with and without ADH. (**A**) Normal blood [ADH]: as blood [H_2O] falls toward its lower normal limit, the hypothalamus and posterior pituitary gland increase their release of ADH; greatly increased reabsorption of water turns kidney faucet down to excreting urine at a slow drip. (**B**) Low blood [ADH]: diabetes insipidus and an uncontrolled high volume of urine excretion from the wide-open kidney "faucet."

hyposecretion of ADH by the brain greatly reduces the reabsorption of water back into the bloodstream (Figure 13.7, B). The ending *symptomatic* (**simp**-tuh-**MAT**-ik)—"referring to" (*-ic*) "symptoms" (*symptomat*)—result is usually diuresis (polyuria).

SUMMARY TABLE 13.1

Some important words and word parts are provided in Summary Table 13.1 for your review.

Summary Table 13.1 Words and Word Parts

Write in the *exact* meaning (literal English equivalent) for up to 10 key terms selected from the preceding block of text. After you are done, check your word meanings with the correct answers, which are given at the end of this chapter.

Key Terms	Prefixes	Roots	Suffixes	Exact Meanings
urinary	(none)	urin "urine"	-ary "pertaining to"	1. ________
renal	(none)	ren "kidney"	-al "pertaining to"	2. ________
glomerulus	(none)	glomerul "little ball of yarn"	-us "presence of"	3. ________
nephron	(none)	nephr "kidney"	-on "presence of"	4. ________
filtrate	(none)	filtr "filtered"	-ate "one that" is	5. ________
reabsorption	re- "again"	absorp "sopping up"	-tion "process of"	6. ________
urocyst	(none)	ur "urine"	-cyst "bladder"	7. ________
polyuria	poly- "much"	ur "urine"	-ia "condition of"	8. ________
hypervolemia	hyper- "excessive"	vol "volume"	-emia "blood"	9. ________
antidiuretic	anti- "against"	diuret "diuresis"	-ic "relating to"	10. ________

THE GENITAL (REPRODUCTIVE) SYSTEM

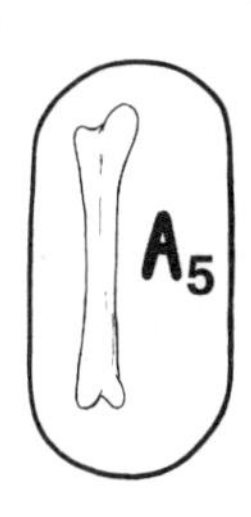

Now that we have dispensed with the *urinary* portion of the genitourinary system, it is time for us to concentrate upon its second part: the *genit* (**JEN**-it). The *genital* (**JEN**-ih-tal) portion literally "refers to" (*-al*) "begetting or producing" (*genit*). Its alternate name is *reproductive* (**ree**-proh-**DUCK**-tiv), which "relates to" (*-ive*) "producing" (*product*) "again" (*re-*). Putting all of this information together, we can conclude that the genital (reproductive) system is the organ system that begets or produces new human beings, again.

Sperm cells and their pathway

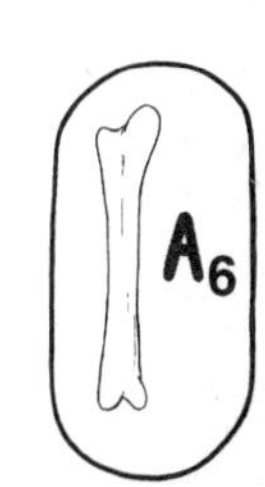

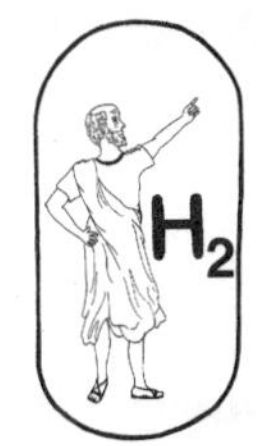

"So, what's it all about, Alfie?" as the old saying goes. It (the genital or reproductive system) is really all about two *sex cells* getting together during *fertilization* (**fer**-tih-lih-**ZAY**-shun). This is the "process of" (*-tion*) getting ready to "bear" (*fertiliz*) a new child. The male sex cell involved in fertilization is the *sperm cell*, which is formally called a *spermatozoon* (sper-**mat**-uh-**ZOH**-un). The *spermatozoa* (sper-**mat**-uh-**ZOH**-ah) are quite colorfully named the "seed" (*spermat*) "animals" (*zoo*). A close look at Figure 13.8 (A) will help explain this unusual identity. Indeed, each spermatozoon (sperm cell) does have a *head piece* with a pointed snout, a *neck* or *midpiece* that contains energy-making mitochondria, and a long *tail piece*. The tail piece acts as a whip, thrashing side to side and helping to propel this tiny dark "seed animal" through the fluid *semen* (**SEE**-men) that is *ejaculated* (e-**JACK**-you-**lay**-ted) with it.

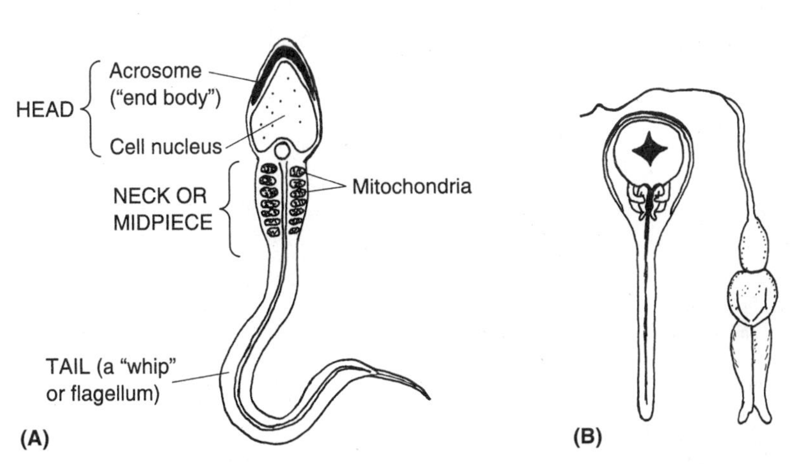

Fig. 13.8 Differing views of the spermatozoon: old versus new. (A) Detailed anatomy of a spermatozoon (sperm cell). (B.) Preformation theory that sperm cell contains a homunculus ("little man")

Adding still more color is the *preformation* (**pree**-for-**MAY**-shun) *theory*, which was believed by many in the 1700s and 1800s. This theory held that each sperm represented a human *embryo* (**EM**-bree-oh) that was already "formed" (*form*) even "before" (*pre-*) fertilization! The primitive microscopes of the day had such poor imaging power that many imaginative observers even thought they saw a *homunculus* (hoh-**MUNK**-kyoo-lus). This was a "little man" (*homuncul*) that was already "present" (*-us*), and all curled up within the sperm cell! (View Figure 13.8, B.)

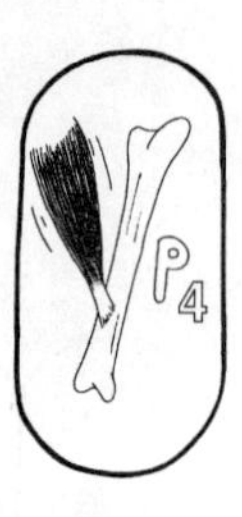

In reality, *spermatogenesis* (sper-**mat**-uh-**JEN**-eh-sis)—the "production of" (*-genesis*) "sperm" (*spermat*) cells—occurs within the two male *testes* (**TES**-tees). Each *testis* (**TES**-tis) is like a small, white, oval "eggshell" (*test*) "present" (*-is*) within the *scrotum* (**SKROH**-tum). The word scrotum, exactly translates to mean a "leathery bag of skin" (Study Figure 13.9).

The actual sites of spermatogenesis (sperm cell production) within each testis are the walls of the *seminiferous* (sem-ih-**NIF**-er-us) *tubules*. These "tiny" (*-ule*), highly coiled "tubes" (*tub*) keep generating new spermatozoa day and night, starting at the time of *puberty* (**PYOO**-ber-**tee**). After they are produced, the spermatozoa are temporarily stored within the *epididymis* (**eh**-pih-**DID**-ih-mus). This is a curved, comma-shaped pouch that lies "upon" (*epi-*) each testis or "eggshell" (*didym*). Following *sexual climax*, the contents of

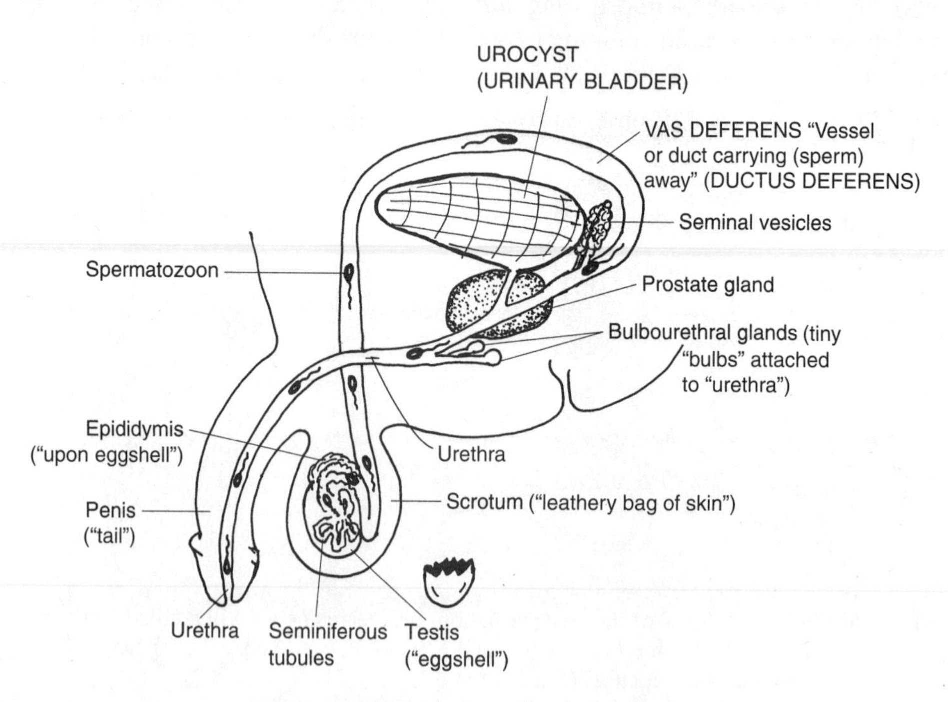

Fig. 13.9 The male reproductive pathway.

the epididymis are ejaculated or "thrown off" (*ejacul*). On their way out, the spermatozoa enter the *vas* (**VAHS**) *deferens* (**DEF**-er-enz). As Figure 13.9 shows, the vas deferens is literally the "carrying away" (*deferens*) "vessel" (*vas*). More correctly, this tube is a hollow duct, rather than a blood vessel. So the alternate name of *ductus* (**DUCK**-tus) *deferens*—"carrying away duct"—is more appropriate.

As the ejaculated spermatozoa travel over the top of the urinary bladder (urocyst), a number of *accessory male reproductive organs* secrete the semen. The semen or *seminal* (**SEM**-ih-nal) *fluid* is a thick, milky, sugar-rich, very alkaline fluid that supports and nourishes the "seeds" (*semin*). The accessory male reproductive organs include the two *seminal vesicles* (**VES**-ih-kls), the two *bulbourethral* (**BUL**-boh-you-**REE**-thral) *glands*, and the single *prostate* (**PRAH**-stayt) *gland*. The bulbourethral glands (Figure 13.9) look like a pair of tiny "bulbs" attached to the sides of the *urethra* (**you-REETH**-rah). Just before the urethra is a short *ejaculatory* (ee-**JACK**-you-lah-**tor**-ee) *duct* (not shown in Figure 13.9).

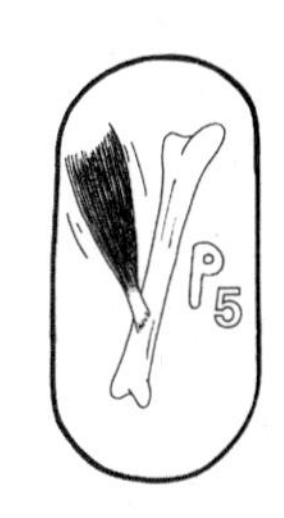

Finally, the long urethra in males passes all the way through the *penis* (**PEA**-nis). The penis, quite interestingly, is named for its resemblance to an anterior "tail" (*pen*). "Standing" (*stat*) "before" (*pro-*) the urethra is the prostate (**PRAH**-stayt) gland. [**Special pronunciation hint:** Please note that this is the *prostate* (**PRAH**-stayt) *gland*, **not** the *prostrate* (**PRAHS**-trayt) *gland*! You often hear people incorrectly make a statement such as: "My Uncle Louie has *prostrate* trouble!" Well, if Uncle Louie is having pro**strate** trouble, then he must be falling down a lot! Why? Because prostrate exactly translates to mean "to stretch out" (*strat*) "before" (*pro-*) something or someone. Proper usage would be reflected in a statement like this one: "Uncle Louie lost his balance and fell *prostrate* (stretched out his full body length) onto the floor!" Such prostrate trouble would be evidence of a neurological disorder, not a genitourinary one! In fact, checking back with Chapter 11, this would likely involve a failure of proprioception, thus possibly reflecting cerebellar _______/_______/_______ ("condition of loss of order"; try to fill in these blanks, then look back and find this term in Chapter 11).]

Male reproductive summary

Summarizing the preceding block of info, we have:

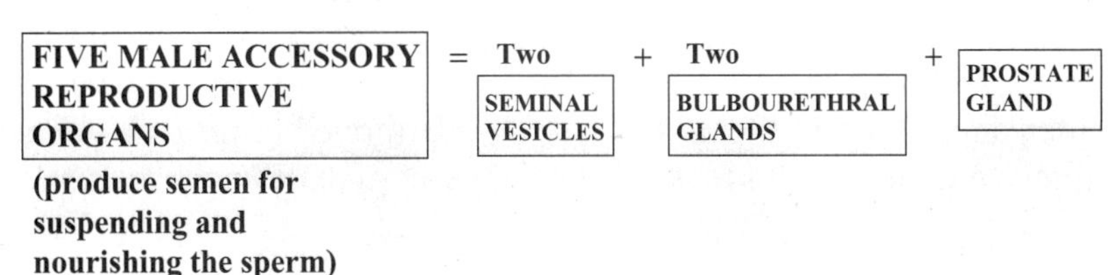

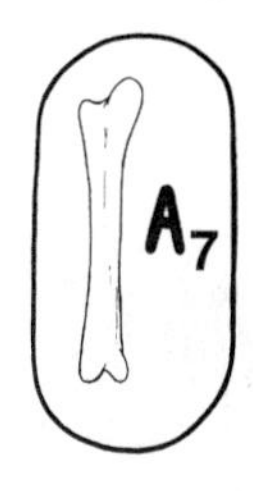

And for the whole male pathway, we state the following sequence:

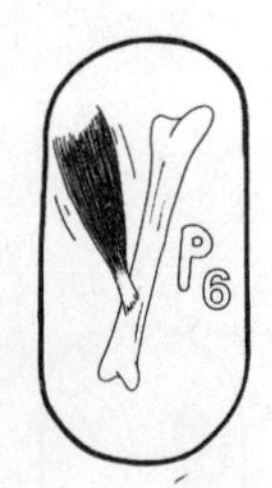

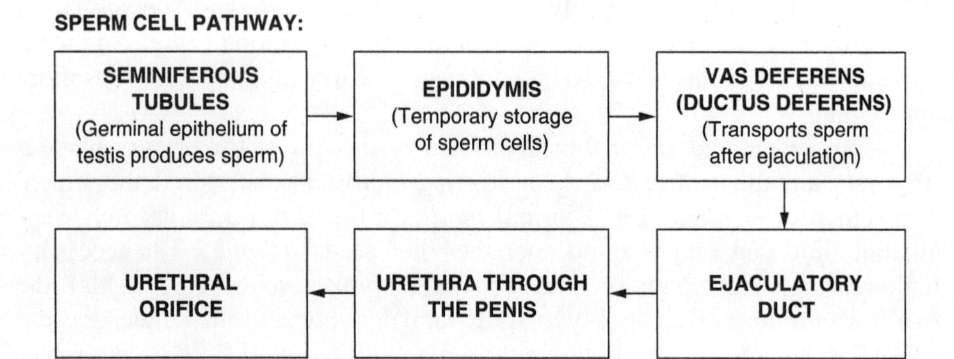

Some male reproductive disorders

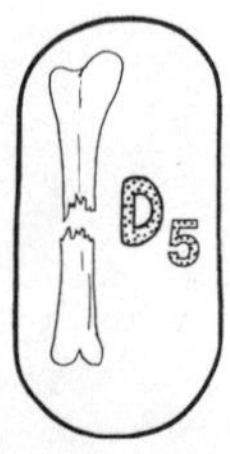

There are many disorders peculiar to the male reproductive pathway. Generally, these fall into three major types: (*1*) disorders of sperm production or transport; (*2*) disorders of sperm pathway structure; and (*3*) disorders of male hormone secretion. In actual life, male reproductive disorders often reflect some combination of the above types.

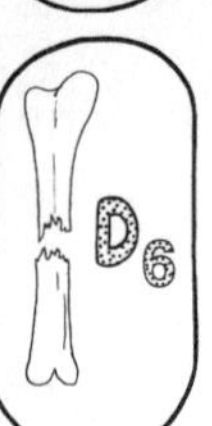

Congenital (kun-**JEN**-ih-tal) difficulties in males "pertain to" (*-al*) problems in "producing" (*genit*) children that are present "with" (*con-*) birth. One such congenital male problem is *cryptorchidism* (**krip-TOR**-kid-**ih**-zum). Cryptorchidism is a "condition of" (*-ism*) "hidden" (*crypt*) "testes" (*orchid*). By hidden, it is meant that one or both testes have failed to descend out of the abdominopelvic cavity and into the *scrotal* (**SKROH**-tal) *sac*. The chief problem occurs when such *undescended testes* remain within the abdominopelvic cavity for too long a period after birth. The high internal body temperature may destroy the *germinal* (**JUR**-mih-nal) or "sprouting" (*germin*) epithelium in the walls of the seminiferous tubules. As a result, the *sperm cell count* after *ejaculation* (e-**JACK**-you-**LAY**-shun) is way below its normal range. Thus, a state of *male infertility* (**in**-fer-**TILL**-ih-tee) exists.

"What good is male fertility, oh Noble Ghost of Hippocrates, if there is no *sex drive* to go along with it?" As you Modern Dwellers in the 21st Century would say, "Right on!" To successfully father children, the modern-day male must have both "the will (sex drive)" and "the way (sperm fertility)." And the hormone critical for stimulating the male sex drive is *testosterone* (tes-**TAHS**-ter-ohn). This is literally a "steroid hormone" (*-sterone*) secreted by certain cells within the testis (*test*). Consider cases of male *hypogonadism* (**high**-poh-**GOH**-nad-izm). Hypogonadism means "an abnormal condition" (*-ism*) of

"deficient" (*hypo-*) secretions by the *gonads* (**GOH**-nads) or "seed-makers." The male testes, of course, are the gonads or seed-makers for spermatozoa. When the endocrine gland cells located within the testes hyposecrete testosterone, an abnormally low male sex drive is often one of the unhappy consequences.

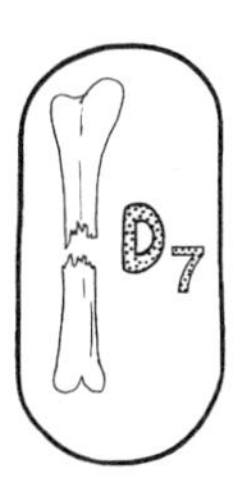

Ova and their pathway to pregnancy

The female reproductive system naturally focuses upon the *ovum* (**OH**-vum), or microscopic "egg" (*ov*) cell "present" (*-um*). There are several hundred thousand primitive, undeveloped *ova* (**OH**-vah) present within a female infant's right and left *ovaries* (**OH**-var-**eez**) at the time of her birth. The real *ovarian* (oh-**VAIR**-ee-an) activity starts at puberty with *menarche* (men-**AR**-kee). Menarche is technically the "beginning" (*—arche*) of the "monthly" (*men*) female cycles.

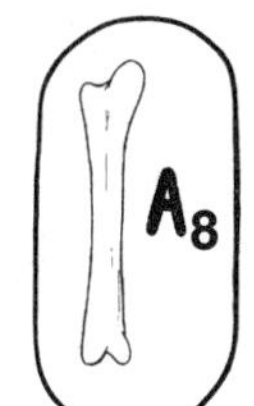

Figure 13.10 reveals why the name *ovary*, which "pertains to" (*-ary*) an "egg" (*ov*), is so appropriate. The ovaries are whitish, oval, egg-like endocrine glands attached to either side of the *uterus* (**YOU**-ter-us). Just as spermatogenesis occurs within the testes, *oogenesis* (oh-oh-**JEN**-uh-sis) occurs within the ovaries. Oogenesis is the "production of" (*-genesis*) mature "egg" (*oo*) cells.

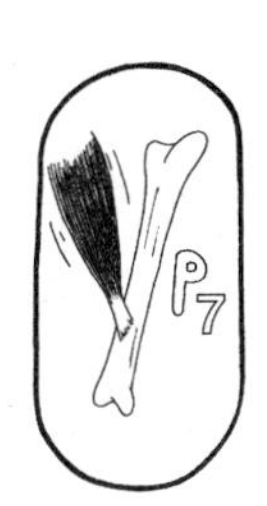

During each *menstrual* (**MEN**-stroo-al) or "monthly" cycle, one or more ova become mature. They are surrounded by a "little bag" (*follicl*) of secreting cells called the *mature ovarian follicle* (**FAHL**-ih-kl). The follicle cells around the

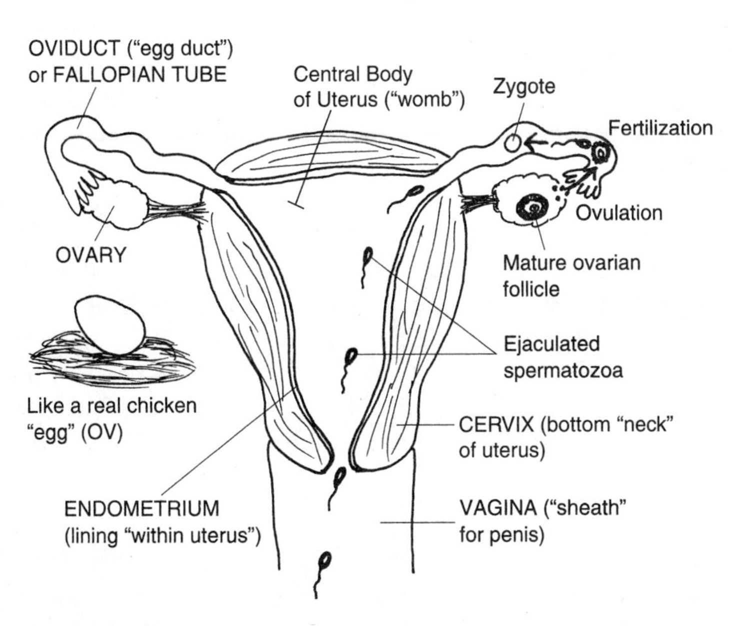

Fig. 13.10 Fertilization and the female reproductive pathway.

mature ovum secrete the two important hormones: *estrogen* (**EHS**-troh-**jen**) and *progesterone* (proh-**JES**-ter-**ohn**). At about Day 14 (halfway through) the typical 28-day menstrual cycle, *ovulation* (**ahv**-you-**LAY**-shun) occurs. Ovulation is the "process of" (*-tion*) releasing a "little egg" (*ovul*) from the surface of an ovary and out into the surrounding abdominopelvic cavity.

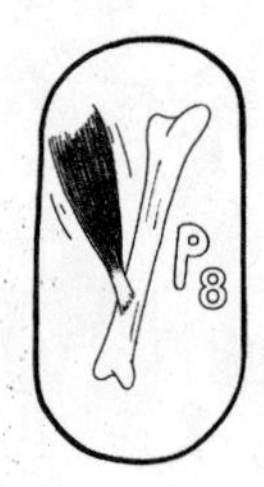

Fertilization and that which follows

Figure 13.10 shows the consequences of a successful *coitus* (**KOH**-ih-tus)—"a" (*-us*) "coming together" (*coit*) of man and woman during sexual intercourse. The penis has been inserted into the *vagina* (vah-**JEYE**-nah)—a "sheath" (*vagin*) that is "present" (*-a*) in the woman. Therefore, the penis releases spermatozoa into this "sheath" during ejaculation. The ejaculated spermatozoa enter a small hole in the tip of the *cervix* (**SIR**-viks). The cervix is the narrow "neck" (*cervic*) at the inferior portion of the uterus. The spermatozoa then swim up through the *body* (large central area) of the *uterus*. The uterus is popularly known as the "womb" (*uter*) "present" (*-us*) in women for developing new life. The *ovulated* (**AHV**-you-**lay**-ted) mature ovum, meanwhile, has usually been swept up into the mouth of a nearby *oviduct* (**OH**-vih-dukt)—"egg duct." The oviduct can also be called a *fallopian* (fah-**LOH**-pea-un) *tube* in honor of its discoverer, an Italian anatomist named Gabriello Fallopio (fah-**LOH**-pea-oh). [**Thinking and application probe:** Perhaps you have heard women make such statements as, "I've just had my *tubes* tied!" In medical terminology, the woman's physician might say, "We've just performed a *tubal* (**TOO**-bal) *ligation* on the patient." Now, try to apply your previous knowledge and your powers of *inference* (**IN**-fur-**ens**) to "bring in" these separate pieces of reproductive info. *What*, specifically, in common English, was being done? And *why* (for what specific clinical reason) is it probably being done?]

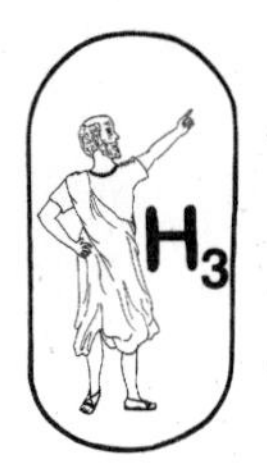

After ovulation, fertilization of the mature ovum by a spermatozoon usually occurs in the first (outer) third of the oviduct (Fallopian tube). Fusion of sperm and ovum together results in a *zygote* (**ZEYE**-goat). The zygote literally represents the single new cell that is created by an ovum nucleus and a sperm cell nucleus being "yoked together" (*zygot*). And the twenty-three chromosomes or "colored bodies" (Chapter 6) of each single sex cell are combined together to create the total of forty-six chromosomes in the nucleus of the zygote:

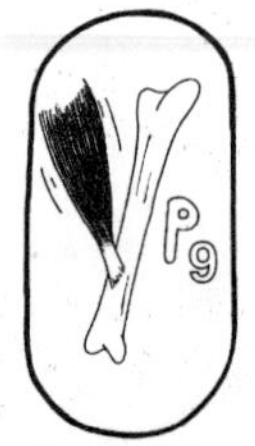

THE ZYGOTE	=	SPERM CELL NUCLEUS	+	OVUM CELL NUCLEUS
(a single *new* cell with *46* chromosomes)		**(A *male* sex cell with *23* chromosomes)**		**(A *female* sex cell with *23* chromosomes)**

Life after the zygote just keeps getting bigger and better!

"How many cells are present in the adult human body, Hippocrates?" Well, there are billions and billions of cells! And they all started with a *single* one, called the _________. [**Study suggestion: You** fill in the correct word in the preceding blank!]

This single zygote started dividing by mitosis (Chapter 6) almost immediately and then just kept going on and on! This single-celled zygote soon becomes a solid mass of many cells called the *morula* (mor-**OO**-lah). The morula is named for its striking resemblance to a "little mulberry" (*morul*) "present" (*-a*) within the oviduct. (See Figure 13.11.)

The morula continues to divide and change as it moves out of the oviduct and enters the large central body of the uterus. Here it becomes a hollow ball of cells named the *blastula* (**BLAS**-chew-lah) or *blastocyst* (**BLAS**-toh-**sist**). These terms are translated into common English as a "little sprouter" (*blastul*) "present" (*-a*) or a "little sprouting bladder" (*blastocyst*). [**Thinking probe:** Since the blastula (blastocyst) is hollow, it doesn't resemble a solid mulberry. What specific kind of fruity, hollow berry would *you* suggest it resembles?]

From Figure 13.11, it becomes obvious that the blastula is a little sprouter, because this is the stage of development in which the blastula embeds itself into the *endometrium* (**en**-doh-**MEE**-tree-um). The endometrium is the "inner" (*endo-*) lining of epithelial tissue present (*-um*) within the "uterus" (*metr*). As it buries itself into the endometrium, the blastula sends out deep roots of cells (much like a "sprouting" plant) that firmly anchor it into place. All the preceding stages (starting with fertilization) are technically called the *embryo* (**EM**-bree-oh)—or "sweller." The reason is that the cells and groups of cells within the embryo keep "swelling" (getting larger) in size.

After the blastula comes the *gastrula* (**GAS**-true-lah) or hollow "little stomach present." The gastrula stage kicks in the real tissue *differentiation* (**dif**-er-en-she-**AY**-shun)—"process of becoming different" (and more specialized). The three *primary germ layers* in the gastrula, for instance, can be thought to "sprout" or "germinate" (*germ*) the rest of the tissue cells that are found in the entire body! The gastrula generally occurs during the second week after fertilization and zygote formation.

A tiny *yolk sac* develops and helps nourish the growing *embryonic* (**em**-bree-**AHN**-ik) body. A protective membrane called the *amnion* (**AM**-nee-un) surrounds the developing body, as if it were gently sheltering a "little lamb." Clear *amniotic* (**am**-nee-**AH**-tik) *fluid* provides shock absorption within the uterus, and tiny *limb buds* poke out from the body surface.

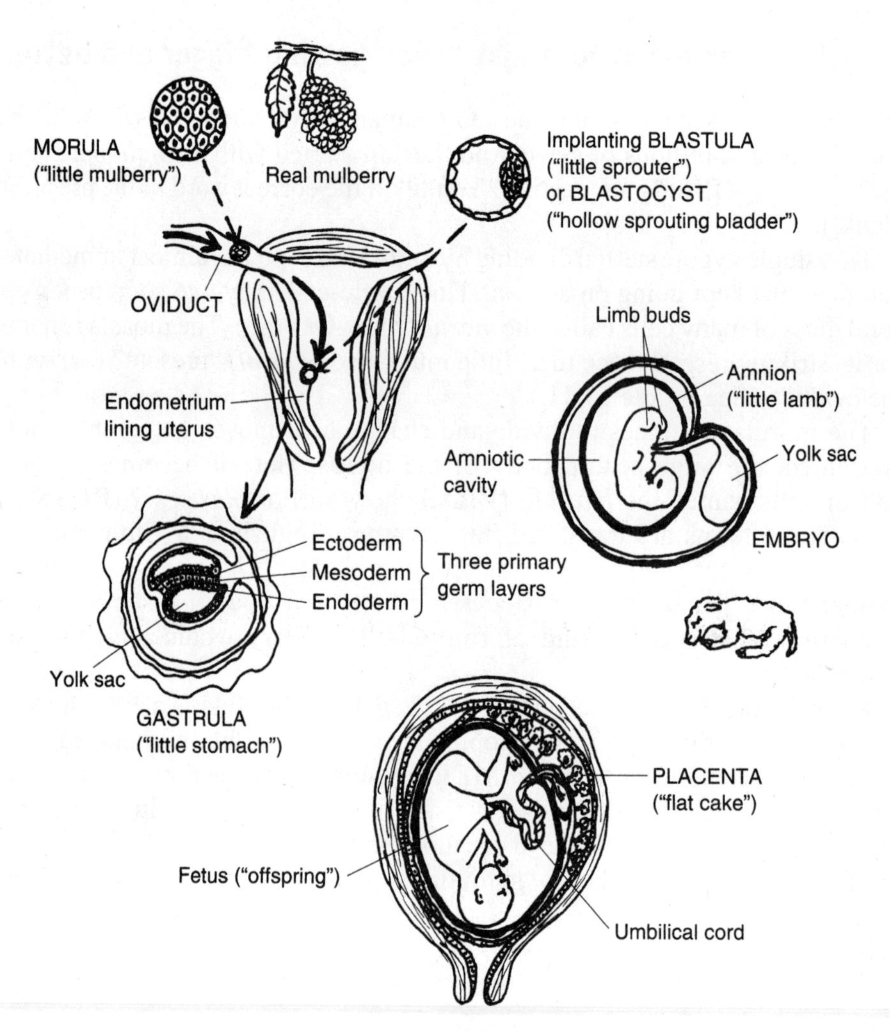

Fig. 13.11 An embryo quickly "swells" into a fetus.

These first 3 months of development, overall, are labeled as the embryo. From 3 months to the time of birth, however, we call these stages the *fetus* (**FEE**-tus), because they represent the fully formed "offspring." A *placenta* (plah-**SEN**-tah) or "flat cake"–shaped temporary organ appears on the inner *uterine* (**YOU**-ter-in) wall. An *umbilical* (um-**BIL**-ih-kal) *cord* attaches the placenta to the "central pit" (umbilicus) of the fetus.

Overall, we can summarize our discussion of embryonic and fetal development in a convenient flow chart.

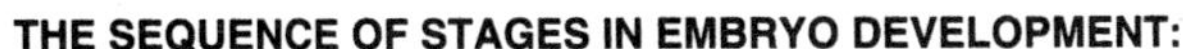

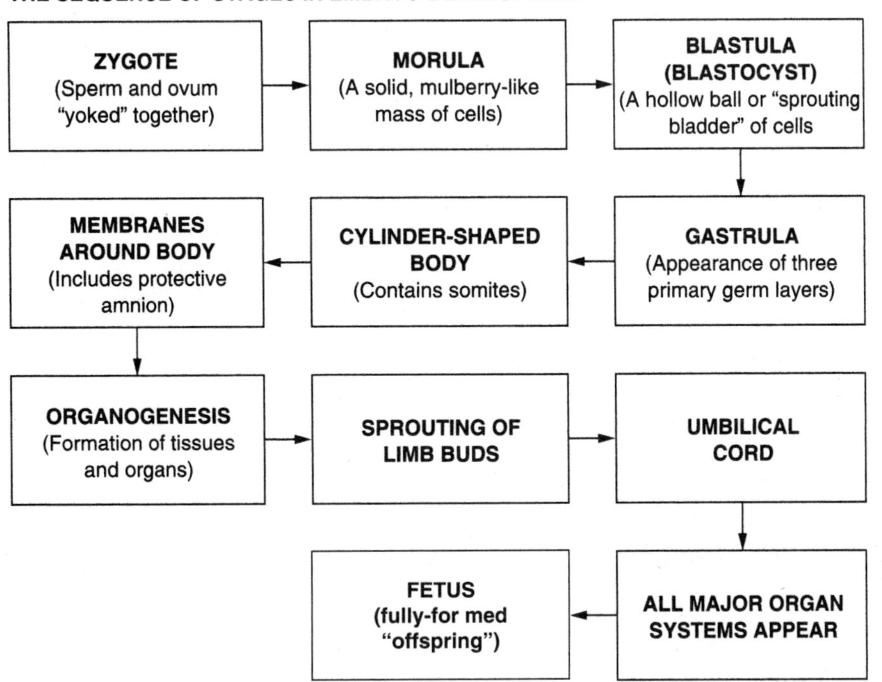

Pregnancy versus birth

In talking about the consequences of fertilization, individual stages like the zygote, embryo, and fetus all occur during pregnancy. The word, *pregnant*, actually translates to mean "before bearing the young." A synonym for pregnant is *gravid* (**GRAV**-id), which also means "laden or filled." Therefore, *pregnancy* and *gravidity* (grah-**VID**-ih-**tee**) are both "conditions of" (*-ity*) being "pregnant, laden, or filled." Now, both of these terms refer to the *woman* as someone who is "laden or filled" with a child before it is born. Therefore, a pregnant woman can be called a *gravida* (**GRAV**-ih-duh).

What we need to realize is that a completely separate set of terms is used to refer to *gestation* (jes-**TAY**-shun), which is the "process of" (*-tion*) "bearing" (*gestat*). "What exactly do we mean by *bearing*, Hippocrates ? Does that mean we're going *bearing*, that is, hunting after *bears*, which are big, furry mammals walking on four feet?" Wrong kind of *bear*, I'm afraid! In ancient Greece we talked about *bearing* as "giving birth to" a child. Hence, words like *gestation* roughly refer to pregnancy, but they are not focused upon the gravida (pregnant woman). Rather, they are focused upon "bearing"—the stages of development

Table 13.2 Terms of Pregnancy and Birth

	Before Birth	Birth	After Birth
	*PRE*NATAL STAGE	NATALITY OR NATIVITY	*POST*NATAL STAGE
THE MOTHER (pregnancy)	Pregnant, gravid	Parturition	Puerpera
THE CHILD (gestation or development)	Embryo, fetus	Neonate	Infant

leading to birth of the child. [**Understanding probe:** From the preceding discussion, would you describe the stages of development from zygote to fetus as most properly called a *pregnancy* or most properly called a *gestation*? Why?]

We can say that gestation focuses upon the development of the *child*—for it is the child, after all, who is *born* (past tense of *bear*). *Nativity* (nuh-**TIV**-ih-tee) is the "condition of" (*-ity*) being "born" (*nativ*). And the related word *natal* (**NAY**-tal) "refers to" (*-al*) "birth" (*nat*). [**Word building:** Using *natal* as the root, add the suffix in *nativity*. The result is: _________/_________, or "a condition of being born.") The *neonate* (**NEE**-uh-nayt), therefore, is a "new" (*neo–*) "born" (*nat*) child who is "present" (*-e*) outside of the uterus. If the natal state refers to birth, then the *prenatal* (**PREE**-nay-tal) *state* "refers to" the period "before" (*pre-*) "birth." The *postnatal* (**POST**-nay-tal) *state* "refers to" the time "after" (*post-*) "birth."

Parturition (**PAR**-choo-**RISH**-en) is the "act of" (*-tion*) "giving birth or delivering" (*parturi*) the young. And a *puerpera* (pyoo-**ER**-puh-ruh) is a woman "giving birth to a child." *Puerperal* (pyoo-**ER**-per-al) "relates to" (*-al*) the "puerpera" or woman "giving birth to a child."

The series of related terms outlined above are quite complex, aren't they? Let's summarize and organize them, as seen in Table 13.2 (See next page).

Some disorders of pregnancy and birth

Breaking of the normal patterns of pregnancy and birth leads to biological disorder associated with the genital (reproductive) system. And this biological disorder, in turn, may result in morbidity or even mortality of the pregnant woman and her child.

Malignant maternity, but benign obstetrics? What if a time of *maternal* (mah-**TER**-nal) or "motherly" joy, becomes one, instead, of death and sorrow? We know that the *maternity* (mah-**TER**-nih-tee) section of a hospital is where professional physicians provide skilled care for the various "conditions of" (*-ity*) "motherhood" (*matern*). What if this maternity section became a dreaded

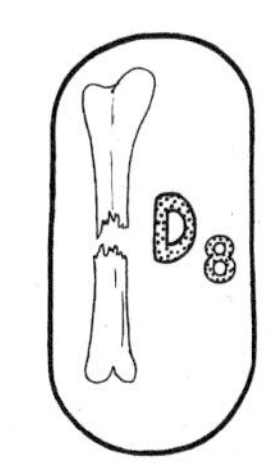

pit of deadly and unsuspected *nosocomial* (**nohs**-oh-**KOH**-me-al) infections? This is really outrageous, isn't it? After all, nosocomial does "pertain to" (*-al*) "hospitals" (*nosocomi*)! There is nothing quite like the tragedy of thousands of young *puerperas* (pyoo-**ER**-puh-rahs) and their neonates dying unnecessarily around the time of nativity, right in maternity hospitals, is there?

If this seems ghastly, then the situation becomes far worse if you compare it to the care received at the same time in *obstetrics* (ahb-**STET**-riks) wards or hospitals run by "midwives"! The word, *midwife*, comes from the Old English word for "with women." A midwife, then, is simply defined as a woman who is "with" other "women" during their time of labor and childbirth, offering assistance.

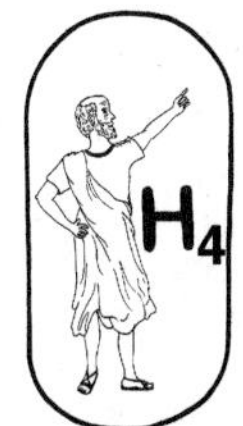

In these modern times, with much less activity by midwives, the original meanings of both obstetrics and *obstetrician* (**ahb**-stuh-**TRISH**-un) have largely been ignored and reinterpreted. An obstetrician literally is "one who specializes in" (*-ician*) "midwifery" (*obstetr*). Nowadays, however, an obstetrician is a *physician* (MD) who specializes in helping women with labor and childbirth.

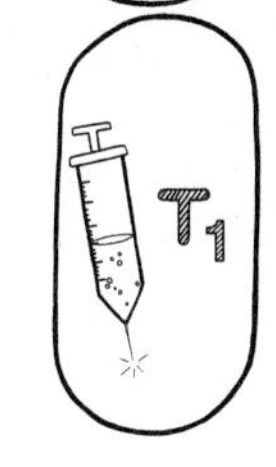

This distinction between modern obstetricians (MDs) and their much more ancient non-MD female counterparts, midwives, may seem merely academic and unimportant. But now, flash back! Flash back over a span of more than 100 years to Central Europe. Flash back to Vienna, Austria, in the year 1846, and to the crowded maternity wards of the Vienna General Hospital. On these maternity wards were pregnant women who did *not* want to be there! The wealthy gravidas stayed away and gave birth safely, at home, often with one or more paid midwives standing by, giving their kind aid and comfort.

Within the Vienna Hospital maternity clinics were the poor gravidas, who had nowhere else to go. Also present were pregnant women with special difficulties or complications. A kindly and wise physician named *Ignaz Philipp Semmelweis* (*SEM*-el-*whys*) became the acting House Officer. He supervised the First Obstetrical Clinic in the Hospital. Here Semmelweis faced a major clinical problem. There was a very high maternal and *neonatal* (**nee**-oh-**NAY**-tal) *mortality rate*, with about 13% of all pregnant patients and their newborns dying! The chief diagnosis was *puerperal* or *childbed fever*. Affected patients in labor became very febrile ("feverish")—hence the name puerperal or childbed *fever*. Other common symptoms were chills, cephalalgia (headache), malaise, and *anorexia* (an-oh-**REK**-see-ah). Anorexia means "loss" (*an-*) of "appetite" (*orexia*). In far too many cases, these symptoms progressed until shock, coma, and death resulted.

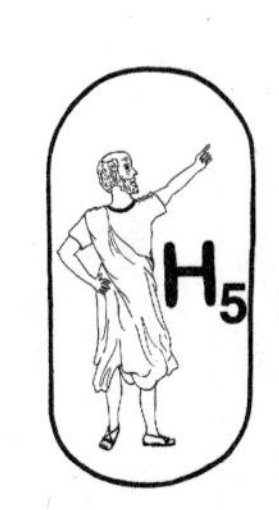

Meanwhile, Dr. Semmelweis noted a dramatic difference in the Second OB (Obstetrical) Clinic of the same hospital. Here the maternal and neonatal mortality rate from puerperal (childbed) fever was only about 2%! "*What* on *earth* accounted for this *huge* difference in morbidity and mortality between two groups of the *same* types of patients, O Good Hippocrates?" Well, even 2,000 years ago in ancient Greece, when I was still alive and becoming known as the Father of Modern Medicine, I, Hippocrates, taught about the importance of cleanliness for preventing illness. And I also observed terrible cases of *sepsis* (**SEP**-sis)—becoming "putrid or rotten"—from dirty wounds full of filth! Not having the proper tools or theory, yet, of course, I was not able to properly identify the actual etiological (causative) agents!

But Dr. Semmelweis was on the right track. He was struck by the fact that the First Clinic, which had such a high incidence of puerperal fever, was staffed by physicians who came directly from doing autopsies (postmortems) with their *bare hands*. The physicians then inserted their filthy hands into the bleeding vaginas of their puerperal patients! Semmelweis strongly suspected that his fellow doctors were making a *fatal error* in their care for expectant mothers! This suspicion was supported by the fact that one of his medical school teachers died of *septic shock* after cutting his finger during an autopsy. Further, his teacher had shown similar symptoms to the poor young mothers with puerperal fever. The Second Clinic, which enjoyed such a low incidence of puerperal fever, was staffed by midwives (not physicians), who did *not* do autopsies before probing their patients' vaginas.

Semmelweis correctly reasoned that some sort of *cadaveric* (kah-**DAV**-er-ik) *material*—chunks of "dead" bodies—was being transferred from the doctors' hands after they performed autopsies. This cadaveric matter was being inserted into the hemorrhaging vaginas of their unsuspecting, helpless, young obstetric patients! Acting on his strong suspicions, the courageous Dr. Semmelweis promptly ordered all physicians and medical students working in his clinics to thoroughly wash their hands with a strong solution of chlorine and lime (View Figure 13.12).

About a month after this rigorous hand-washing regimen was implemented, the mortality rate from puerperal fever declined sharply, to 2%! *Eureka!* Semmelweis was right! So, did he receive universal acclaim, honor, and recognition from his fellow doctors? Hardly! The chief of his clinic didn't *like* the fact that Semmelweis was basically blaming the doctors for killing their own patients. Most of his other fellow doctors didn't like it, either! Further, the *germ theory of disease* had not yet been proposed. Hence, poor Dr. Semmelweis was a little too far ahead of his time. As a result, Dr. Semmelweis was fired from his position and forced into poverty and disgrace. Cracking under the pressure (and perhaps stricken with Alzheimer's disease or senile dementia), the good doctor was finally sent to an asylum for the insane. Only 2 weeks after his admission to the asylum, he was severely beaten by the caretakers, and he died soon after.

Over 150 years later, we now realize that the unthinking doctors were infecting the vaginas of their pregnant patients. They were *cross-contaminating* their bloodstreams with *tuberculosis* (tyoo-**ber**-kyoo-**LOH**-sis) bacilli and various other nasty pathogenic bacteria carried on their hands from the rotting flesh

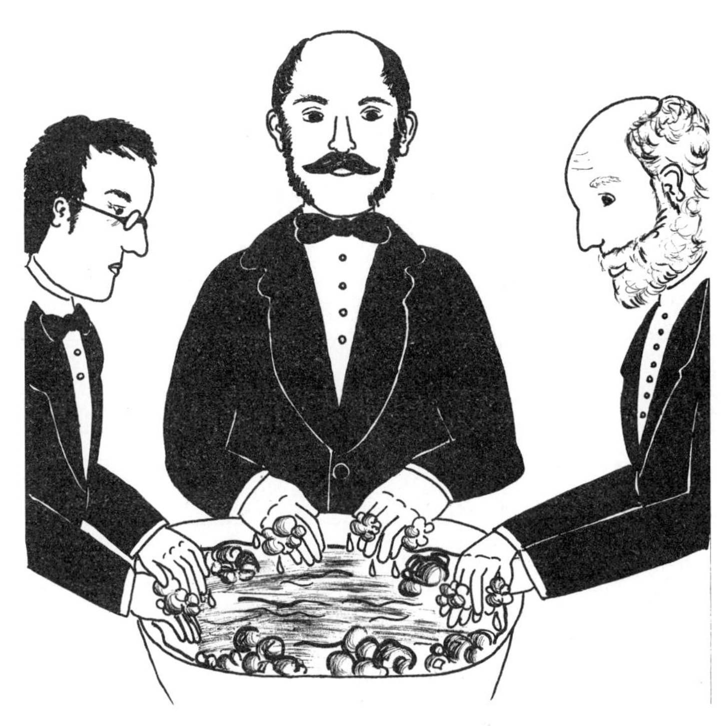

Fig. 13.12 The good Dr. Semmelweis and his associates wash their hands.

of cadavers! They were basically causing *bacteremia* (**bak**-ter-**EE**-me-ah)—a "condition of" (*-ia*) "bacteria" (*bacter*) in the "blood" (*em*). The infectious bacteria and their toxins (poisons), after they had entered the maternal bloodstream from cut vessels in the vagina, went on to create a severe *puerperal sepsis*. In modern times, this condition can be effectively treated with penicillin and other antibiotics. But back in Semmelweis's day, many afflicted young ladies and their neonates perished from untreated puerperal fever that was brought on by the filthy hands of their own stubbornly unenlightened physicians!

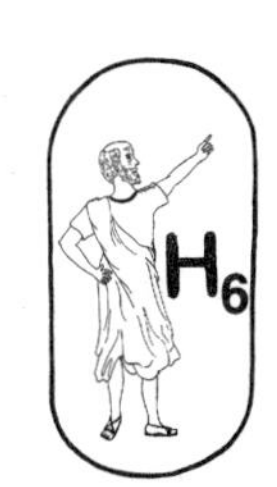

SUMMARY TABLE 13.3

Some important words and word parts are provided in Summary Table 13.3 for your review (See next page).

Medical Case History: Modern-Day Toxemia of Pregnancy

Jennifer W. was a 23-year-old *primigravida* (**prim**-ih-**GRAV**-ih-dah)—in her "first" (*primi-*) "pregnancy" (*gravida*). She came for a routine visit to her local OB-*gyn* or obstetrician-*gynecologist* (**guy**-neh-**KAHL**-oh-jist). Dr. Suzanne S.,

Summary Table 13.3 Words and Word Parts

Write in the *exact* meaning (literal English translation) for up to 10 key terms selected from the preceding block of text. After you are done, check your word meanings with the correct answers, which are given at the end of this chapter.

Key Terms	**Prefixes**	**Roots**	**Suffixes**	**Exact Meanings**
spermatogenesis	(none)	spermat "sperm"	-genesis "production of"	1. ________
epididymis	epi- "upon"	didym "eggshell"	-is "presence of"	2. ________
penis	(none)	pen "tail"	-is "presence of"	3. ________
prostate	pro- "before"	stat "standing"	-e "presence of"	4. ________
congenital	con- "with"	genit "producing"	-al "pertaining to"	5. ________
cryptorchidism	(none)	crypt "hidden"; orchid "testes"	-ism "condition of"	6. ________
oogenesis	(none)	oo "eggs"	-genesis "production of"	7. ________
menstrual	(none)	menstru "month"	-al "relating to"	8. ________
ovulation	(none)	ovul "little egg"	-tion "process of (releasing)"	9. ________
endometrium	endo- "within"	metr "uterus"	-um "presence"	10. ________

in other words, was a trained expert in obstetrics, as well as "one who studies" (*-ologist*) the diseases of "women" (*gynec*).

Jennifer's BP, upon routine examination, was found to have skyrocketed to over 162/100 mmHg. (Her previous resting blood pressure had been normotensive: 118/78 mmHg.) In addition, the patient had severe bilateral edema in both calves and feet. Her pulse was *tachycardic* (**tak**-ih-**KAR**-dik) and bounding.

Dr. Suzanne S. became very concerned. She could have made a diagnosis of *toxemia of pregnancy*, but she knew that this old, outdated disease label was really a *misnomer* (**miss-NOH**-mer) or "wrong" (*mis-*) "name" (*nomer*). In fact, Jennifer was *afebrile* (**ay-FEB**-ril), and showed no other signs of bacterial infection. Thus, a tentative diagnosis of *pregnancy-induced hypertension*, etiology unknown, was made.

A *urinalysis* (**you**-rih-**NAL**-ih-sis)—"breakdown or analysis" (*-lysis*) of the "urine" (*urin*) was done in follow-up. It revealed a dramatic *proteinuria* (**proh**-tuh-**NUR**-ee-ah). This exactly translates as an "abnormal condition of" (*-ia*) "proteins" (*protein*) being excreted in the "urine" (*ur*). Thus, Jennifer wasn't really afflicted with any known *toxic* (**TAHK**-sik) substance. Rather, her own body was having a highly negative reaction to the fetus within her uterus, almost *as if* she were being "poisoned" by it! The urinalysis results confirmed a suspected *preeclampsia* (**pree**-e-**KLAMP**-see-ah). This term literally translates as "a condition" (*-ia*) "before" (*pre-*) "eclampsia." The word *eclampsia* (eh-**KLAMPB**-see-ah) comes from the ancient Greek for "a sudden development." Stated more directly, eclampsia basically represents the "sudden development" of convulsions in the gravid woman. Such convulsions are extremely dangerous, because they may lead to coma and death! In Jennifer W's case, however, her initial preeclampsia and essential hypertension was gradually *abated* (uh-**BAY**-ted) or "beaten down" spontaneously. Her healthy fetus was delivered soon after, full-term, by the normal *vaginal* (**VAJ**-ih-nal) route. She was observed carefully for some time in the *postpartum* (**pohst-PAR**-tum) ward to ensure that the danger of eclampsia had passed.

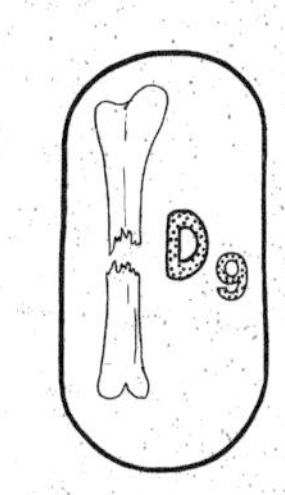

Probe of case history

(**A**) Why wasn't the patient afflicted with a "real" toxemia? What makes the label *toxemia of pregnancy* a misnomer? (**B**) Dissect *postpartum* into its prefix, root, and suffix by inserting slash marks. Now, the root in *postpartum* has the same meaning as the root we previously identified in *parturition*. Taking this fact into account, utilize your knowledge of medical terminology to write the exact common English translation of *postpartum*. [Check your short answers with the key near the end of this chapter.]

A Final Farewell

Well, Dear Reader, I truly hope you have enjoyed your all-too-brief visit with me, the Ghost of Hippocrates, in the pages of *MEDICAL TERMINOLOGY DEMYSTIFIED*. As the Father of Modern Medicine, I have tried to serve as your guide. Surely, we must feel for the noble men and women in the Healing Arts, some of whom we have discussed in this book. They, like me, have helped build a Great Monument to human understanding and compassion, and have framed it in the Ancient Terminology of Greece and Rome. I trust that this is only the beginning, and that you will work to expand your knowledge of the medical language much farther. As for me, I must now return to the Island of *Cos* (**KOHS**), off the Greek coast. This is where I was born, and where I practiced medicine for most of my natural life. I firmly believed that facts and reason should govern our treatment of human disease and injury. But you know, Dear Reader, I still have this nagging suspicion that a rotten little kid named Baby Heinie has been following me around, popping up here and there in the oddest places in this book!

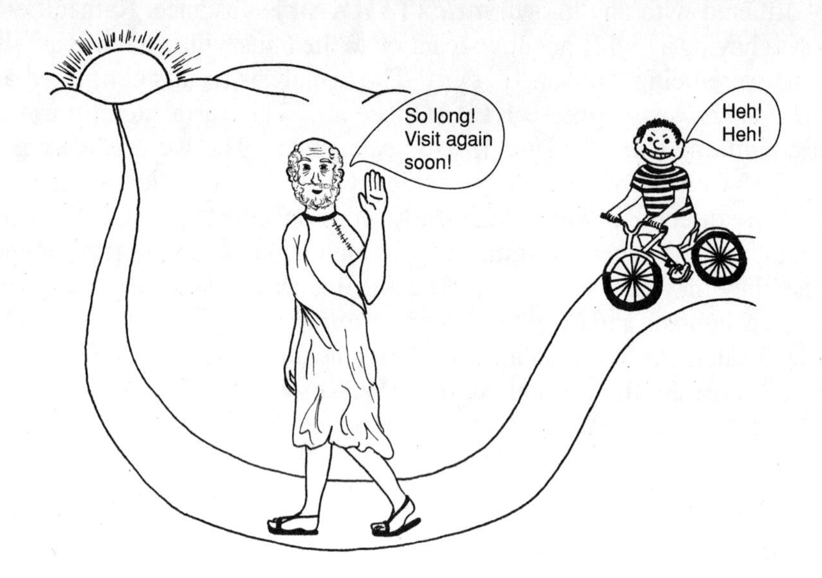

Quiz

Refer to the text in this chapter if necessary. A good score is at least 8 correct answers out of these 10 questions. The answers are listed in the back of this book.

1. Two roots that mean "kidney":
   (a) Ur and cyst
   (b) Ren and nephr
   (c) Cyt and urin
   (d) Dia and phoret
2. The alternate name for the genitourinary system:
   (a) Digestive
   (b) Gastrointestinal

(c) Endocrine-exocrine
(d) Urogenital

3. The broad middle zone of each kidney:
(a) Renal cortex
(b) Glomeruli
(c) Renal medulla
(d) Renal pelvis

4. The proper dissection of glomerular is:
(a) Glomerul/ar
(b) Gl/omer/ul/ar
(c) Glomer/ular
(d) Glom/er/u/lar

5. *Glomerular* literally translates to mean:
(a) "A red bird present"
(b) "A little ball of yarn"
(c) "Tiny hairs"
(d) "Pertaining to a little ball of yarn"

6. The formal term for the urinary bladder is:
(a) Urethra
(b) Prostate
(c) Ureter
(d) Urocyst

7. If a woman is described as *gravid*, she can also be called:
(a) Obese
(b) Pregnant
(c) Preeclampsic
(d) Postpartal

8. The "womb" is technically known as the:
(a) Fallopian tubes
(b) Endometrium
(c) Uterus
(d) Fundus

9. Can rightfully be called the Father of *Antisepsis* (**an**-tih-**SEP**-sis):
(a) Florence Nightingale
(b) Philippe Fourneau
(c) Ignaz Philipp Semmelweis
(d) Calvin Coolidge

10. The word *obstetrics* literally refers to:
    (a) "Study of women"
    (b) "Helpful physicians"
    (c) "Childbirth and labor"
    (d) "Midwives"

Memory Pillboxes for Chapter 13

Several key facts were tagged with numbered icons in the page margins of this chapter. Write a short summary of each of these key facts into a numbered cell or compartment within the appropriate type of *Memory Pillbox* that appears below:

Background and History **Pillboxes for Chapter 13:**

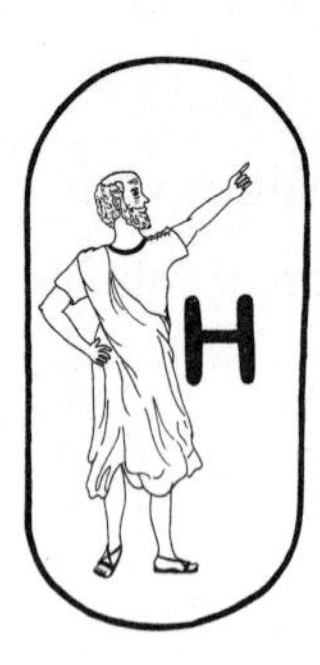

1	2

3	4

5	6

***Anatomy* Pillboxes for Chapter 13:**

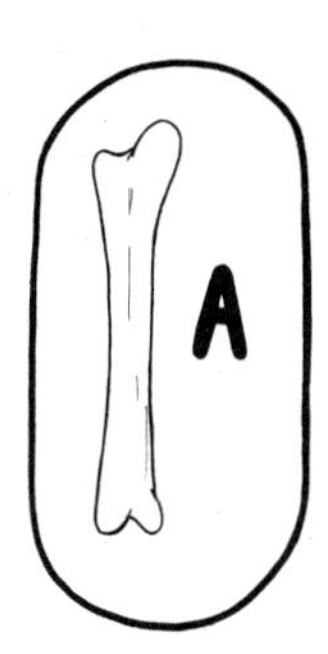

1	2

3	4
5	6
7	8
9	

***Physiology* Pillboxes for Chapter 13:**

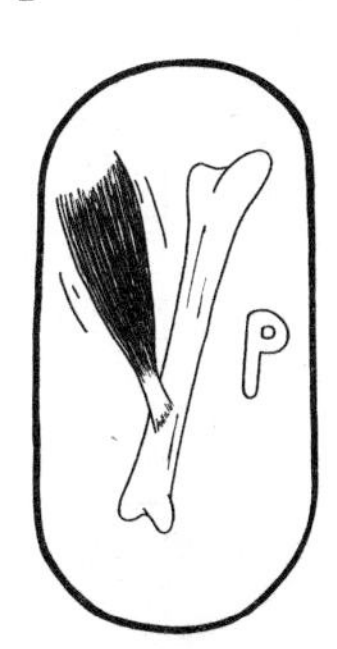

1	2
3	4
5	6

7	8
9	10

Disease/Injury **Pillboxes for Chapter 13:**

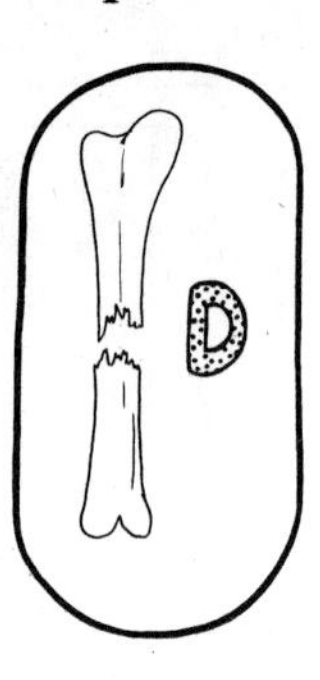

1	2

3	4
5	6
7	8
9	

***Treatment/Therapy* Pillboxes for Chapter 13:**

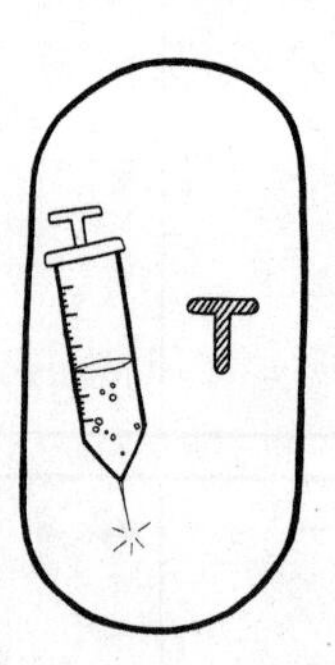

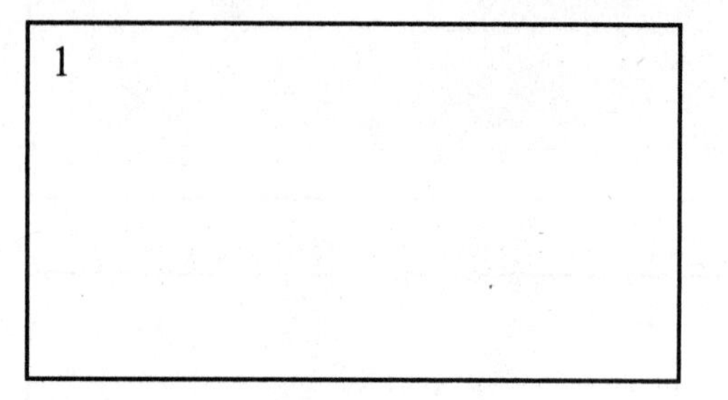

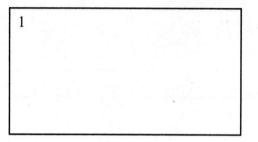

Answers for Chapter 13 Summary Tables

FOR SUMMARY TABLE 13.1

1. "pertaining to urine"
2. "pertaining to kidney"
3. "presence of a little ball of yarn"
4. "presence of kidney"
5. "one that (is) filtered"
6. "process of sopping up again"
7. "urine bladder"
8. "condition of much urine"
9. "condition of excessive blood volume"
10. "relating to (something) against diuresis"

FOR SUMMARY TABLE 13.3

1. "production of sperm"
2. "presence of (something) upon an eggshell"
3. "presence of a tail"

4. "presence of a standing before"
5. "pertaining to producing with"
6. "condition of hidden testes"
7. "production of eggs"
8. "relating to a month"
9. "process of (releasing) a little egg"
10. "presence of (something) within the uterus"

Answers to Probe of Case History

(**A**) Preeclampsia and eclampsia are not really toxemia, because there are no "poisons" (*tox*) actually present within the bloodstream. (**B**) post (prefix)/part (root)/um (suffix) = "presence of (something) before birth."

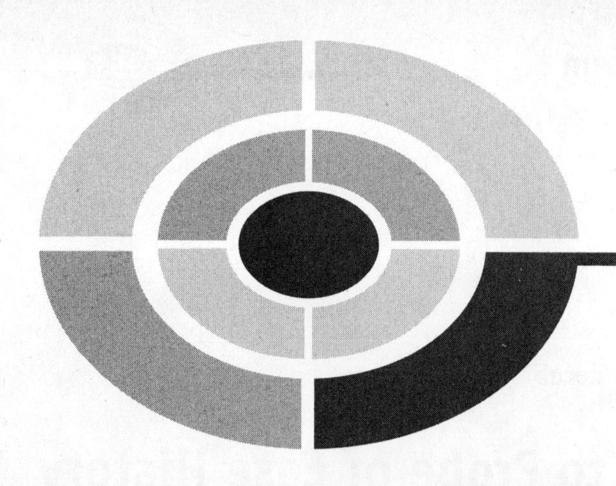

Test: Part 6

DO NOT REFER TO THE TEXT WHEN TAKING THIS TEST. A good score is at least 18 out of 25 questions correct. The answers are in the back of the book. It's best to have a friend check your score the first time so you won't memorize the answers if you want to take the test again.

1. The cardia is the:
   (a) Region of the stomach just below the esophagus
   (b) Middle zone of the kidney
   (c) Front, but not the back, of the seminiferous tubules
   (d) Distal portion of the stomach that touches the duodenum
   (e) S-shaped portion of the large intestine

2. Ingestion is the exact opposite of:
   (a) Digestion
   (b) Absorption
   (c) Ventilation
   (d) Respiration
   (e) Defecation

3. The root in *ileum:*
   (a) Il
   (b) le
   (c) Um
   (d) Ile
   (e) Ileu

4. The accessory digestive organ located within the oral cavity:
   (a) Pancreas
   (b) Salivary gland
   (c) Cholecyst
   (d) Beta cells
   (e) Seminal vesicles

5. *Cecum* is correctly analyzed as:
   (a) Ce/cu/m
   (b) Cec/u/m
   (c) Cecu/m
   (d) Ce/cum
   (e) Cec/um

6. *Cecum* exactly translates to mean:
   (a) The "presence of (something) blind"
   (b) "Referring to (something you can) see"
   (c) "*Seek*, and ye shall *find* 'um!"
   (d) The "presence of (something) empty"
   (e) "Relating to the body hip or flank"

7. Abnormal condition that is nicknamed "heartburn":
   (a) Septicemia
   (b) Pyrosis
   (c) Psychosis
   (d) Pyromania
   (e) Hyperthyroidism

8. A term like *vermitis* (**verm-EYE**-tis) would probably translate to mean:
   (a) "Removal of the appendix"
   (b) "Inflammation of a worm"
   (c) "Perforation of the uterus"
   (d) "Cutting around the stomach"
   (e) "A full heart bypass operation"

9. An edematous body part is one that is:
   (a) "Painful"
   (b) "Dried up"
   (c) "Hot," but not red
   (d) "Red," but not hot
   (e) Swollen
10. The most common bacillus in the human GI tract:
   (a) *Staphylococcus aureus*
   (b) *Clostridium tetani*
   (c) Tuberculin bacilli
   (d) *Escherichia coli*
   (e) Amoebic dysentery
11. Hydrochloric acid donates or gives off lots of:
   (a) Sodium bicarbonate
   (b) Strong base
   (c) Salt particles
   (d) Alkali
   (e) H+ ions
12. "Instrument used to examine the abdomen":
   (a) Otoscope
   (b) Laryngoscopy
   (c) Peritonitis
   (d) Laparoscope
   (e) Gastric lavager
13. *Urogenital* has the same English translation as:
   (a) Uroabdominal
   (b) Spermatogenesis
   (c) Genitonephron
   (d) Genitourinary
   (e) Leukocytosis
14. The shallow "bowl" of the "kidney":
   (a) Renal medulla
   (b) Nephric pyramid
   (c) Renal pelvis
   (d) Glomerulus
   (e) Nephrolith
15. The force causing fluid to be pushed out of the glomerulus:
   (a) Peristalsis
   (b) Oogenesis

(c) Normotension
(d) Hyperthermia
(e) Defecation

16. "How is it that about 180 L of fluid enter the renal tubules every day, yet only about 1 L is urinated?" The best answer is that:
    (a) Most of the filtrate is secreted
    (b) Plasma cholesterol levels are excessive
    (c) Nephrons stop functioning after sundown!
    (d) Nearly all of the glomerular filtrate is reabsorbed back into the bloodstream
    (e) The collecting ducts just keep taking the urine round and round in a circle

17. A schoolgirl with polyuria probably couldn't sit in class for a full hour because:
    (a) Diuresis would have her leaving the room frequently
    (b) Urinalysis results might prove inconclusive
    (c) She was suffering from a gangrenous appendix
    (d) Renal compensation was operating perfectly
    (e) Bile secretion was nearly lacking

18. A temporary organ during pregnancy named for its resemblance to a "flat cake":
    (a) Placenta
    (b) Ovary
    (c) Endometrium
    (d) Zygote
    (e) Liver

19. Also known as the "gullet":
    (a) Pylorus
    (b) Esophagus
    (c) Trachea
    (d) Stomach
    (e) Small intestine

20. Scientific name for the "large intestine":
    (a) Vermiform appendix
    (b) Jejunum
    (c) Pyloric sphincter
    (d) Rectum
    (e) Colon

21. Alexis St. Martin was valuable as a subject for GI study, owing to his unique:
    (a) Attitude toward science
    (b) Accidental creation of a permanent gastric fistula
    (c) Reflux esophagitis
    (d) Practice of hypoventilation without acidosis
    (e) Irritation of the duodenal mucosa

22. The intestinal neutralization equation:
    (a) $NaCl + H_2O \longrightarrow HCl + H_2CO_3$
    (b) $CO_2 + H_2O \longrightarrow H_2CO_3$
    (c) $NaHCO_3 + HCl \longrightarrow NaCl + H_2CO_3$
    (d) Amino acids + Energy $\longrightarrow$ Protein
    (e) $H + + Cl - \longrightarrow HCl$

23. The use of a Magic "mini-" Hand, rather than a "macro-" one, to symbolize tubular secretion is appropriate, since:
    (a) Macrophages don't exist in the renal tubular system
    (b) This process involves the active addition of only tiny quantities of particles to the urinary filtrate
    (c) Ovarian activity is little (if any) affected
    (d) Such a huge BP is pushing fluid across the walls of the glomerular capillaries
    (e) The cholecyst reabsorbs practically *everything* that the liver sends it!

24. In *menarche*,______ is a root for "monthly."
    (a) Mena
    (b) Arche
    (c) Rche
    (d) Arc
    (e) Men

25. A "little bag" of secreting cells that forms around a maturing ovum:
    (a) Urocyst
    (b) Hydrocele
    (c) Follicle
    (d) Seminal vesicle
    (e) Mucosal sac

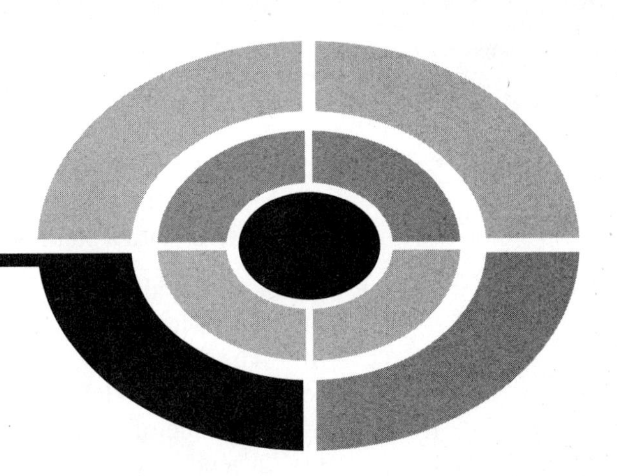

Final Exam

DO NOT REFER TO THE TEXT WHEN TAKING THIS EXAM. A good score is at least 75 correct. The answers are in the back of the book. It's best to have a friend check your score the first time so you won't memorize the answers if you want to take the test again.

1. Hippocrates (really, his ghost) was chosen as our noble host for *MEDICAL TERMINOLOGY DEMYSTIFIED* because he:
   (a) Was the first to perform dissections of human cadavers
   (b) Maintained that medical practice should be based upon reason, nature, and logic, rather than superstition and magic
   (c) Carried out most of the pioneering experiments in animal physiology
   (d) Developed early cures for brain cancer
   (e) Founded a novel School for Ancient Nurses
2. The traditional symbol for Modern Medicine:
   (a) Two hanging gourds, pierced by a single arrow
   (b) A flying fish with bright wings

(c) A sacred snake of healing coiled around a wooden staff
(d) Mercury, the winged Messenger of the Gods
(e) An MD with a stethoscope hanging around his or her neck

3. *Medic/al* literally translates to mean:
(a) "One who is practiced in"
(b) "The study of treatments and cures"
(c) "Referring to healing"
(d) "Absence of pain"
(e) "A tendency to snore"

4. The _____ of a word is its main idea, in a sense "anchoring" it into the ground:
(a) Prefix
(b) Combining vowel
(c) Suffix
(d) Synonym
(e) Root

5. In *arthrometer* (**arth-RAH**-meh-ter), the letter *o* serves as:
(a) A combining vowel
(b) A former of the word's plural
(c) A vital part of the total word's meaning
(d) An indicator of connection to the world of the "heart"
(e) A suffix for "an instrument used to measure"

6. The Father of Anatomy:
(a) Galen
(b) Hippocrates
(c) Florence Nightingale
(d) Vesalius
(e) Rudolf Hesselmeyer

7. ___/___ "pertains to the skull":
(a) Cephal/ic
(b) Dors/al
(c) Crani/um
(d) Epi/gastric
(e) Crani/al

8. Cocaine is most accurately classified as a _____ type of drug:
(a) Narcotic
(b) Antibiotic
(c) Anesthetic

(d) Analgesic
(e) Diaphoretic

9. *Trepanation* has exactly the same common English meaning as:
(a) Dehydration
(b) Obfuscation
(c) Trephination
(d) Craniotomy
(e) Narcolepsis

10. An analgesist (**an**-al-**JEE**-zist) is literally "one who . . .":
(a) "Specializes in removing tumors"
(b) "Loves to pop ugly comedos and blackheads"
(c) "Becomes unconscious, automatically"
(d) "Specializes in lack of feeling or sensation"
(e) "Specializes in the lack of pain"

11. A curette "scrapes," while a cautery (**KAW**-ter-ee):
(a) "Burns"
(b) "Ties up"
(c) "Scoops up"
(d) "Throws down"
(e) "Stitches"

12. _____ takes tissue samples from a *dead* person, while _____ takes them from a *living* person:
(a) Defecation; urination
(b) Necropsy; supination
(c) Autopsy; biopsy
(d) Anesthesia; depression
(e) Ligation; cauterization

13. We humans, all animals, and all plants are properly classified as:
(a) Tissues
(b) Organs
(c) Geologica
(d) Protozoa
(e) Organisms

14. *Macroscopic* is accurately analyzed as:
(a) Ma/cro/scop/i/c
(b) Mac/ro/scopic
(c) Macr/o/scop/ic

(d) Macro/sco/pic
(e) M/crosco/pic

15. *Macroscopic* exactly translates as:
(a) "Tiny bodies present"
(b) "Referring to the examination of large (things)"
(c) "An instrument used to examine tiny (things)"
(d) "Pertaining to yummy Big Mac sandwiches!"
(e) "An instrument used to examine big (things)"

16. The type of bacteria that resembles slender "rods":
(a) Ancylostomas
(b) Spirilla
(c) Cocci
(d) Bacilli
(e) Spirochetes

17. A pathogen is literally a:
(a) "Disease-producer"
(b) "Destroyer of cells"
(c) "Mating insect"
(d) "External invader"
(e) "Cell eater"

18. The plural word, *traumata* (traw-**MAH**-tah), like *lesions*, means:
(a) "Treatments"
(b) "*Draw* Mah? *Duhhhh*!"
(c) "Operations"
(d) "Stresses and strains"
(e) "Wounds"

19. A "condition of" a "flame within":
(a) Inflammation
(b) Pyrosis
(c) Hyperthermia
(d) Hypogonadism
(e) Electrofirosis

20. A ___/___ is "one who studies drugs," while a ___/___ is "one who specializes in drugs":
(a) Psych/iatrist; phys/ician
(b) Neur/ology; phys/iatrist
(c) Pharmac/ologist; pharmac/ist

(d) Anesthesi/ologist; anesthet/ist
(e) Bi/ologist; techn/ician

21. The major active ingredient in OTC (over-the-counter) aspirin tablets:
(a) Barbituric acid
(b) HCl
(c) ADH
(d) $NaHCO_3$
(e) Acetylsalicylic acid

22. Baby Heinie gets bitten by his pet cobra, Black Bart. A trip to the local ER would probably result in him receiving therapeutic dosages of:
(a) Depressants
(b) Tranquilizers
(c) Antitoxins
(d) Narcotics
(e) Amphetamines

23. A word root frequently used to indicate "violent tearing or shaking":
(a) Convuls
(b) Deliri
(c) Hallucin
(d) Ambul
(e) Muscul

24. A clinical _____ is a problem or complaint noticed by the *patient*, whereas a clinical _____ is a problem uncovered during examination by a *health professional*:
(a) Ginsing; gensong
(b) Depression; elevation
(c) Pustule; papule
(d) Sign; symptom
(e) Symptom; sign

25. "Don't worry about your husband's heart problem, Mrs. Facquat! We'll find the cause during the *postmortem*!" your family MD tries to assure you. But this would not be very helpful to Mr. Facquat, since his:
(a) Morbid etiology would be established after his death
(b) Big toe was really aching!
(c) Life insurance premiums remained unpaid
(d) Pathogenic sequelae would likely be discovered, but then be transfused into his wife!
(e) Cephalalgia did not justify his early death to perform an autopsy!

26. Deep massage therapy would be part of a total treatment program in ____:
    (a) Narcosis
    (b) Cryosurgery
    (c) Chemotherapy
    (d) Physiatrics
    (e) Psychotherapy

27. An injection given _____ is made "into a vein":
    (a) Intramuscularly
    (b) Extracorporeal
    (c) Intravenously
    (d) Endoarterially
    (e) Transrectally

28. "You just told a really *morbid* joke!" Thus, the joke was:
    (a) "Healthy"
    (b) "Disgusting"
    (c) "Dumb"
    (d) "Nonsense"
    (e) "Sick"

29. A prophylactic agent is one that:
    (a) Cures illnesses
    (b) Guards against diseases
    (c) Helps destroy healthy tissues
    (d) Promotes pregnancy as well as sexual intercourse
    (e) Confuses and overwhelms the trusting patient

30. We can build a single term that means "clear spring water lover" by combining:
    (a) *hemat* with *doormat*
    (b) *lymph* with *phil*
    (c) *aque* with *ptosis*
    (d) *hydro* with *phob*
    (e) *ectomy* with *spring*

31. Two acceptable alternative medical terms for the common cold:
    (a) Coryza and esophagitis
    (b) Rheumatoid and arthritis
    (c) Diabetes mellitus and diabetes insipidus
    (d) Acute coryza and rhinitis
    (e) Influenza and gastroenteritis

32. A syndrome differs from a prodrome in that it:
    (a) Requires a careful set of clinical observations before being stated
    (b) Includes a bunch of signs and symptoms that "run together" in the same patient, at the same time
    (c) Only involves clinical symptoms, rather than signs
    (d) Represents a group of signs and symptoms that occur "before" a particular disease
    (e) Is very "synful" or "naughty," versus being more "professional"

33. P & A is sometimes used as an abbreviation for *posterior and anterior* but also for:
    (a) Poppa & Alberto
    (b) Penis & anus
    (c) Percussion & auscultation
    (d) Peritonitis & adenoma
    (e) Putrid & alkaline

34. A ___ */o/scope,* like a *steth/o/scope*, is an instrument used to examine the "chest":
    (a) Lapar
    (b) Ot
    (c) Proct
    (d) Thorac
    (e) Cervic

35. Radio*gram* differs from radio*graphy* in that it is:
    (a) An instrument used to record songs played on radio
    (b) An actual record of rays, rather than the process of recording them
    (c) The study and testing of rays
    (d) A person who records the rays
    (e) A process for removing the lethal effects of radiation

36. "Your breast cancer is idiopathic, I'm afraid," your local oncologist gravely informs you. This means that your breast cancer:
    (a) Is in a late stage that's always fatal
    (b) Was caused by an "idiot"
    (c) Will progress in measured phases that can be treated
    (d) Has an unknown etiology
    (e) Will probably be benign

37. A prediction made "before" a disease actually occurs:
    (a) Prognosis
    (b) Case history

(c) Diagnosis
(d) Cecum
(e) Immunity

38. A "condition of not serving" disease:
(a) Tuberculosis
(b) Fertility
(c) Immunity
(d) Lymphatics
(e) Cybernetics

39. Chemical markers on the surfaces of cells that label them as foreign or "non-self":
(a) Antibodies
(b) Cholesterols
(c) Maculas
(d) Antigens
(e) Leukospheres

40. *Cell* and *cellular* are different names for:
(a) "Little chambers or boxes"
(b) "Big bladders"
(c) "Sacs in the middle"
(d) "Heavy droplets"
(e) "Bladders that burst"

41. The level of body organization lying just below the cell level:
(a) Molecules
(b) Atoms
(c) Organelles
(d) Tissues
(e) Organs

42. "Control of sameness":
(a) Hemostasis
(b) Autolysis
(c) Steady as she goes!
(d) Homeostasis
(e) Normothermia

43. __ is a root in *lysosome* for "breakdown":
(a) Lys
(b) Yso
(c) Som

(d) Lysos
(e) Some

44. *Aerobic* has the exactly opposite meaning of:
(a) Oxidative
(b) Intracellular
(c) Anaerobic
(d) Mitochondrion
(e) ATP

45. The primary carbohydrate fuel for cell metabolism:
(a) Protein
(b) Glucose
(c) Lipid
(d) Hemoglobin
(e) Sodium bicarbonate

46. ATP is an abbreviation for:
(a) A Tee-Pee (where Indians live!)
(b) Aldosterone Triester Phosphadine
(c) Always Trust People!
(d) Adenosine triphosphate
(e) Adenosine diphosphate

47. By definition, intercellular material is always found "____ cells":
(a) "Within"
(b) "Around"
(c) "Upon"
(d) "Outside"
(e) "Between"

48. If a *fibr/o/blast* is a "fiber former," then an *oste/o/blast* is a "____ former":
(a) Skin
(b) Grass
(c) Bone
(d) Gristle
(e) Blood

49. Biological *dis*order has what literal relationship to biological *order*?
(a) "Twice"
(b) "Not"
(c) "Supporting"
(d) "Building"
(e) "Stimulates"

50. A *histologist* is to *histology* as a *biologist* is to:
    (a) Dermatology
    (b) Biology
    (c) Physiologist
    (d) Biological
    (e) Registered nurse

51. Using the root and suffix in *epithelial* and the prefix in *subatomic*, we can build the following new term:
    (a) Epithelic
    (b) Subthelial
    (c) Subatomal
    (d) Epiatomic
    (e) Subpithelial

52. In Latin, our body's outer "covering" is called its:
    (a) Endoskeleton
    (b) Dermis
    (c) Integument
    (d) Muscle fibers
    (e) Valve coat

53. The prefix *hypo-* is appropriate to use whenever some body parameter is:
    (a) Relatively constant
    (b) Way below its normal range
    (c) Consistently above its normal range
    (d) Following homeostasis
    (e) Right at its average long-term level

54. *Necrosis* is properly dissected as:
    (a) Nec/ro/sis
    (b) Ne/crosi/s
    (c) Necros/is
    (d) Ne/c/r/osis
    (e) Necr/osis

55. *Necrosis* exactly translates as:
    (a) "Condition of life"
    (b) "Fairly constant condition"
    (c) "Abnormal condition of death"
    (d) "Removal of the spleen"
    (e) "Tissue cells destroyed"

56. "A process of changing over" to another "place" in the body (as for a tumor):
    (a) Tumorigenesis
    (b) Hyperplasia
    (c) Osmosis
    (d) Metastasis
    (e) Lysis

57. A *malignant carcinoma* is literally a(n):
    (a) "Evil growth of a Carson"
    (b) "Cool race car in Oklahoma"
    (c) "Deadly tumor of the flesh"
    (d) "Mean and carsick in Omaha"
    (e) "Wicked crab tumor"

58. A "joining place":
    (a) Heart
    (b) Trachea
    (c) Joint
    (d) Oviduct
    (e) Melanocyte

59. "Battle lines of soldiers" in the fingers and toes:
    (a) Carpals
    (b) Metacarpals
    (c) Humeri
    (d) Phalanx
    (e) Phalanges

60. "Quit your *carping*!" approximately means, "Stop your *complaining*!" If we take the root out of *carping* and replace it with its body part name, we can create this nonsense sentence:
    (a) "Quit your *thigh*ing!"
    (b) "Stop your *mouth*ing!
    (c) "Stop *butt*ing in!
    (d) "Please cease your *wrist*ing!"
    (e) "Give me some *skin*, Jack!"

61. The "shoulder blade":
    (a) Sternum
    (b) Clavicle
    (c) Scapula

(d) Mandible
(e) Fossa

62. Fractures are basically a result of severe bone:
(a) Hypostrain
(b) Myopia
(c) Hyperstress
(d) Tensile strength
(e) Hypostress

63. *Osteoporosis* is properly dissected with slash marks as:
(a) Oste/o/por/osis
(b) Ost/eo/po/rosis
(c) Os/teoporo/sis
(d) Ost/e/o/por/osis
(e) Oste/o/po/rosis

64. *Osteoporosis* means ______ in common English:
(a) "Abnormal condition of soft gristle"
(b) "Referring to holey bones"
(c) "Inflammation of crispy bone cells"
(d) "Say *Ahs*, tee yoh *poor* ol' *Sis*!"
(e) "Abnormal condition of pores (in) bones"

65. If your kid brother joins the Army *Delta* Force, then that suggests he really likes:
(a) Squares
(b) Ovals
(c) Circles
(d) Rectangles
(e) Triangles

66. "I'm gonna break your *brachi*!" a Mafia hit man threatens you. You better try to protect your:
(a) Leg
(b) Teeth
(c) Soft face
(d) Arm
(e) Hip

67. "I wouldn't *fibula*, Mom!" Baby Heinie pleads (trying to be clever with his growing knowledge of anatomy). The fibula is actually a:
(a) Way of fashioning bone tissue out of gold dust
(b) Sheet of connective tissue fascia in the thigh

(c) Long bone in the lower leg
(d) Cube-shaped bone of the ankle
(e) Slender skeletal muscle supporting the buttocks

68. An orthopedist would most likely be called to consult on what general type of medical problem?
(a) Severe cephalalgia
(b) An addiction to smoking
(c) A ruptured appendix
(d) Chronic patellar pain
(e) Frequent constipation

69. The exactly opposite movement of flexion is:
(a) Elevation
(b) Extension
(c) Contraction
(d) Abduction
(e) Inversion

70. A cicatrix is a:
(a) Bony outgrowth
(b) Scar
(c) Area of ischemia
(d) Amputation
(e) Type of cancer

71. *Myocardial* is correctly subdivided as:
(a) Myo/ca/rdi/al
(b) My/o/cardia/l
(c) My/o/cardi/al
(d) My/o/car/dial
(e) My/o/card/ial

72. *Myocardial* technically translates to mean:
(a) "Inflammation of the heart wall"
(b) "Removal of a mushy brain growth"
(c) "Referring to skeletal muscle"
(d) "Relating to heart muscle"
(e) "Involving the cardia but not the atria"

73. The "little plates" or "clot cells" that stick together and assist in achieving hemostasis:
(a) Bucketoblasts or clotocytes
(b) Platelets or thrombocytes

(c) Leukocytes and lumpectocytes
(d) Erythrocytes and lymphocytes
(e) Macrophages and thromboblasts

74. "A graphical record of the electrical activity of the heart":
(a) Electroencephalogram
(b) Electrocardiography
(c) Echocardiogram
(d) Myomectomy
(e) Electrocardiogram

75. "Difficult breathing" is called:
(a) Tachypnea
(b) Endocarditis
(c) Dyspnea
(d) Bradycardia
(e) Normotension

76. Both *pneumon* and *pulmon* are roots for:
(a) "Head"
(b) "Drinking"
(c) "Lungs"
(d) "Stomach"
(e) "Testes"

77. The "windpipe" is formally called the:
(a) Bronchiole
(b) Trachea
(c) Alveolus
(d) Pharynx
(e) Esophagus

78. A rhinovirus is named for its ability to infect the:
(a) Nasal mucosa
(b) Abdominal peritoneum
(c) Base of the brain
(d) Sheath around muscles
(e) Loose connective tissue below the skin

79. *Respiration* is correctly dissected as:
(a) Re/spir/ation
(b) Resp/i/rat/ion
(c) Re/spir/a/tion

(d) R/espirati/on
(e) Resp/ira/tion

80. In a poetic sense, if one were literally picking "little acorns" within the human body, you would really be harvesting groups of:
(a) Pulmonary alveoli
(b) Glands
(c) Muscle fibers
(d) Renal pyramids
(e) Connective tissue fibers

81. Dehydration is the exact opposite of:
(a) Normohydration
(b) Diuresis
(c) Hyperglycemia
(d) Hyperhydration
(e) Urination

82. A synonym for diaphoresis:
(a) Alimentation
(b) Hyperhidrosis
(c) Normoperfusion
(d) Dermostasis
(e) Edema

83. The endocrine glands that secrete insulin:
(a) Parathyroids
(b) Pineals
(c) Ovarian follicles
(d) Pancreatic islets (Islets of Langerhans)
(e) Mammary bodies

84. *Hyperglycemia* is properly broken down as:
(a) Hyper/glyce/mia
(b) Hyp/ergl/ycemia
(c) Hyper/glyc/emia
(d) Hy/perglycem/ia
(e) Hypergl/y/cemi/a

85. *Normoglycemia* exactly translates to mean:
(a) "A condition of deficient blood glucose"
(b) "Relating to normal blood glucose"
(c) "Lowering blood glucose below its range"

(d) "A condition of normal blood glucose"
(e) "No more glucose!"

86. The CNS equals the:
(a) Encephalon plus spinal cord
(b) Nerves and sensory receptors
(c) Motor nerve fibers only
(d) Both afferent and efferent nerve fibers
(e) Cerebrum plus cerebellum

87. "Refers to farsightedness":
(a) Paranoia
(b) Schizophrenia
(c) Myopic
(d) Hyperopic
(e) Hyperopia

88. Intraocular pressure occurs:
(a) "Around the eyes"
(b) "Below the ears"
(c) "Through the forehead"
(d) "Under the nose"
(e) "Within the eyes"

89. A nail is indigestible. This means it:
(a) "Cannot be separated or carried apart"
(b) "Will be sopped up"
(c) "Has been secreted again"
(d) "Shall be chewed through"
(e) "Loves cigarettes"

90. A brownish-green detergent substance from the liver that emulsifies fats:
(a) $NaHCO_3$
(b) Pancreatic juice
(c) Bile
(d) Kickapoo juice
(e) GH

91. Alkalosis represents the exact opposite of:
(a) Reabsorption
(b) Acidosis
(c) Glycosuria
(d) Hematuria
(e) Hemoglobin saturation

92. Epigastric pain would be localized:
    (a) “Upon the stomach”
    (b) “Within the duodenum”
    (c) “Perpendicular to the cecum”
    (d) “Inside of the stomach”
    (e) “Below the belt”

93. The prefix in *endometrium*, the root in *gynecologic*, and the suffix in *oogenesis* are used to build this term:
    (a) Engynesis
    (b) Endogynecis
    (c) Metrogyneendo
    (d) Endogynecogenesis
    (e) Ooendogenesis

94. Where in the body would the protein in the word *proteinuria* literally be found?
    (a) Digestive tube
    (b) Ureter
    (c) Pineal gland
    (d) Vermiform appendix
    (e) Rectum

95. Puerperal fever only occurs in:
    (a) Young boys before puberty
    (b) Cases of gunshot wounds
    (c) Pregnant women who have suffered bacterial sepsis
    (d) Older men with prostrate trouble
    (e) Middle-aged individuals of both sexes

96. In the human body, each glomerulus consists of a:
    (a) Throwback to the Stone Age
    (b) Little red ball of kite string
    (c) Collection of looping blood capillaries
    (d) Large group of urinary sphincters
    (e) Destroyed group of nephrons

97. The “kidney flower cups”:
    (a) Nephrons
    (b) Renal calculi
    (c) Renal cortices
    (d) Renal tubules
    (e) Renal calyces

98. Produces estrogen and progesterone within the female ovary:
    (a) Mature ovarian follicle
    (b) Placenta
    (c) The immature ovum
    (d) Endometrium
    (e) Islet

99. Fallopian tubes are alternately called:
    (a) Oviducts
    (b) Uteri
    (c) Cervices
    (d) Ureters
    (e) Ejaculatory ducts

100. Sexual intercourse:
    (a) Zygotism
    (b) Coitus
    (c) Pruritus
    (d) Defecation
    (e) Neutralization

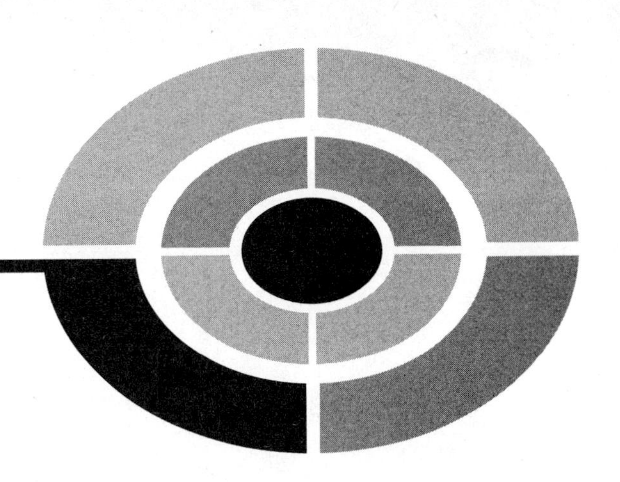

Answers to Quiz, Test, and Exam Questions

Chapter 1

1. D	2. B	3. C	4. A	5. D
6. D	7. D	8. C	9. A	10. B

Chapter 2

1. C	2. B	3. D	4. D	5. D
6. A	7. D	8. B	9. D	10. C

Chapter 3

1. B	2. B	3. D	4. A	5. D
6. C	7. B	8. D	9. B	10. C

Chapter 4

1. C	2. D	3. D	4. A	5. B
6. C	7. D	8. B	9. D	10. C

Test: Part 1

1. B	2. D	3. C	4. D	5. B
6. A	7. C	8. C	9. D	10. E
11. D	12. E	13. D	14. B	15. C
16. D	17. E	18. D	19. B	20. D
21. C	22. A	23. C	24. E	25. A

Chapter 5

1. C	2. A	3. D	4. C	5. A
6. C	7. D	8. C	9. A	10. D

Chapter 6

1. C	2. B	3. A	4. D	5. B
6. D	7. A	8. C	9. C	10. B

Test: Part 2

1. C	2. B	3. A	4. A	5. D
6. A	7. C	8. E	9. A	10. D
11. B	12. B	13. E	14. C	15. E

16. D	17. E	18. A	19. C	20. B
21. C	22. A	23. B	24. E	25. C

Chapter 7

1. D	2. B	3. A	4. D	5. C
6. C	7. A	8. C	9. A	10. C

Test: Part 3

1. E	2. B	3. C	4. A	5. E
6. B	7. A	8. C	9. D	10. C
11. D	12. A	13. A	14. D	15. A
16. A	17. C	18. E	19. C	20. B
21. C	22. E	23. B	24. A	25. D

Chapter 8

1. C	2. A	3. A	4. B	5. D
6. B	7. C	8. D	9. C	10. D

Chapter 9

1. A	2. B	3. D	4. C	5. D
6. B	7. C	8. B	9. D	10. A

Test: Part 4

1. B	2. C	3. D	4. E	5. A
6. C	7. D	8. C	9. D	10. D
11. A	12. C	13. A	14. D	15. A
16. C	17. B	18. B	19. A	20. D
21. A	22. E	23. D	24. A	25. B

Chapter 10

1. C	2. C	3. D	4. D	5. A
6. D	7. C	8. A	9. B	10. D

Chapter 11

1. C	2. D	3. A	4. C	5. A
6. D	7. D	8. D	9. B	10. A

Test: Part 5

1. C	2. E	3. C	4. D	5. E
6. A	7. E	8. B	9. B	10. C
11. B	12. D	13. C	14. C	15. E
16. E	17. A	18. D	19. C	20. A
21. A	22. C	23. E	24. D	25. B

Chapter 12

1. C	2. A	3. D	4. A	5. C
6. B	7. C	8. D	9. A	10. C

Chapter 13

1. B	2. D	3. C	4. A	5. D
6. D	7. B	8. C	9. C	10. D

Test: Part 6

1. A	2. E	3. D	4. B	5. E
6. A	7. B	8. B	9. E	10. D
11. E	12. D	13. D	14. C	15. C

16. D	17. A	18. A	19. B	20. E
21. B	22. C	23. B	24. E	25. C

Final Exam

1. B	2. C	3. C	4. E	5. A
6. D	7. E	8. A	9. C	10. E
11. A	12. C	13. E	14. C	15. B
16. D	17. A	18. E	19. A	20. C
21. E	22. E	23. A	24. E	25. A
26. D	27. C	28. E	29. B	30. B
31. D	32. B	33. C	34. D	35. B
36. D	37. A	38. C	39. D	40. A
41. C	42. D	43. A	44. C	45. B
46. D	47. E	48. C	49. B	50. B
51. B	52. C	53. B	54. E	55. C
56. D	57. E	58. C	59. E	60. D
61. C	62. C	63. A	64. E	65. E
66. D	67. C	68. D	69. B	70. B
71. C	72. D	73. B	74. E	75. C
76. C	77. B	78. A	79. A	80. B
81. D	82. B	83. D	84. C	85. D
86. A	87. D	88. E	89. A	90. C
91. B	92. A	93. D	94. B	95. C
96. C	97. E	98. A	99. A	100. B

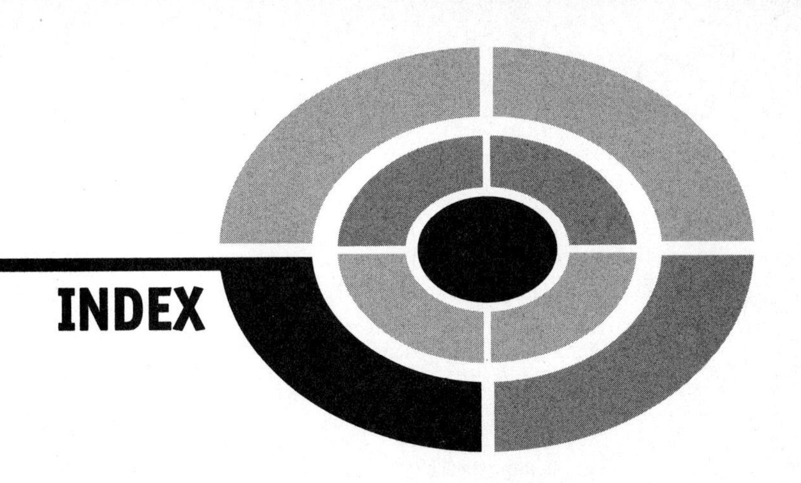

INDEX

ABOUT THE AUTHOR

Dr. Dale Layman is a Professor of Biology, Human Anatomy, Physiology, and Medical Terminology at Joliet Junior College. A resident of Joliet, Illinois, he is a frequent author with many international honors and awards. Dr. Layman has more than 30 years of experience in the field of biological sciences. He is the first Grand Doctor of Philosophy in Medicine for the United States. He is a multiple-year honoree in *Who's Who Among America's Teachers*, which lists the best teachers in the United States as selected by the best students. Dr. Layman previously wrote McGraw-Hill's *Biology Demystified*, *Anatomy Demystified*, and *Physiology Demystified*.